USMLE STEP 2 *EDGE*

USMLE STEP 2 *EDGE*

MAXWELL UHAKHEME M.D.

Shamans Publishing

Maxwell Uhakheme is a member of the House Staff at Einstein/Jacobi Medical Center, Department of Medicine, Bronx, New York.

Published by:

Shamans Publishing
78 Rockport drive
Riverdale, Georgia, 30274
muhakheme@shamanspublishing.com

Disclaimer

Although every effort has been made to make the information in this book as accurate and complete as possible, the author is aware that medicine is an ever-changing field and that there will be mistakes both in the content and typography of this manual. The author and Shamans Publishing shall not be held responsible in any way for any injury or dissatisfaction caused directly or indirectly by the information contained herein.

ISBN 10 digits: 0989266508
ISBN 13 digits: 9780989266505

Editor: Barb Every
Cover Designer: Robert Howard
Interior Design and Layout: Ghislain Viau

This book is dedicated to my wife
and all the 4th year medical students.

Contents

Preface

This book was written to fill the gaps left by most Step 2 review books. Most of these review books are either too large to read within the time frame allotted to study for the exam, or they do not contain enough information for medical students to perform beyond merely a passing mark. Fourth-year medical students have only about 6 weeks or less to study for the exam.

This book has been written in a concise format that highlights crucial facts for the Step 2 to provide medical students enough time to study for it and enough information to conquer it. This third edition of *USMLE Step 2 Edge* can be used solely to effectively study for the USMLE Step 2 Exam.

Studying tips

When I first started studying for the Step 2, I did not set out to achieve a mark of 99, but my aim was to score a high enough mark to match my specialty of choice. My intention at the time was to go into Ophthalmology, one of the most competitive fields around. I finally did achieve a 99, and I interviewed for Ophthalmology. So, how did I do it?

You are probably feeling excited to read this and anxious to know how to achieve such a high score. I say this because I felt the same way when I went to several USMLE Step 2 forums and saw some students post their score as 99. My heart would jump with anticipation and I wished that I were in their position. Why is it important to have such a high score? Well, it is if you are aiming to match a highly competitive specialty, or to match a less competitive specialty but in a top program. The first thing you need to understand is that preparation is the key. Think of this as a heavyweight championship or a big football game and you are the underdog. The timing, resources, and mental psyche are part of the preparation process, all of which I will discuss in detail, followed by my method for studying for the Step 2.

Timing

Most programs will give you at least 6 weeks off for the exam, so use the time wisely. I had about the same time to study, and so I scheduled my exam accordingly. This is the first thing you need to do because spots fill up very quickly. In addition, even if you are given more time, you should probably take the exam in 6 weeks because your recall may not be as effective. The longer you wait to take the test, the more difficult it will be to recall concepts and facts. I will revisit this issue in the "Approach to Studying" section below. Make sure to count the number of pages and the number of days you have to study. Then divide the number of pages by the number of days to get an estimate of how many pages per day you need to study. In this way, you will not run out of time, and you will have a realistic approach to a completion date.

Resources

You need books and MCQ banks that are easy to read, concise, and high yield. As an author, I have had the opportunity to review many Step 2 review books and MCQ banks. My recommendations are a complete but easily readable Step 2 text such as *USMLE Step 2 Edge* or Kaplan books, First Aid, or an equivalent. Finally, buy an MCQ bank such as Kaplan Q bank or USMLE World Q bank or an equivalent.

Mental psyche

It is helpful to have a positive attitude. Even if you have not done well in your past exams, forget all about that and think only about the Step 2. Tell yourself that you are starting afresh, that you have a score of 100%, and that you are trying to maintain that great score. Eat healthy, sleep well, and typically do not study the day before the exam. Instead, have a light, quiet evening.

Approach to studying

Before you open any books, the first thing to do is a diagnostic test (e.g., NBME questions) to identify your weaknesses. You should then tailor studying to your weaknesses; for example, if the NBME exam shows that you are weak in OB/GYN, you should start off by reading that topic.

The most important part of achieving a high score is the way that you study. We all study differently for exams, but the approach I will be sharing with you emphasizes reinforcement, which is the key to the recall and understanding of concepts needed for the Step 2. I have divided questions in the Step 2 into recall and reasoning questions, as you will need to memorize concepts, as well as be able to reason your way through questions.

The way to conquer the Step 2 is to find books that can aid memorization as well as enhance reasoning. For example, a book that describes the pathophysiology behind a condition will help you figure out its possible management. The books mentioned earlier will do this very well, as the concept of reinforcement was taken into account in suggesting them. Further, reading properly will allow for more retention of information.

So how do you read to retain most of the information from these books? Study the material concurrently. What I mean is that topics in the review text (e.g., *USMLE Step 2 Edge*) should be studied concurrently with questions in the MCQ bank. For example, after studying pediatrics in the *USMLE Step 2 Edge* review book, use a question bank to reinforce the same topic (pediatrics). You can do one or two question sets (48 questions each) per day with this method. If you are using USMLE World, you can choose "tutor mode" for the first 4 weeks. In this way, you will reinforce what you learn, from one resource to the other, and you will be less likely to forget the material 6 weeks later.

In addition, take constructive breaks while studying. Most people have an attention span of about 2 hours, after which brain fatigue no longer allows the retention of as much information. After studying for 2 hours, take a short 10-minute break to eat a high-calorie snack, and then continue for another 2 hours.

It will probably take you 4 weeks to complete studying this way, after which you will probably have some MCQ banks left to finish. After you have finished studying the content (books and reinforcement with an MCQ bank), you should concentrate only on the questions during the remaining 2 weeks.

In addition, after completing the content in the first 4 weeks, you should complete your second NBME test, and then continue doing questions with Q bank and work on your weaknesses according to the NBME. At the end of the fifth week, do your third NBME and fourth NBME test 3 days later. Continue to do Q bank questions 2 days before your exam.

And remember on the day before the exam: eat well, sleep well, and no studying (absolutely not)! Tell me afterward how you scored. I used this method, as did several of my colleagues. We obtained high scores, and you can, too. Even if you do not score as high, you should definitely score above average.

Chapter 1

Cardiovascular System

1. How is chest pain differentiated?

Chest pain can be visceral or non-visceral (localized).

2. What is the objective of a chest pain differential diagnosis?

The aim is to differentiate less serious causes from life-threatening causes such as aortic dissection, heart failure (HF), and acute coronary syndrome.

Risk factors for coronary artery disease (CAD) are age >50, male sex, diabetes, smoking, hypertension, hyperlipidemia, and inflammatory diseases.

The first step is to obtain an electrocardiogram (EKG), especially if the patient is >50 and has some of these risk factors. A stress test is used to evaluate patients with chest pain who have an intermediate probability of CAD based on age, sex, and symptoms.

3. In patients with a normal baseline EKG who can tolerate exercise, what is the preferred type of stress test?

The preferred test is an exercise stress test using EKG to evaluate for ischemia.

4. In patients with an abnormal baseline EKG, or in patients who cannot exercise what type of stress test is preferred?

The preferred tests are a pharmacological stress test with adenosine or dipyridamole, which cause vasodilation, or with dobutamine, which mimics exercise. In addition, radionuclide imaging; or echocardiogram to

When is a stress test indicated?

detect ischemia is usually combined with pharmacologic stress test.

5. How do patients present with pleuritis?

The patient may present with localized sharp pain that is worse with inspiration. Why? Inflamed membranes (visceral and pleural) are rubbing against each other.

Examples of pleuritic pain include pericarditis, pneumonia and pneumothorax, and pulmonary embolus.

6. How do patients present with pericarditis?

The patient presents with sharp pain that is exacerbated by inhalation and relieved by sitting forward. The examination reveals a pericardial rub (squeaky, scratchy, or whooshing sound heard best at the left sternal border during inspiration while leaning forward).

Lack of jugular venous pressure depression with inspiration is know as Kussmaul's sign. It is seen in constrictive pericarditis and restrictive cardiomyopathy.

7. How is pericarditis evaluated?

The first step is to obtain an EKG, which shows ST elevation in all leads and PR depression in limb leads (except aVR) and some chest leads(V5, V6). Use levels of cardiac enzymes to rule out myocardial infarction (MI); an echocardiogram may reveal pericardial effusion with or without cardiac tamponade. Evaluate for viral, bacterial, and mycobacterial causes; systemic inflammatory diseases; and malignancy.

8. What are the treatment options for pericarditis?

A nonsteroidal anti-inflammatory drug (NSAID) or colchicine is used to treat pericarditis. But if it is caused by kidney failure (uremia), dialysis should be used.

A history of pericarditis, trauma, or disease that affects the pericardium (TB, malignancy) favors the diagnosis of constrictive pericardium over restrictive cardiomyopathy.

9. A patient presents with dyspnea, fatigue, elevated jugular venous pressure, ascites, and absence of pulmonary edema in the setting of recurrent pericarditis. What is this suggestive of?

These are signs of right heart failure suggestive of constrictive pericarditis, a complication of acute pericarditis.

10. Differentiate constrictive pericarditis from restrictive cardiomyopathy.

Patients with these conditions will present with right heart symptoms/signs. Echocardiogram or magnetic resonance imaging (MRI) can differentiate pericardial disease (fibrotic pericardium) from ventricular disease.

11. List some causes of restrictive heart disease.

- Infiltrative diseases (amyloidosis, sarcoidosis)

- Storage diseases (hemochromatosis, glycogen storage diseases, scleroderma)
- Drugs (anthracycline such as doxorubicin)
- Carcinoid
- Radiation
- Eosinophilic syndrome
- Endomyocardial fibrosis

12. How do patients present with pulmonary embolus (PE)?
The patient presents with pleuritic chest pain, in addition to shortness of breath, cough, and hemoptysis. Massive PE can cause pulmonary infarction, leading to right bundle branch block on the EKG. Chest X-ray (CXR) may show Westermark sign ("cut off" sign of the pulmonary artery).

13. What are the risk factors for PE?

- Deep vein thrombosis (DVT)
- Drugs (oral contraceptives, hormone replacement therapy)
- Surgery
- Prolonged immobilization
- Hypercoagulable state (e.g., Factor V Leiden, in which factor V is resistant to protein C inactivation)

14. What is the first step in the evaluation of patients with PE?
Obtain a V/Q scan if you are not sure of the diagnosis and the patient has a high pretest probability; an alternative is the spiral computed tomography (CT) scan. If you are absolutely sure of the diagnosis, start intravenous (IV) or subcutaneous heparin right away. The fibrin splits detection test (D-dimer) is used to diagnose patients with low pretest probability. Why? D-dimer has high specificity.

Treatment: IV heparin or low-molecular-weight (LMW) subcutaneous heparin immediately, followed by oral warfarin. An inferior vena cava filter is used only when anticoagulants are contraindicated or have failed.

15. How do patients present with DVT?
The patient presents with thrombus formation in the deep vein in the extremities, especially in the lower extremity deep veins (e.g., superficial femoral vein). The patient may present with calf pain. On examination,

Which imaging modality has less radiation, and thus preferred during pregnancy to diagnose pulmonary embolus? CT scan

Wells criteria is a point scoring system used to assess for the risk of PE, and it consists of symptoms of DVT, HR >100, previous surgery within 4 weeks, previous DVT/PE, immobilization ≥3 days, hemoptysis and malignancy.

When is a V/Q scan indicated vs. a D-dimer test?

the area of involvement is tender, edematous, hyperpigmented, and warm to the touch.

Proximal DVT (e.g., thigh) is more of a risk factor for PE than is distal DVT (e.g., calf). The first step is to obtain a venous duplex ultrasound to confirm the diagnosis by checking blood flow.

Treatment: Treat the same as PE.

16. How can DVT be prevented?

Postoperative patients: Postoperative pneumatic compression devices are used for low-risk patients. LMW heparin or unfractionated heparin is used for postoperative orthopedic surgical patients or medical patients with chronic illnesses that are hospitalized.

17. How do patients present with visceral chest pain?

Visceral pain is characterized by burning, crushing, or squeezing that is not localized and radiates to the arm, jaw, shoulder, and back. The pain may be associated with nausea, vomiting, and diaphoresis. An example is coronary artery syndrome.

Nitrates such as nitrogylcerin are mainly venodilators with little effect on arterioles (afterload reduction) while hydralazine is mainly a vasodilator (with little effect on the veins).

18. In CAD syndromes, oxygen demand outmatches supply, causing ischemia with any stress. True or false?

True

19. How do patients with stable angina present?

The patient presents with visceral chest pain that lasts 5-10 minutes with exertion and is relieved with rest. The diagnosis is clinical.

Treatment: Aspirin, nitroglycerin, beta-blockers

20. Beta-blockers and calcium channel blockers reduce oxygen demand by reducing HR and contractility. True or false?

True

21. Nitroglycerin reduces stress on the myocardium by reducing preload and causing coronary artery dilation. True or false?

True

22. How do patients present with unstable angina?

The patient presents with previously stable angina that has progressed or with chest pain at rest.

Treatment: Aspirin, clopidogrel, nitroglycerin, beta-blockers, heparin. Consider a GIIb/IIIa inhibitor if pain is persistent despite medical treatment.

Definitive treatment: Consider performing coronary angiography in patients with high-risk factors or if chest pain is persistent.

23. How do patients present with Prinzmetal angina?

The patient presents with chest pain at rest that is secondary to vasospasm. The patient may present with visceral chest pain at rest occurring in the morning. Why in the morning? Vasospasm occurs especially in the morning.

Treatment: Calcium blockers

Why is Prinzmetal angina worse in the morning?

24. How do patients present with MI?

The patient may present with sudden onset of visceral chest pain, associated with shortness of breath, diaphoresis, nausea, and vomiting. The patient may also present with signs of HF such as S3 and S4 heart sounds, elevated jugular venous pressure, and rales. Laboratory tests may reveal elevation of CK and troponin levels.

Treatment: Thrombolysis within 30 minutes of onset for ST elevation MI, or percutaneous transluminal coronary angioplasty (PTCA) within 90 minutes if thrombolysis is contraindicated. Oxygen, aspirin, clopidogrel, beta-blockers, angiotensin-converting enzyme (ACE) inhibitors, and morphine are also used for treatment in stabilizing thrombosis, alleviating oxygen demand, supplementing oxygen, and treating HF. Consider ACE inhibitors when cardiac function has decompensated and ejection fraction (EF) is <50%.

Definitive treatment: Coronary angioplasty is preferred in patients with non-ST elevation MI (NSTEMI) and high-risk factors and those with ST elevation MI. Thrombolysis is contraindicated in NSTEMI.

When is percutaneous coronary intervention preferred in MI?

25. In diabetic patients with stable angina or acute coronary syndrome, classic angina symptoms may not occur. True or false?

True. Patients with neuropathy may present with no symptoms (silent MI); however, their EKG is often indicative of ischemia.

26. The first manifestation of myocardial ischemia is chest pain. True or false?

False. Ischemia usually first manifests as acidosis or hyperglycemia, as shown with biochemical testing, and

ST elevation in what lead suggests right sided infarct?

then as diastolic/systolic dysfunction, EKG changes, and chest pain.

27. Do not treat cardiac arrhythmias in the first 24-48 hours after revascularization of MI. True or false?

True. Why? Arrhythmias within this time frame are thought to be due to reperfusion injury and usually manifest as transient accelerated idioventricular rhythm or nonsustained ventricular tachycardia. They do not have long-term prognostic implications.

28. How do patients present with right/inferior wall MI?

The patient presents with sudden onset of visceral chest pain in addition to hypotension, elevated JVD, and absent pulmonary edema. Right-sided EKG may reveal ST elevation in lead V4.

Treatment: IV fluids replenishment. Do not use furosemide or nitroglycerine. Why? They will deplete the already hypotensive patient.

29. What may an EKG reveal in patients with acute coronary syndrome (MI and unstable angina)?

EKG in MI may reveal ST elevation and reciprocal ST depression, depressed Q waves, and inverted T waves. Unstable angina/NSTEMI may reveal ST depressions or T-wave inversions.

30. What may biochemical tests reveal in acute coronary syndrome?

These tests may reveal elevated creatine kinase-MB that peaks in 4-6 hours (lasts 2 days) and troponin-I elevation in 3-6 hours (lasts 1 week) in MI and usually are not present in unstable angina.

31. New-onset S4 is a classic sign of MI. True or false?

True. It indicates an incompliant left ventricle.

32. What EKG finding may reveal inferior wall MI

ST elevation in leads II, III, and aVF and reciprocal ST depression in leads V1 and V2 may reveal inferior wall MI.

33. Which anti-anginal drugs reduce mortality rate in patients with a history of MI?

Only beta-blockers prevent reinfarction and increase survival rate in patients with a history of MI.

34. When is coronary angiography performed?

Coronary angiography is performed when medical therapy has failed for CAD, when there is prolonged chest pain (>20 minutes) in the setting of acute coronary syndrome, or when there is associated pulmonary edema. Why? These are signs of evolving ischemia. Those with positive stress test results will also undergo coronary angiography.

When is coronary intervention indicated?

35. What is an ominous complication of coronary angioplasty (arterial reconstruction)?

During coronary angioplasty, a thrombus (cholesterol emboli) can embolize to multiple arteries, including the popliteal artery, renal artery, and retinal artery. This can present as a triad of **acute renal failure, livedo reticularis rash**, and **eosinophilia**. A funduscopic examination may reveal **Hollenhorst plaques** (cholesterol plaques). Popliteal artery involvement leads to digital stenosis, leading to gangrenous toes (discoloration of the digits or blue toe syndrome).

What is the triad of cholesterol emboli that occurs during coronary intervention?

36. What are some complications of MI?

- Hypotension
- Arrhythmia
- Pericarditis
- Mechanical complications (ventricular wall rupture, left ventricular free wall rupture, papillary muscle rupture)
- HF

37. What is the most common early cause of death in MI?

Arrhythmia is the most common cause, but do not give an antiarrhythmic agent for prophylaxis if arrhythmia is absent. Why? It may cause the heart to stop working (asystole).

38. What are the risk factors for mechanical complications of MI?

Risk factors include first MI, female sex, advanced age, delayed recognition, and prolonged physical activity during an MI.

39. Papillary muscle rupture may present with pulmonary edema and acute mitral regurgitation. True or false?

True. An echocardiogram is diagnostic.

Why does rupture of the ventricular wall occur within the first few days of an MI?

Why are beta-blockers effective in hypertropic cardiomyopathy?

Why are beta-blockers or calcium channel blockers contraindicated in acutely decompensated heart failure?

40. Free ventricular wall rupture can lead to pericardial tamponade. Which test is diagnostic?

Right-sided cardiac catheterization or echocardiogram may reveal equalization of all pressures in all chambers of the heart.

41. How do patients present with rupture of the interventricular septal wall?

The patient presents with chest pain, sudden pulmonary edema, and a new murmur. Rupture occurs within the first 2-7 days. Why? The wall is at its earliest stage of healing.

42. What is the pathogenesis of HF?

HF is characterized by the inability of the myocardium to meet oxygen demand, whether by decompensation of the heart muscles or inability of the muscles to relax.

43. What are the different types of HF?

- Acute versus chronic
- Systolic versus diastolic
- Right versus left
- High output

44. What is the pathogenesis of diastolic HF?

The pathophysiology of diastolic failure is the lack of heart muscle compliance. Major causes are hemochromatosis, amyloidosis, hypertension, hypertrophic cardiomyopathy, and sarcoidosis.

Treatment: Beta-blockers in hypertrophic cardiomyopathy. Why? They block the hypercontractile state of this disease.

45. What is the pathogenesis of systolic HF?

The pathophysiology of systolic failure is reduced ejection fraction (EF), leading to low systolic volume. Why? The contractile heart muscles are weak.

46. Do not give beta-blockers or calcium channel blockers to those in acute severely decompensated heart failure. True or false?

True. This may further decrease contractility and make HF worse.

47. What is the definition of EF?

EF = stroke volume/end diastolic volume.

48. What are some major causes of systolic HF?

Systolic HF is caused by ischemia and cardiomyopathy such as dilated cardiomyopathy. Dilated cardiomyopathy can be caused by ischemia, viral or infectious agents (coxsackievirus A and B virus), toxins (ethanol), and drugs (doxorubicin), or it can be idiopathic.

49. What are some causes of cardiomyopathy?

- Idiopathic dilated cardiomyopathy
- Restrictive cardiomyopathy
- Alcoholic cardiomyopathy
- Chemotherapy-induced cardiomyopathy (anthracycline)
- Drug-induced cardiomyopathy (cocaine, stimulants)
- Tachycardia-induced cardiomyopathy

50. Avoid beta-blockers in cocaine-induced heart failure/ ischemia. Why?

Unopposed alpha agonists can worsen ischemia.

Why are beta-blockers contraindicated in cocaine-induced heart failure/ ischemia?

51. What is common to both diastolic and systolic HF and what is the consequence?

Since both diastolic and systolic HF results in low cardiac output, this stimulates the renin-angiotensin system and beta receptors as a compensatory response. Later overcompensation ensues and, as a result, both types of HF are characterized by elevated **end-diastolic pressures**.

52. How do patients present generally with acutely decompensated HF??

The patient presents with low cardiac output and elevated heart rate (HR), peripheral fluid accumulation (pitting edema), tissue fluid accumulation (pulmonary edema, paroxysmal nocturnal dyspnea), pleural effusion, and ascites.

On the physical examination, S3 and hepatojugular reflux are present. Serum pro-BNP levels are elevated. An echocardiogram should be performed to ascertain systolic versus diastolic dysfunction and valvular abnormalities. Cardiac catheterization or endomyocardial biopsy can be performed to rule out CAD or infiltrative diseases as the cause of HF.

S3 is a classic sign of heart failure.

LMNOP is a mnemonic for the treatment of HF.

53. How do patients present with right-sided HF (cor pulmonale)?

The patient presents with peripheral edema, ascites, hepatomegaly, and pleural effusion with underlying chronic obstructive pulmonary disease.

54. What are some causes of high-output HF?

High-output HF can be caused by hyperthyroidism and arterial venous malformation.

55. **What may a** CXR reveal in patients with HF?

CXR may reveal pulmonary edema, cardiomegaly, and Kerley B lines (Figure 1-1).

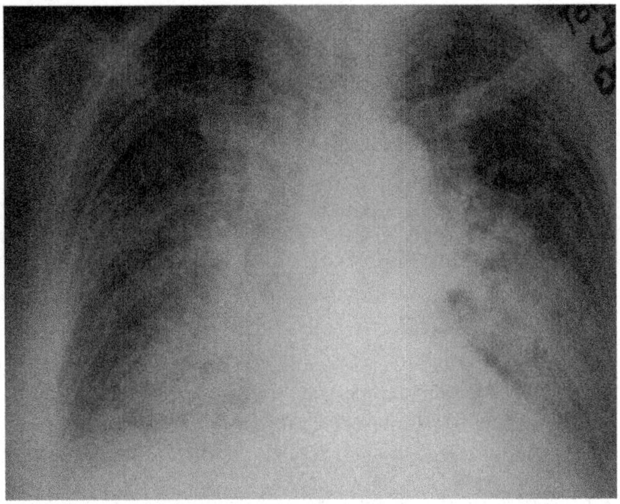

Figure 1-1. *Chest X-ray of pulmonary edema.*

56. What are the treatment options for HF?

Treatment is directed against activated renin and beta receptors and accumulation of fluid. The first step in the treatment of acute HF (i.e., patients with signs of pulmonary edema) can be recalled with the mnemonic LMNOP (Lasix [**furosemide**], morphine, nitroglycerin (a vasodilator), oxygen, and positive pressure [BiPAP]). Why? Lasix, morphine, and nitroglycerine reduce the preload (filling pressure) to reduce pulmonary edema. Supplemental oxygen and positive pressure ventilation improve dyspnea, acidosis, and heart rate. Inotropes can be used in cardiogenic shock.

57. What are the treatment options in chronic HF?

ACE inhibitors and beta-blockers are given to reverse the renin-angiotensin, beta-receptor stimulated compensatory response system. Make sure beta-blockers are given only after stabilizing the patient who has pulmonary edema.

Other treatment options: nitrates, hydralazine, digoxin, and spironolactone.

58. How do patients present with digoxin toxicity?

The patient presents with nausea, vomiting, and altered visual perception. EKG may reveal atrioventricular (AV) nodal block and **ventricular tachycardia**. A low threshold of toxicity should be taken into account in patients with kidney failure and atrial fibrillation (A-fib).

Treatment: Discontinue the drug. The indication for anti-digoxin antibody is a serum potassium level >5 mg/dl and life-threatening arrhythmias.

59. What drugs reduce the mortality rate in HF?

Only ACE inhibitors, beta-blockers, and spironolactone increase the survival rate in patients with HF. Hydralazine or a direct nitrate agonist can increase the survival rate in African Americans.

How do ACE inhibitors reduce mortality rate?

60. When are ACE inhibitors useful in HF?

ACE inhibitors are particularly useful in **systolic** HF, as they reduce cardiac remodeling (remodeling increases susceptibility to recurrent HF). Thus, use ACE inhibitors when the EF is low.

When is an ACE inhibitor indicated?

61. Which devices may reduce mortality in patients with HF?

Implantable cardioverter-defibrillators (**ICDs**) can reduce the death rate in those with systolic HF who meet certain selection criteria by preventing sudden death. Cardiac resynchronization therapy with a biventricular pacemaker can be used to improve mortality rates in those with atrial fibrillation and interventricular conduction delay.

62. What is the definition of bradyarrhythmia?

In bradyarrhythmia, the impulse is <60 beats/minute. The patient can present with hypotension, syncope, and lightheadedness.

Know the various therapies for arrhythmias.

63. What does a normal sinus rhythm on an EKG look like?

See Figure 1-2.

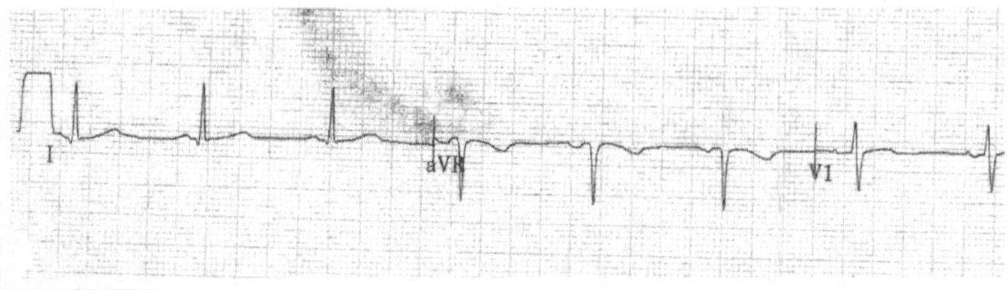

Figure 1-2. *Normal sinus rhythm. Note the discernible P waves before every QRS and the regular rhythm.*

64. What are the types of heart block and treatment?

- First-degree AV nodal block: PR elongation. No treatment if no symptoms; if symptomatic, administer atropine (Figure 1-3).

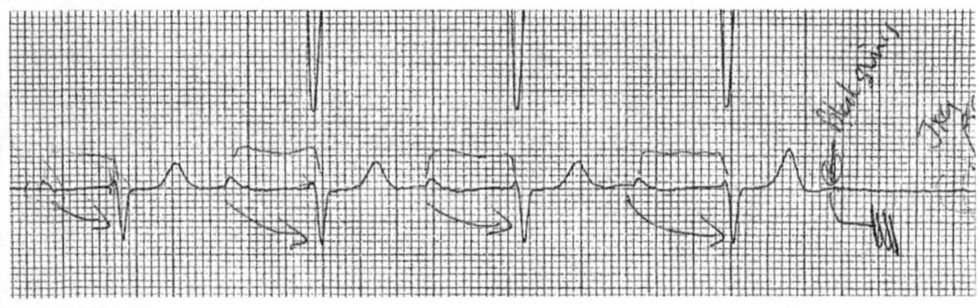

Figure 1-3. *PR elongation. Arrows show P wave and its conducted QRS. Do not pay attention to the blocked sinus.*

- Second-degree AV blocks type I and type II. Mobitz type I: PR is elongated until there is a dropped QRS beat.

  Type II: QRS beat is dropped suddenly without any PR elongation.

Treatment for type I that is symptomatic or type II is atropine first and then a pacemaker if this fails. Why? They prevent progression to complete heart block. Atropine would not be effective in those with a type II block because the heart block is below the AV node.

- Third-degree complete block: Independent atria and ventricle causing independent P wave and QRS complexes.

  Treatment: Pacemaker

65. What is the definition of tachyarrhythmia?

In tachyarrhythmia, the impulse is >100 beats/minute. The patient can present with shortness of breath, chest pain, and lightheadedness.

66. What is the definition of A-fib/atrial flutter (A-flutter)?

No P waves are distinguishable in A-fib. Saw-tooth P waves are present in A-flutter.

Causes of A-fib: Hyperthyroidism, mitral stenosis (these two are common on the boards), and mitral valve prolapse (Figure 1-4)

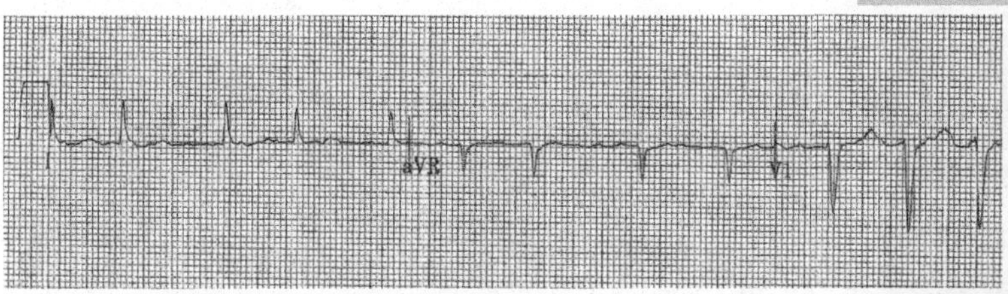

Figure 1-4. *Atrial fibrillation. Take note of the nondiscernible P waves and irregular rhythm.*

67. What are the treatment options for acute A-fib/A-flutter?

First reduce the rate, if it has been <24 hours since onset, with beta-blockers, calcium blockers, or digoxin. Use cardioversion in hemodynamically unstable patients.

68. If a patient presents with chronic A-fib or A-flutter (>48 hours after onset), what is the first step?

Anticoagulate first before cardioversion (warfarin or aspirin). Why? The chance of having an embolism is increased compared with the acute scenario.

Why are patients with chronic A-fib anticoagulated?

69. In asymptomatic/minimally symptomatic patients with chronic/paroxysmal Afib, rate control is preferred over rhythm control. True or false?

True. There is no need for rhythm control in these patients. Rate control and anticoagulation is the key to reducing mortality.

70. Lifelong anticoagulation treatment with warfarin is needed for those with high-risk factors such as HF, age >65, diabetes, and stroke. True or false?

True.

Paroxysmal episodes of palpitation with EKG showing tachycardia with a narrow QRS complex is diagnostic of SVT.

71. Catheter ablation is indicated for patients with refractory symptomatic Afib despite medical therapy. True or false?

True

72. What is the definition of supraventricular tachycardia?

This is tachycardia produced above the ventricles. The most common type is secondary to reentrant loop (AV nodal reentrant tachycardia). On the EKG, P waves can be inverted, indistinguishable (buried in QRS), or come after QRS with a heart rate of >150 beats/minute.

Treatment: Vagal-stimulating techniques (place ice on the face, massage the carotid sinus). If that does not work, administer IV adenosine, which is quick acting and inhibits the AV node. Radiofrequency ablation is curative.

73. What are the usual rates (beats/minute) for supraventricular tachycardia, atrial flutter, and fibrillation?

Supraventricular tachycardia: 150-250
Atrial flutter: 250-350
Atrial fibrillation: 350-450

74. What is the definition of ventricular tachycardia/fibrillation?

Ventricular tachycardia is organized wide-complex tachycardia, whereas ventricular fibrillation is disorganized wide-complex tachycardia.

Wide-complex runs of <30 seconds are considered non-sustained ventricular tachycardia. **Asymptomatic non-sustained ventricular tachycardia should not be treated; instead, correct the electrolyte abnormality and review the patient's medications. Treat non-sustained and symptomatic tachycardia with beta-blockers or amiodarone.**

75. What are the treatment options for acute sustained ventricular tachycardia?

For sustained ventricular tachycardia, treat with antiarrhythmic drugs (amiodarone, lidocaine); treat hemodynamically unstable patients with synchronized defibrillation and antiarrhythmic drugs; and use ICD to prevent sustained ventricular arrhythmia.

76. Multifocal atrial tachycardia (MAT) suggests what chronic condition?

MAT occurs as multiple p-wave morphology (≥3) and causes a variable PR interval with tachycardia. It is seen in patients with chronic obstructive pulmonary disease (COPD) in the setting of acute illness.

77. What is the definition of torsade de points?

Torsade de points is twisting, wide-complex tachycardia, a polymorphic ventricular tachycardia associated with prolonged QT. First-line therapy is with magnesium and potassium. Why? It can be caused by electrolyte disturbances. Cardioversion/defibrillation should be considered for hemodynamically unstable patients.

78. What is the definition of Wolff-Parkinson-White syndrome (WPW)?

WPW is an **accessory tract** that bypasses the AV node and can cause a short circuit that depolarizes (pre-excites) a portion of the left ventricle (delta wave). EKG will show a **short PR interval** and a slurred QRS (**delta wave**)

Treatment: Procainamide or cardioversion. Do not treat A-fib in patients with underlying WPW syndrome with AV nodal blocking drugs (e.g., adenosine); they will precipitate tachycardia.

Why is A-fib in WPW syndrome not treated with AV-nodal blocking drugs?

WPW is a type of SVT.

79. List the adverse effects of amiodarone.

- Pneumonitis
- Hepatitis
- Cirrhosis
- Hypo/hyperthyroidism
- Photosensitivity
- AV block
- Bradycardia

80. What are the various definitions of hypertension?

Prehypertension: 120-139/80-89

Stage 1: 140-159/90-99

Stage 2: ≥160/≥100. Stage 1 and 2 hypertension are diagnosed only after two or more separate measurements confirm diagnosis at two or more visits after the initial screen.

81. What are the risk factors for hypertension?

- Obesity (modifying this risk is the biggest payback)
- Smoking

Differentiate hypertensive retinopathy from diabetic retinopathy.

- Alcohol
- Stress
- Diabetes
- Oral contraceptives

82. What type of diet is recommended for cardiovascular health and management of hypertension?

One similar to the DASH diet (combination diet rich in fruits, veggies, and low-fat dairy products; low in saturated and total fats; low in sodium [1.5 g/day])

83. What are some microvascular complications of hypertension?

Retinopathy: Signs of **mild retinopathy** include vessel constriction (mild increased luminal pressure), silver and copper wiring (arteriolar wall thickening or arteriosclerosis), and AV nicking (thickening of basement membrane and media of arteriole impinging on vein). Signs of **moderate retinopathy** are exudates, cotton wool spots (retinal ischemia), and flame- or dot-shaped hemorrhages and microaneurysms. **Severe retinopathy** includes all of the above signs, as well as optic disc edema (papilledema).

84. What are macrovascular complications of hypertension?

Complications are hypertrophy of the heart, peripheral arterial disease, and coronary artery disease.

85. What are the treatment options for complications of hypertension?

Prehypertension, stage 1 hypertension, and stage 2 hypertension should be treated with exercise, weight loss, and smoking cessation as the initial treatment. Stage 1 should be treated with pharmacological therapy if the initial non-pharmacology treatment fails.

Stage 2 hypertension is treated with pharmacological therapy after two or more measurements confirm diagnosis. Starting with two drugs should be considered in stage 2 hypertension.

86. What are the types of pharmacological treatment for hypertension?

Diuretics, especially low-dose thiazide, are the mainstay of treatment. Why? Studies have confirmed that they have the fewest side effects.

Calcium blockers: Initial treatment in patients with peripheral arterial disease, and black and elderly population (dihydropyridine type). Why? They are used because of the vasodilatation effects.

Beta-blockers: Initial treatment for patients with coronary heart disease and baseline HF. Why? They have a protective effect on mortality.

ACE inhibitors and angiotensin receptor blockers: Initial treatment in patients with diabetes and chronic kidney disease (CKD) and younger patients. Why? These drugs have a protective effect on the kidneys.

87. What is the goal of blood pressure (BP) treatment?

The goal is <140/90 for most patients and <130/80 for patients with diabetes and CKD. Why? This is thought to protect the kidneys.

Always work on modifiable risk factors such as losing weight, discontinuing oral contraceptives, and quitting smoking before initiating treatment with pharmacological therapy.

Why is the goal of BP management in diabetes or CKD 130/80?

88. What is the pathogenesis of mitral stenosis?

Mitral stenosis is most commonly caused by rheumatic fever. Know the consequences of pressure in the heart: The left atrium is enlarged and pulmonary artery pressure is increased, which leads to pulmonary venous congestion. This is logical. The physical examination reveals a diastolic rumble in the apex.

Treat pulmonary edema with diuretics and use beta-blockers to reduce HR (elevated HR will increase pulmonary pressure, causing pulmonary edema) and anticoagulants against atrial dilation and Afib.

Percutaneous mitral valve repair is preferred. Surgical valve replacement is used if repair is not possible.

89. What is the pathogenesis of acute rheumatic fever?

Acute rheumatic fever occurs weeks after having streptococcal pharyngitis as a result of autoimmune mimicry. The patient may develop carditis, rash (erythematic marginatum), migratory arthritis, and chorea. The patient may present acutely with mitral regurgitation.

The five major criteria are carditis, arthritis, rash, Sydenham chorea, and subcutaneous nodules.

Diagnosis: Only two of the major criteria are needed for diagnosis. One major and two minor criteria with

What is a mnemonic for major criteria in acute rheumatic fever? J♥nes criteria.

Joints, carditis, nodules, erythema marginatum, Sydenham chorea

evidence of a prior streptococcal infection can be used as an alternative. Minor criteria are arthralgia (joint pain), fever, elevated ESR, antistreptolysin O antibody, and a previously documented streptococcal infection.

Treatment: Penicillin

Complication: A long-term complication of acute rheumatic fever is mitral stenosis, which can lead to atrial fibrillation.

90. What is the pathogenesis of mitral regurgitation?

The most common **chronic** cause is mitral valve prolapse and then rheumatic disease, ischemic heart disease, and heart failure. The physical examination reveals a holosystolic murmur in the apex. The patient's heart undergoes the same consequences as for mitral stenosis except that left ventricle dysfunction presents later on.

Treat mitral regurgitation with diuretics (to reduce pulmonary edema), and vasodilators to decrease afterload, and use anticoagulation therapy in patients with atrial fibrillation. Mitral valve repair is preferred for severe cases.

91. What is the most common cause of acute mitral regurgitation?

The most common cause is **connective tissue valve disease** (e.g., Marfan syndrome) causing rupture of the chordae tendineae, or endocarditis causing rupture of the chordae tendineae. Papillary muscle rupture from MI is also a known cause.

92. Syncope, angina or CHF, or exertional dyspnea are manifestations of AS. True or false?

True. Patients can present with symptoms similar to those of angina and will have similar risk factors.

Know the different causes of AS in elderly vs young adults.

93. What is the pathogenesis of aortic stenosis (AS)?

The most common cause in the elderly is calcification of the valves. The most common cause in young individuals is bicuspid aortic valve or hypertrophic cardiomyopathy. The physical examination may reveal a midsystolic ejection murmur in the second right interspace. Aortic stenosis can lead to elevated left ventricular (LV) pressure, and then an enlarged ventricle, leading to LV dysfunction later on.

Treatment: No effective medical treatment. Surgery (aortic valve replacement) is better.

94. The magnitude of delayed carotid upstroke (carotid pulse is closer to S2 rather than to S1) corresponds to the level of severity in AS. True or false?

True.

95. Differentiate hypertrophic cardiomyopathy from AS.

Anything that reduces volume, such as the Valsalva maneuver, or that increases contraction usually increases the severity and the intensity of the murmur of hypertrophic cardiomyopathy. Squatting and hand grip both increase ventricular volume and systemic vascular resistance and therefore will reduce the intensity of the murmur of hypertrophic cardiomyopathy.

Use different maneuvers to differentiate AS from hypertrophic cardiomyopathy.

96. What is the evaluation of aortic regurgitation (AR)?

The physical examination will reveal a harsh blowing diastolic murmur in the second right interspace. Murmur can be accentuated by having the patient lean forward at the end of expiration or by performing a handgrip maneuver. Aortic regurgitation can lead to LV enlargement. Common causes are bicuspid valve or ascending aorta aneurysm and Marfan syndrome. A wide pulse pressure of >60 is present (e.g., BP of 160/55 has a pulse pressure of 105, which is high).

Treatment: ACE inhibitors to reduce afterload. Why? They improve forward progress. Surgical aortic valve replacement is preferred in severe AR.

In general, inspiration increases the intensity of the murmurs from the right side of the heart and diminishes the intensity of the murmurs from the left side of the heart.

97. What are some drugs that can cause mitral regurgitation?

Anorexic drugs such as fenfluramine and phentermine (fen-phen) can cause MR and other valvular diseases.

98. Aortic stenosis in the setting of GI bleed suggests what syndrome?

It suggests **Heyde's syndrome**, bleeding due to arteriovenous malformations in the gastrointestinal tract, and acquired VWD where VWF passes through the aortic valve and becomes dysfunctional.

99. What is the most common cause of tricuspid regurgitation?

The most common cause is **pulmonary hypertension**; others are endocarditis (intravenous drug use), carcinoid, drugs (fen-phen), and Marfan syndrome.

What are the indications for endocarditis prophylaxis?

100. Which murmurs require prophylactic antibiotics prior to invasive procedures (e.g., dental extraction)?

The following murmurs require prophylactic antibiotics: prosthetic heart valves; those with a history of infectious endocarditis; unrepaired congenital heart defects; and repaired congenital heart disease with residual defects; the first 6 months in those with repaired congenital defects.

101. How may patients present with mitral valve prolapse (MVP)?

Patients may be asymptomatic or have chest pain with mild systolic murmur and midsystolic click in the apex. Adults with MVP can present with A-fib or nonspecific symptoms.

102. What prophylactic antibiotics are used in patients with heart valve dysfunction prior to surgical procedures to prevent endocarditis?

Amoxicillin is the first choice. Clindamycin is administered to individuals who are allergic to amoxicillin.

103. What types of valves are used for valve replacement?

Valves are either mechanical or biological (porcine).

104. When are mechanical and biological valves used?

Mechanical valves are coagulation prone but last longer, whereas porcine valves last about 10 years but are not prone to thrombus development. Thus, mechanical valves are contraindicated in patients with coagulation susceptibility (pregnancy, elderly) and biological valves are excellent for the elderly population. Why for the elderly? The elderly have a shorter life expectancy.

105. What are the major causes of cardiogenic shock?

The major causes are congestive heart failure, tension pneumothorax, and cardiac tamponade.

106. Why is cardiac output decreased in cardiogenic shock?

Cardiac tamponade or tension pneumothorax compresses the inferior vena cava and atria, leading to low outflow and decreased preload and venous return, while congestive heart failure causes pump failure (Table 1-1).

107. What is the definition of vasovagal (neurogenic) syncope?

Vasovagal syncope is caused by paradoxical vagal-stimulating effects, leading to generalized vasodilation. This may cause sweating and a feeling of hot flushes. Several factors can cause this syncope, such as micturition, the Valsalva maneuver, and cough.

Vasovagal syncope is the same as neurogenic syncope.

What is the most common type of syncope? Vasovagal

108. What is the differential diagnosis of syncope?

Consider true syncope (global hypoperfusion) versus pseudosyncope (no true loss of consciousness).

109. What are the causes of true syncope?

- Arrhythmia
- Vertebrobasilar transient ischemic attack (TIA)
- Seizures
- Orthostatic hypotension
- Vascular steal syndrome
- Carotid hypersensitivity
- Massive pulmonary embolism
- Structural valvular disease

110. What are the causes of pseudosyncope?

- Hypoglycemia
- Carotid TIA
- Psychogenic disorder
- Cataplexy (drop attacks with narcolepsy)

111. What is the definition of orthostatic syncope?

This syncope can be due to autonomic dysfunction, antihypertensive medications, low intravascular volume secondary to hemorrhage, and gastrointestinal losses. The patient will present with syncope from sitting to standing. On the physical examination, BP will decrease by at least 20 mm Hg in systolic BP and 10 mm Hg in diastolic BP within 3 minutes of standing.

112. What is the mechanism of orthostatic hypotension?

The sympathetic system is unable to maintain cerebral perfusion in the upright position because of autonomic dysfunction, volume depletion, blockade of receptors used by the sympathetic system, or downregulation of these receptors due to their chronic exposure to natural agonists (epinephrine, norepinephrine).

The deadliest type of syncope is cardiogenic.

113. What is the definition of carotid hypersensitivity syncope?
Hypersensitivity syncope is neurogenic syncope secondary to carotid dysfunction, leading to vagus stimulation in the carotid sinus because of its compression by neck bending. The patient will present with syncope associated with movement of the neck.

114. How does arrhythmic syncope present?
Many types of arrhythmia can cause sudden onset of syncope with no warning. Palpitations, chest pain, and dizziness may precede this type of syncope. An EKG may reveal an arrhythmia.

115. How do patients present with valvular syncope?
This type of syncope can occur in young adults with hypertrophic cardiomyopathy or in the elderly with calcification of the aortic valve, leading to AS. The patient may present with exercise-induced syncope. Lightheadedness may precede syncope.

Table 1-1. *Types of Shock*

Shock	SVR	JVP	CO	PCWP
Cardiogenic	Increased	Increased	Decreased	Increased
Hypovolemic	Increased	Decreased	Decreased	Decreased
Septic	Decreased early on	Decreased	Increased early on	Decreased

SVR, systemic vascular resistance; JVP, jugular venous pressure; CO, cardiac output; PCWP, pulmonary capillary wedge pressure.

116. What is the differential diagnosis of acute dyspnea?
Acute dyspnea can present in patients with MI, asthma exacerbation, COPD exacerbation, pulmonary embolus, decompensation of HF, pneumothorax. Lung parenchymal diseases such as pneumonia and pleural effusions are acute but progressive causes of dyspnea.

117. What is the differential diagnosis of chronic dyspnea?
Chronic dyspnea is usually due to **chronic lung diseases** such as COPD (associated with clubbing) and interstitial pulmonary fibrosis, or deconditioning, anemia, thyroid diseases, valvular disorders, or psychogenic disorders (associated with periorbital and peripheral paresthesia).

118. What are the cardiac manifestations of Chagas disease?
Manifestations include conduction system abnormalities, apical aneurysm, left ventricular dilation, and congestive heart failure. It is treated with benznidazole.

Chapter 2
Vascular Diseases

1. How do patients present with carotid artery disease?

Carotid artery disease can lead to an acute embolic episode. This disease may present asymptomatically as a carotid bruit or symptomatically as a transient ischemic attack and a cerebrovascular accident.

2. How do patients present with acute peripheral artery disease (PAD)?

The patient may present with acute arterial peripheral occlusion and have sudden onset of lower extremity pain, pallor, pulselessness, poikilotherm, and paresthesia. Why? These symptoms result from ischemia.

The first step is to order an arterial ultrasound, or a magnetic resonance angiogram (MRA), or an angiogram for diagnosis.

Treatment: Anticoagulants, embolectomy plus thrombolysis with or without vascular reconstruction surgery.

3. How do patients present with chronic peripheral arterial disease?

What is Buerger's symptom?

The patient presents with long-term lower extremity pain while walking (intermittent claudicating), which is relieved at rest. On examination, the foot will become pale while the patient is lying down but red while the foot is hanging down (Buerger's symptom).

The first step is to obtain an ankle brachial index, a ratio of measured ankle and arm BP. The normal ratio is 1. If the ratio is <1, it means that there is abnormal blood flow, suggesting ischemia. ABI <0.4 indicates severe ischemia. Treatment is exercise; smoking cessation;

weight loss; diabetes, dyslipidemia, and hypertension management; and antiplatelet therapy (aspirin, clopidogrel, ticlopidine).

4. What is the most common intervention that leads to limb salvage in PAD?

The most common intervention is smoking cessation.

5. What cause of leg pain should be differentiated from PAD?

Spinal stenosis, unlike PAD ischemic pain, **occurs while standing**, but is relieved by bending forward.

6. What are the complications of chronic peripheral arterial disease?

The complications are ischemic ulcer and leg pain at rest. These are indications for arterial reconstructive surgery (PTCA or bypass procedure).

Differentiate types of extremity ulcers.

7. Differentiate ischemic ulcer from venous insufficiency ulcers and diabetic ulcers.

Venous ulcer (a complication of varicose veins): The patient presents with an ulcer at the lateral or medial malleolus. Why? Superficial and deep veins of the lower extremities cross at these locations. It is the incompetency of the superficial veins that causes venous insufficiency (varicose veins).

Diabetic ulcer: The patient presents with an ulcer in the plantar or lateral aspect of the foot. Why? There is a lack of sensation in this location.

Ischemic ulcers from PAD: These ulcers are located **distally on the dorsum of the foot**. They are associated with hair loss, cool skin, and lack of distal pulses.

8. How do patients present with acute mesenteric ischemia?

This is mostly caused by an embolus that creates an obstruction of the mesenteric arterial vessels; other causes are thrombus occlusion and nonobstructive causes (associated with cocaine use, digoxin, hypotension, and venous occlusion). The patient presents acutely with **history of atrial fibrillation**, heart murmur, anorexia, and diarrhea; later on with obstipation, abdominal distention, and gastrointestinal bleed; and finally with metabolic and lactic acidosis, sepsis, and shock.

9. How are patients with suspected acute mesenteric ischemia evaluated?

The first step is to order an abdominal X-ray and a chest X-ray (CXR) to rule out bowel obstruction and perforation. A computed tomography (CT) scan is typically used for diagnosis, but angiography is the gold standard for diagnosis.

10. What are the treatment options for acute mesenteric ischemia?

Treatment: Look for necrotic bowel and resect as needed; consider embolectomy plus thrombolysis, balloon angioplasty and stenting, or revascularization surgery.

11. What is the pathogenesis of chronic mesenteric ischemia?

This is mostly caused by a thrombus obstructing the mesenteric artery. The patient may present with a history of A-fib, abdominal pain out of proportion to the physical examination, postprandial epigastric pain, early satiety, and a rectal bleed. Diagnostic evaluation and treatment is similar to that for acute mesenteric ischemia.

Postprandial epigastric pain within the first hour is suggestive of chronic mesenteric ischemia.

12. What is the most common cause of intestinal ischemia?

The most common cause is **ischemic colitis**, which usually presents as **left lower quadrant** abdominal pain in older patients with risk factors for CAD and hypotension. Colonoscopy may be diagnostic by revealing segmental ulcerations in the region of the splenic flexure (areas with limited blood supply).

13. What are the risk factors for aortic aneurysm?

Patients that present with aortic aneurysm are usually **older than 60** and are **smokers** with hypertension and hyperlipidemia. In younger patients, consider **Marfan syndrome**, especially in aortic root dilation.

14. List the risk factors associated with aortic dissection.

Those that present with aortic dissection are usually **older than 70** and have hypertension, diabetes, aortic aneurysm, and vasculitis (Takayasu arteritis, giant cell arteritis, syphilitic aortitis). In younger patients, consider **Marfan syndrome** or cocaine use.

Trans-esophageal echocardiogram is preferred in confirming the diagnosis of patients with aortic dissection.

15. What is the significance of Takayasu arteritis?

This is vasculitis of unknown cause seen in young women from Japan and parts of Asia. It can present as ischemia of several organs due to stenosis of major arteries.

16. How do patients present with abdominal aortic aneurysm?

The patient presents with dull abdominal pain. Most patients present asymptomatically. On the physical examination, a pulsatile mass is felt. The first step is to obtain an ultrasound or a CT scan.

Treatment: Surgery when the mass is >5.5 cm or increases at a rate of >0.5 cm/year; otherwise, a follow-up CT scan is scheduled based on the size of the aneurysm.

17. What is an ominous complication of aneurysm surgery?

Colonic ischemia is an ominous complication. Why? During surgery, the inferior mesenteric artery could be transected, leading to hypoperfusion to the splenic flexure (an area with a less than stellar blood supply).

18. How do patients present with aortic dissection?

The patient presents with severe tearing chest pain radiating to the back. Most patients will have elevated BP. Associated symptoms include neurological symptoms (syncope and hypovolemia from excessive vagal tone), peripheral nerve symptoms (numbness from ischemia of branch vessels), cardiovascular symptoms (congestive heart failure from aortic regurgitation and hypotension from cardiac tamponade), and renal symptoms (flank pain and renal failure from renal ischemia).

19. What might the physical examination reveal in aortic dissection?

The physical examination might reveal a **diastolic murmur** (aortic regurgitation).

20. What is the diagnostic imaging method of choice for aortic dissection?

A CXR may show a **widened mediastinum**, but it is not diagnostic. A **CT scan** of the chest/abdomen/pelvis with contrast can be performed in hemodynamically stable patients. A **transesophageal echocardiogram** is preferred in hemodynamically unstable patients because, in addition to having better diagnostic accuracy compared with a transthoracic echocardiogram, it can be performed at the bedside, unlike a CT scan.

21. What is the first step in the treatment of aortic dissection?

The first step is treatment with **surgery** if the tear is at the **ascending aorta** (involving the aortic valve, causing a murmur) or **beta-blockers** to reduce BP if the tear is at the **descending aorta**.

22. How do patients present with renal stenosis?

In the elderly, renal stenosis may present as a periumbilical bruit in patients with risk factors for atherosclerosis. In young individuals, renal stenosis may present as a periumbilical bruit in patients with no risk factors for vascular disease. The latter case is usually due to fibromuscular dysplasia.

Renal stenosis can be diagnosed with a renal ultrasound, a spiral CT scan of the kidneys (also known as a CT urogram), or conventional angiography.

Treatment: Balloon angioplasty/stenting or other revascularization surgery

Causes of renal stenosis differ, depending on the age of the patient.

23. How do patients present with arterial venous malformation?

The patient may present with an elevated cardiac output, and on the physical examination, a thrill is felt. Risk factors can be congenital or traumatic in origin.

24. What is the pathogenesis of subclavian steal syndrome?

This syndrome is a proximal occlusion of the subclavian artery, causing diversion of blood flow via the contralateral vertebral artery to the other vertebral artery, compromising the subclavian artery branch distribution.

The patient may present with dizziness, headache, and arm pain with exercise or exertion.

This syndrome is usually caused by atherosclerosis disease; thus, treat it with antiplatelet drugs.

25. What is the pathogenesis of thoracic outlet syndrome?

Subclavian artery and brachial plexus are compressed in the costoclavicular space, leading to paresthesias and lack of radial pulse on raising the ipsilateral arm.

Treatment is based on the underlying cause.

Chapter 3

Emergency Medicine

1. When is the Glasgow coma scale (GCS) most useful?
The GCS is most useful in trauma patients. If GCS <8, it indicates severe head injury; if it is between 9 and 12, it indicates moderate head injury; if it is between 14 and 15, it indicates mild head injury.
Why use the GCS? Patients with moderate to severe injury and those with loss of consciousness will need a computed tomography scan.

2. The mnemonic for GCS is MVp 6, 5, 4. True or false?
True. See Table 3-1.

Table 3-1. *GCS Scale* Motor Verbal Eye Opening

Score (6)	**M**otor response (6)	**V**erbal response (5)	Eye O**p**ening (4)
6	Obeys command		
5	Localizes pain	Oriented	
4	Flexion-withdrawal	Disoriented	Spontaneously
3	Decorticate (flexion abnormal)	Inappropriate words: -cries	To verbal commands
2	Decerebrate	Incomprehensible sounds	To pain
1	No response	No response	No response

The GCS score is most useful in trauma patients with traumatic brain injury (TBI).

For all patients with coma, always perform ABCs, intubate if GCS ≤8, give thiamine, glucose, treat seizures with phenytoin, and consider other empiric treatments for infection, ingestion (naloxone), elevated ICP(mannitol) and nonconvulsive status epilepticus.

3. If the GCS score is <9 with increased intracranial pressure (ICP), ICP monitoring may be warranted. True or false?

True. This can be done by ventriculostomy. Cerebral brain perfusion = mean arterial pressure (MAP)–ICP. The autoregulation mechanism in the normal brain is at play when MAP is between 50 mm Hg and 150 mm Hg and a constant amount of blood flow to the brain is maintained regardless of blood pressure (BP). In TBI, autoregulation ceases to exist in injured areas, and blood flow is entirely dependent on BP.

4. What is the definition of concussion?

Concussion is a physiological injury to the brain without any structural dysfunction. Patients may present with loss of consciousness for 5-10 minutes or more, confusion, and memory changes.

Treatment: Supportive care

5. Define post-concussive syndrome (PCS).

This is characterized by the persistent constellation of symptoms after a head injury: emesis, headaches, blurry vision, dizziness, emotional disturbances. PCS usually lasts 2-4 months.

Treatment: CT scan of the brain. If it is a mild head injury and the CT scan is normal, send the patient home after 8 hours of observation. Ancillary support with an occupational therapist, social worker, or mental health professional can be offered on an outpatient basis if symptoms are refractory. Patients with moderate to severe head injury are admitted for observation.

6. What is the significance of Battle's sign (postauricular ecchymosis)?

Ecchymosis in the postauricular area (mastoid bone) indicates a traumatic blow to the temporal bone. It suggests an underlying fracture of the temporal bone, which is part of the basilar bone. A CT scan should be obtained for diagnosis.

Unilateral, clear rhinorrhea is usually a sign of CSF leak.

7. What is the significance of raccoon eyes (periorbital ecchymosis)?

This suggests a fracture of the frontal bone, which is part of the basilar bone. Clear rhinorrhea, Battle's sign, and raccoon eyes suggest a basilar bone fracture.

8. What is the first step in evaluating a trauma patient?

Always assess airway, circulation, and breathing (ABC) first.

9. What is the first step in evaluating patients with gunshot wounds?

All patients with gunshot wounds should be assessed for ABC and then taken to the operating room for an exploratory laparotomy.

10. What is the first step in evaluating patients with stab wounds?

Patients should be assessed for ABC, and for those with deep wounds involving the viscera or unstable vitals, an exploratory laparotomy is the preferred treatment. If the wounds are shallow, local wound debridement is preferred.

11. What differential diagnosis is considered in patients with blunt chest trauma?

Consider contusion of the lungs or heart, pneumothorax, pneumomediastinum, flail chest, pericardial effusion, pericardial tamponade, and hemothorax.

First step: A chest X-ray (CXR) should be obtained.

12. What could a CXR show in patients with pulmonary contusion?

A CXR could show unilateral hyperdensities. The patient may also present with hemoptysis and respiratory distress. On the physical examination, an ipsilateral breath sound is absent. Why? Pulmonary edema may be present. Treatment is to focus on ventilation and possible intubation.

Pulmonary contusion is usually due to blunt chest trauma.

13. What are the physical examination findings in pneumothorax?

A large pneumothorax may present with **decreased breath sounds, hyperresonance** to percussion, and decreased chest excursion on the affected side. A tension pneumothorax involves sudden-onset dyspnea caused by increased intrapleural pressure that can lead to cardiovascular compromise. Symptoms suggestive of hemodynamic compromise such as tachycardia and hypotension suggest a tension pneumothorax, and emergency decompression is indicated.

On what position on the chest is a thoracostomy done?

Tube thoracostomy is preferred over needle drainage for a large pneumothorax.

14. What could a CXR show in patients with a pneumothorax?

A CXR could show a **hyperlucent hemithorax, with the ipsilateral side larger** than the contralateral hemithorax, and a flattened diaphragm on the ipsilateral side. A white visceral **pleural line** and a **deep sulcus sign** are seen on CXR. In a large pneumothorax, the first step is to decompress with a **needle thoracostomy** (second intercostal space, midclavicular line) and to perform a **tube thoracostomy** (chest tube in fifth intercostal space, midaxillary line) (Figure 3-1).

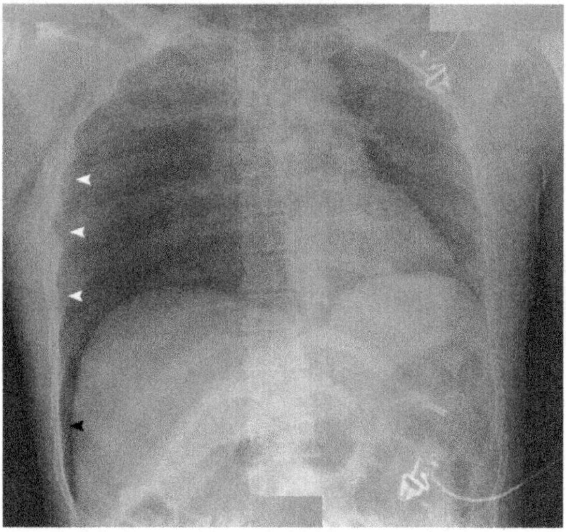

Figure 3-1. *White arrowheads show pleural line of pneumothorax. Deep sulcus sign of pneumothorax (black arrowhead).*

15. What could a CXR show in patients with a pneumomediastinum?

A CXR could show bilateral hyperlucency and subcutaneous emphysema.

Suspect rupture of the esophagus or bronchus. Esophagoscopy and bronchoscopy will confirm the diagnosis.

16. What could a rib radiograph show in patients with a flail chest?

A rib radiograph could show >2 consecutive rib fractures with multiple fractures in each rib. The patient may present with paradoxical movement of the chest wall.

Treat pain with analgesics and adequate ventilation.

17. What could a CXR and an electrocardiogram (EKG) show in patients with cardiac tamponade?

A CXR will show, in addition to a widened mediastinum, a hemi-dense region, and an EKG will show low voltage and electrical alternans (beat-to-beat variation of the QRS axis). Why? The heart is swinging in fluid.

18. AMPLE is a mnemonic for the first step in evaluating patients with blunt abdominal trauma. True or false?

True: Allergies, Medications, Past medical history, Last meal, Events leading to incident

19. How do patients present with cardiac tamponade in general?

Patients present with low cardiac output, tachycardia, Beck triad (hypotension, muffled heart sounds, increased central venous pressure), and pulsus paradoxus (>10 mm Hg drop in systolic BP with inspiration). Treatment is **pericardiocentesis** (needle thoracotomy) initially; definitive treatment is immediate surgical **pericardial drainage.**

20. What are some causes of cardiac tamponade?

Aortic dissection, pericarditis, and aortic rupture are all causes of pericardial effusion, which can lead to tamponade.

21. What is the pathophysiology of cardiac tamponade?

It is caused by intrapericardial accumulation of fluid that compresses the cardiac chambers, causing reduced ventricular filling, stroke volume, and cardiac output.

22. What is the characteristic echocardiogram finding in cardiac tamponade?

The characteristic finding is **elevated intrapericardial pressure** with right ventricular or atrial free wall invagination.

23. The first step in imaging the hemodynamically unstable patient with blunt abdominal trauma is obtaining a focused assessment sonography for trauma (FAST) or a diagnostic peritoneal lavage (DPL). True or false?

True. FAST is equivalent in accuracy to DPL. A CT scan can be considered for stable patients.

24. What is the definition of a hemothorax?

A hemothorax is the presence of blood in the pleural space, usually caused by blunt or penetrating trauma

When is a thoracotomy indicated in patients with cardiac tamponade and hemothorax?

What is the difference between thoracotomy and thoracostomy?

or systemic diseases. Injury to the great vessels, chest wall, lung parenchyma, or heart can cause a hemothorax. A thoracotomy to drain the collection of blood is the preferred treatment.

25. What is the most common cause of aortic rupture?

Aortic rupture is mostly caused by a deceleration injury (e.g., fall from a building, a motor vehicle collision, or a motor cycle injury). A CXR will show widening of the mediastinum.

26. Why is abdominal blunt trauma ominous?

Abdominal blunt trauma is very dangerous because the damage to the internal organs is not seen.

27. What is the objective of the FAST technique?

The FAST technique is used to look for free fluid in the hepatorenal recess, pouch of Douglas, spleen recess, and thorax. If fluid is present in any of these places, the next step is to take the patient to the operating room for an emergency exploratory laparotomy.

28. What is the objective in the DPL technique?

DPL is a method used to rapidly determine the presence of intraperitoneal blood. A syringe and needle is used to withdraw fluid from the abdomen, which is then lavaged. DPL is positive if 10 ml of gross blood is obtained before the lavage fluid, or if the withdrawn lavage fluid consists of >100,000 red blood cells (RBCs)/ml, >500 white blood cells (WBCs)/ml, elevated amylase, bile, and bacteria. An emergency exploratory laparotomy is indicated for positive DPL; otherwise, conservative management is recommended.

29. What is the next step in patients with blunt abdominal trauma accompanied by peritonitis?

The patient may present with generalized abdominal rebound, rigidity, and distention. The next step is to perform an emergency exploratory laparotomy.

30. What is the pathogenesis of compartment syndrome?

The upper and lower extremities have thick fascia, in which vessel leakage and accumulation leads to increased intracompartmental pressure on the nerve, eventually causing ischemia.

Remember: Patients do not have to be pulseless to be diagnosed with compartment syndrome.

31. How do patients present with compartment syndrome?

Patients can present with a trauma-related upper or lower extremity injury (fracture) associated with severe pain, numbness, weakness, and discoloration. On the physical examination, the involved extremity pulse may be intact. Treatment is to decompress the nerve involved by fasciotomy.

Note: Do not wait until the pulse is absent to diagnose compartment syndrome.

32. Where do physicians always look in patients with burns?

Physicians should check the nares and pharynx to rule out inhalation injury. The first step is to maintain airway ventilation if inhalation thermal injury is present.

The preferred treatment for partial thickness burn (associated with blisters, pain, and blanches with pressure) is to apply topical silver nitrate or silver sulfadiazine and to administer an analgesic.

Differentiate treatment of partial thickness burn from full thickness burn.

33. If circumferential full-thickness burn injuries (involves the dermis and are usually anesthetic or hypoesthetic) on the extremities are present in patients, what is the first step?

Check for pulses with a Doppler pulse probe and then perform an escharotomy. However, overall goal should be to maintain perfusion and prevent shock by administering IV fluids. In addition, excision and coverage of wound, antibiotics prophylaxis, and nutritional support should be part of treatment.

34. Fern-like pattern skin injuries are pathognomonic for lightning strikes. True or false?

True. They are also called Lichtenberg figures and usually fade away within hours.

35. What are types of spinal fractures?

- Central cord syndrome
- Anterior cord syndrome
- Hemi-transection

36. What is the pathogenesis of central cord syndrome (syringomyelia)?

Syringomyelia is central cord cavitation that can occur in patients with degenerative arthritis who have sustained

What malformation is associated with nontraumatic syringomyelia?

What is the most common cause of anterior spinal artery infarct? ***Atherosclerosis***

forced hyperextension, as in a whiplash that occurs in a motor vehicle accident, especially in the elderly. Why central cord syndrome? Buckling and consequent contusion occurs to the central region of the cord. The cause of nontraumatic syringomyelia is idiopathic and commonly associated with Arnold Chiari malformation type 1.

37. How do patients present with syringomyelia?

Patients present with damage to the decussating cervical lateral spinothalamic axons leading to bilateral loss of pain and loss of temperature sensations in the upper extremities. Lower motor neuron (ventral or anterior horns) lesions can result in flaccid paralysis of the hands. The lower extremities are spared. Why? Most lesions involve the cervical cord.

38. What is the pathogenesis of anterior cord syndrome?

Anterior cord syndrome is due to a diving injury (flexion of the cervical vertebrae), anterior spinal artery thrombosis, and vertebral herniation. The complete anterior portion of the cord (anterior horns, lateral spinothalamic, corticospinal tracts) is affected, but not the posterior portion (dorsal columns and horns). The patient presents with bilateral loss of motor control and of ability to feel pain and temperature, and bilateral spastic paresis and pyramidal signs (Babinski), but a preserved sense of balance and ability to feel light touch.

39. What is the pathogenesis of Brown-Séquard syndrome (hemi-transection)?

Brown-Séquard syndrome is caused by a shearing injury of the spinal cord, usually by a knife. Half of the spinal cord is affected, leading to deficits of contralateral pain, temperature sensation, ipsilateral motor function, and proprioception. Remember that lateral spinothalamic tract is the only major tract that decussates in the spinal cord.

40. What is the pathogenesis of subdural hematoma?

Subdural hematoma is a rupture in the bridging veins caused by stretching of the atrophied cerebral cortex. It causes an intracranial hemorrhage that is crescent-shaped. Patients may present acutely with a "lucid" interval or chronically with insidious headaches and cognitive impairment that may not occur until weeks after the initial head injury. If there is no midline shift or neurological deterioration, treatment is observation.

41. What is the pathogenesis of epidural hematoma?

Epidural hematoma is an intracranial hemorrhage that has a biconvex shape (lens-shaped pattern) on a CT scan, usually after head trauma in young adults or adolescents. The patient initially loses consciousness, then regains consciousness, then loses it again; this sequence is called a lucid interval. The patient should be observed, except if there is a midline shift or focal neurological defect that would require surgery. Non-decompressed hematoma can lead to signs of increased intracranial pressure such as ipsilateral pupillary dilation (uncal herniation with oculomotor compression) or Cushing reflex (bradycardia, hypertension, and respiratory depression) (Figure 3-2).

Epidural hematoma is convex shaped and subdural hematoma is concave shaped

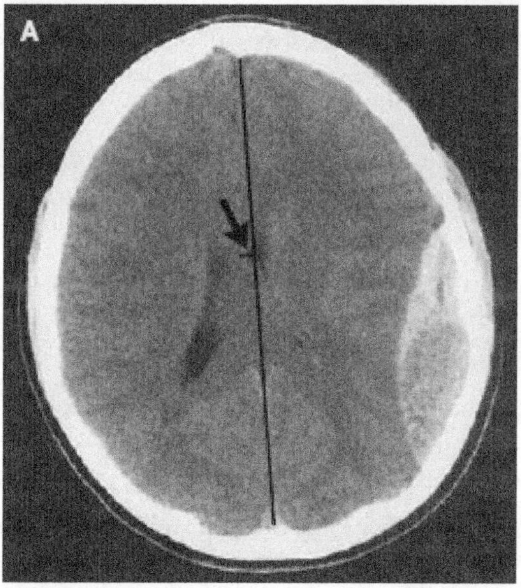

Figure 3-2. *Epidural hematoma with midline shift (arrow).*

42. What is the pathogenesis of transtentorial (uncal) herniation?

In uncal herniation, the medial portion of the temporal lobe (uncus) is pushed down over the tentorium as a result of increased intracranial pressure, causing midline shift and compression of the brainstem and its structures, such as the third cranial nerve and the ascending arousal tracts. As a result, patients may present with contralateral hemiparesis, ipsilateral eye dilation, and coma.

What is the difference between threatened and missed abortion?

All patients with suspected abortion should obtain serum human chorionic gonadotropin (HCG), blood type and cross and hematocrit.

Women with missed abortion may have noticed signs of early pregnancy (e.g., nausea, breast tenderness) that no longer exist.

What is the difference between incomplete and complete abortion?

43. What is the most common cause of subarachnoid hemorrhage in children?

The most common cause is an arteriovenous malformation.

44. What is the first step in the management of all patients with spinal injury or compression?

Administer high-dose intravenous (IV) steroids within the first 8 hours of injury. The best test after stabilization is magnetic resonance imaging (MRI). Why? It shows soft tissue better than a computed tomography scan does.

45. What differential diagnosis is considered in patients with vaginal bleeding in the first trimester?

In the first trimester, rule out threatened, missed, and inevitable abortion.

46. How do patients present with threatened abortion?

Patients may present with vaginal bleeding or spotting, with or without mild abdominal cramps. On the physical examination, the cervix is closed. The treatment is to administer RhoGAM (anti-Rh antibody) to patients who are Rh negative and follow up with an obstetrician/gynecologist.

47. How do patients present with missed abortion?

Patients present with vaginal bleeding, with or without abdominal cramps. On the physical examination, the cervix is closed and intrauterine pregnancy is present, but no fetal heart rate is heard (in utero death). The treatment is to administer RhoGAM to patients who are Rh negative and follow up with an obstetrician/gynecologist.

48. How do patients present with inevitable abortion?

Patients present with vaginal bleeding, with or without abdominal cramps. On the physical examination, the cervical os is open. The treatment is to administer RhoGAM to patients who are Rh negative and follow up with an obstetrician/gynecologist.

49. How do patients present with incomplete abortion?

Patients present with vaginal bleeding, with or without abdominal cramps. On the physical examination, retained tissue is present and the cervix is dilated. The treatment is to perform dilation and curettage and administer RhoGAM to patients who are Rh negative.

50. How do patients present with complete abortion?

Patients present with vaginal bleeding, with or without abdominal cramps. On the physical examination, no fetal tissue is seen. The products of conception have been completely passed out and the cervix is closed and uterus is contracted. The treatment is to administer RhoGAM to patients who are Rh negative and follow up with an obstetrician/gynecologist.

Spontaneous, missed, inevitable or incomplete abortions are managed medically (misoprostol), surgically (dilation and curettage) or expectantly, but surgical management is recommended for those that are unstable.

51. How do patients present with ectopic pregnancy?

Patients present with lower abdominal pain, vaginal bleeding, and fever. Always do a beta-human chorionic gonadotropin (B-HCG) pregnancy test in all sexually active women of reproductive age presenting with abdominal pain and or vaginal bleeding to rule out pregnancy. Ultrasound should be done to locate ectopic pregnancy and to rule out a tubo-ovarian abscess.

Risk factors for ectopic pregnancy are previous pelvic inflammatory disease and scarring of the fallopian tubes.

Give RhoGAM to Rh-negative patients in ectopic pregnancy. An ultrasound can detect an intrauterine pregnancy when B-HCG is >1500 IU/ml. Absence of an intrauterine pregnancy at this level of B-HCG is diagnostic of ectopic pregnancy.

52. When patients present with a third-trimester vaginal bleed, what differential diagnosis should be considered?

Placenta previa and placenta abruptio are the most common causes.

53. How do patients present with placenta previa?

Placenta previa is defined as placenta overlying the internal cervical os.

Risk factors include age >35 years, multiparity, prior uterine surgery, smoking, cocaine use, and digital examination. Patients usually present with bright red blood, little to no abdominal pain, and no fetal distress. Ultrasound is used for diagnosis. Treatment is expectant (scheduled cesarian section [C-section] if stable). A C-section is the delivery method of choice. Why? A C-section prevents aggravated bleeding.

Abortion >12 weeks of gestation usually causes retained products of conception.

Fetal cardiac activity is usually detected at 5-6 weeks of gestation.

A serum HCG less than 1500IU should be followed up by repeat HCG in 72 hours, since HCG levels usually doubles every 2 days in viable pregnacy.

What is the difference between placenta previa and placenta abruptio?

Non severe placenta abruptio (reassuring fetal heart rate) >34 weeks of gestation should still be treated with delivery. Only minor placenta abruptio (cessation of bleeding, minimal signs and symptoms) >34-36 weeks are eligible for watchful waiting.

Nonsevere placenta abruptio with <34 weeks of gestation can be treated with conservative expectant management and steroids for lung maturity.

A caesarian delivery is indicated in placenta abrutio if vaginal delivery is not possible.

If bleeding is minimal and fetal reassurance is normal, expectant management is considered for fetal maturity if the patient is remote from delivery, for example, at 36-37 weeks.

54. How do patients present with placenta abruptio?

Placenta abruptio is the premature separation of the placenta from the uterus. Risk factors are cocaine use, smoking, trauma, coagulopathy, and others (hypertension, prior placenta abruptio). Patients usually present with abdominal pain and dark red blood. Fetal distress may be present. If fetal distress occurs, delivery of the fetus is the ultimate treatment, regardless of the maturity of the lungs.

Placenta abruptio can be treated with prompt vaginal delivery in most cases except when the mother is unstable or fetal heart rate is non-reassuring and vaginal delivery is not imminent.

55. How do patients present with velamentous bleeding or vasa previa?

Vasa previa is the insertion of the fetal vessel between the chorion and the amnion located in the membranes covering the internal cervical os, where they are subjected to compression and rupture. The patient may present with vaginal bleeding and rapid fetal distress. Why rapid fetal distress? Fetal blood is being lost. The treatment is the rapid delivery of the fetus, regardless of the maturity of the lungs.

56. What is the definition of bloody show?

Bloody show is blood-stained mucus released from the cervix, which signals the onset of labor. This sign is normal and should be a diagnosis of exclusion after ruling out more ominous causes of third-trimester bleed.

57. What are third-trimester complications?

- Preeclampsia
- Eclampsia
- Chronic hypertension

58. What is the definition of preeclampsia?

Preeclampsia is hypertension and proteinuria of ≥300 mg/24 hours.

59. What is the definition of chronic hypertension in pregnancy?

Chronic hypertension in pregnancy is blood pressure (BP) ≥140/90 with a history of hypertension before pregnancy. Treat with bed rest and reduced salt diet; if BP ≥160/110, consider alpha 2 agonists (methyldopa), beta-blockers (metoprolol), or alpha and beta agonists (labetalol) as treatment options.

60. What is the definition of mild preeclampsia?

Mild preeclampsia is BP ≥140/90 at ≥20 weeks and proteinuria ≥300 mg/24 hours without other evidence of end-organ damage. Treatment is labetalol for BP and magnesium sulfate for prophylaxis of seizure during labor.

61. What is the definition of moderate-to-severe preeclampsia?

Moderate-to-severe preeclampsia is BP ≥160/100 and proteinuria ≥5 g/24 hours. Patients with associated neurological signs, or HELP (hemolysis, elevated liver enzymes, and low platelets) syndrome, have severe preeclampsia. The definitive treatment of severe preeclampsia is the delivery of the fetus, regardless of gestational age.

In general, in mild to moderate preeclampsia, if the patient is ≤37 weeks, treatment is expectant management (admit patient, treat severe hypertension, administer magnesium sulfate, and perform a non-stress test and a biophysical profile). Labor induction is indicated at ≥37 weeks. If the patient is ≤32 weeks and has severe preeclampsia, give a course of steroids before delivery.

62. All patients with preeclampsia should receive magnesium sulfate for seizure prophylaxis. True or false?

False. Magnesium sulfate prophylaxis for mild preeclampsia is controversial. However, prophylaxis is recommended for all patients with severe preeclampsia.

63. Magnesium sulfate is recommended for both prophylaxis and treatment of eclampsia. True or false?

True. Seizures in preeclampsia (eclampsia) are prevented and treated with IV magnesium sulfate.

64. When is a patient admitted against his or her will?

A patient is admitted against his or her will when there is a threat to harm self (e.g., acute manic episode, agitation, homicidal or suicidal ideations) or others.

Severe hypertension in preeclampsia is treated with IV labetalol, hydralazine or oral nifedipine.

Why is sodium bicarbonate administered to patients with anticholinergic toxicity?

When is the right time to treat acetaminophen toxicity?

Osmolal gap is the difference between calculated and measured serum osmolality.

65. How do patients with cholinergic toxicity present?

The patient may be exposed to insecticides (organophosphates bind cholinesterase, releasing choline) and may present with rhinorrhea, diarrhea, lacrimation, and meiosis. The antidote is atropine and pralidoxime.

66. How do patients with anticholinergic toxicity present?

The patient may present with ingestion of tricyclic antidepressants. The patient may progress from cardiac arrhythmias to concussion to coma (three Cs). Anticholinergic effects may also present as dry mouth and blurry vision. An EKG will show a prolonged QRS >100 ms and a terminal right axis (R wave in aVR >3 mm). The first step is to give sodium bicarbonate. Why? It binds the sodium channel, relieving QRS prolongation.

67. How do patients with sympathomimetic toxicity present?

An example is cocaine toxicity. The patient may present with hypertension, tachycardia, and seizures or arrhythmias. Treat hypertension with a short-acting benzodiazepine. Why? If hypertension is treated with a beta-blocker, it will stimulate unopposed alpha agonist activity.

68. How do patients with acetaminophen (APAP) toxicity present?

When APAP is ingested, in the first 24 hours the patient will present with nausea and vomiting, with some right upper quadrant tenderness and elevated serum transaminases. Seventy-two hours later, the patient can present with encephalopathy, liver necrosis, and renal failure, but have complete resolution of symptoms and organ dysfunction in 4 days to 3 weeks.

69. What is the treatment option for acetaminophen toxicity?

Treat with N-acetylcysteine (NAC) only if, after 4 hours, APAP serum levels are ≥150 mg/L. If ingestion occurred ≥8 hours ago, give NAC while awaiting the serum acetaminophen level results. The treatment is based on the Rumack-Matthew nomogram, which is also used to predict hepatotoxicity. NAC binds glutathione to convert the toxic intermediate, NAPQI, to the soluble, nontoxic products cysteine and mercapturic acid. Note that the APAP nomogram is based on a single ingestion and does not apply to chronic ingestion. Treat all symptomatic patients with NAC.

70. How do patients with ethylene glycol toxicity present?

Ethylene glycol can cause kidney failure in addition to central nervous system (CNS) disturbances.

Ethylene glycol causes metabolic acidosis with anion gap and osmolal gap > 10 mosmol/kg. It fluoresces on a wood lamp examination. Crystalluria (presence of needle-shaped crystals) is seen on urine microscopy as a result of calcium oxalate accumulation. The antidote is fomepizole or ethanol.

71. How do patients present with methanol toxicity?

Methanol toxicity causes CNS disturbances and blurry vision. Methanol causes metabolic acidosis with anion gap. The treatment is similar to that for ethylene glycol toxicity.

72. How do patients present with heroin (opioid) withdrawal symptoms?

Patients present with piloerection, nausea, vomiting, diarrhea, and chills. Treat with a long-acting opioid (e.g., methadone). Reverse acute opioid toxicity symptoms (respiratory depression or coma) with naloxone.

73. How do patients present with phencyclidine hydrochloride (PCP) abuse?

PCP is a hallucinogen. PCP causes pupillary constriction, nystagmus, and aggressive behavior. The treatment is supportive care.

74. How do patients present with lead toxicity?

The patient may present with nonspecific signs and symptoms: nausea, vomiting, abdominal pain, constipation, and encephalopathy. Burton's line (a blue line along the gums) is suggestive of lead toxicity. If the lead level is between 10 and 20 mg/dl, treat with removal from exposure and repeat testing with follow-up. Treat with chelation if the lead level is >60 mg/dl (potentially encephalopathic). The recommended chelator at this level is dimercaprol (BAL) because it crosses the blood-brain barrier rapidly. If edetate calcium disodium (EDTA) is desired, the recommended use is in combination with BAL because

Calculated serum osmolality= (2x serum [Na]) + [glucose, in mg/dL]/18 + [blood urea nitrogen, in mg/dL/2.8].

Isopropyl alcohol can present with altered mental status and elevated osmolar gap, but unlike methanol or ethylene gycol will not present with metabolic acidosis.

Tests to obtain after poisoning in all patients are: fingerstick for hypoglycemia, acetaminophen and salicylate levels, EKG for QRS or QTc intervals, and pregnancy tests in all women of child bearing age.

When are fractures closed vs. left open?

parenteral EDTA has been shown to increase brain lead levels in the first few days.

75. How may patients present with arsenic toxicity?

Arsenic is usually found in soil and rocks and gets into drinking water from underground drilled wells. In the United States, arsenic is present in low levels in fish. Acute toxicity from inhalation of high levels can present in workers (e.g., miners) with gastrointestinal symptoms and signs such as nausea, vomiting, diarrhea, QTc prolongation, and severe cardiac arrhythmia. Chronic toxicity presents as skin and neurological symptoms, including skin cancer, Bowen's disease (squamous cell cancer), and peripheral neuropathy.

76. How do patients present with sudden infant death syndrome (SIDS)?

Patients who are 3 months to 1 year old present with sudden death. By law, all infants with SIDS must undergo an autopsy to confirm this diagnosis.

77. How is SIDS prevented?

To prevent SIDS, avoid prone sleeping in infants, promote supine sleeping, and decrease smoking exposure. Recall prevention technique with the mnemonic "back to sleep".

78. What is the definition of open fractures?

Open fractures are fractures in contact with the outside environment in which the skin is not intact. Treat with emergency debridement, IV antibiotics, and immobilization in the operating room. Never close open fractures after debridement. Why? Not closing them prevents infection.

79. What is the definition of closed fractures?

Closed fractures are fractures with intact skin. They can be treated with closed reduction and immobilization with a cast or splint.

80. Tibia shaft fractures are the most common long bone fractures. True or false?

True. Most patients will present with an associated fibular fracture.

81. Blunt trauma is the most common cause of fat emboli. True or false?

True. A surgical technique, **intramedullary nailing** (a

form of external fixation), can be helpful in reducing the volume of fat embolization.

82. How may patients present with fat emboli?

Patients may present **12-72 hours** after a long bone fracture with tachycardia, **dyspnea**, hypoxia, **petechial rash**, and CNS dysfunction. Treatment of fat emboli is supportive care.

83. When there is a fracture from trauma (fall or motor vehicle accident), what is a necessary step in the patient's evaluation?

A fracture from trauma is an alert to probe for fractures in other joints. Why? Occult fracture is more likely to be present.

84. Falling on an outstretched arm is a risk for what type of fracture?

It is a risk for scaphoid fracture. On the physical examination, pain is localized to the radial aspect of the wrist and the anatomical "snuffbox" is tender. Any tenderness in snuffbox should be treated as a scaphoid fracture even in the absence of normal radiograph findings because scaphoid fractures are usually occult. Treatment is a thumb spica splint or cast; pain is controlled with analgesics.

85. In elderly female patients, falling on an outstretched arm can also lead to what type of fracture?

It can lead to a Colles' fracture, a distal radius fracture that can be diagnosed with a wrist X-ray. This type of fracture can be complicated by a median nerve injury. Other complications are compartment syndrome and neurovascular compromise. Treatment is based on whether it is an opened or a closed fracture.

What is the first step in evaluating patients with urethral injury?

86. How do patients with urethral injury present?

The patient may present with blood in the urethral meatus or a high-riding prostate on rectal examination. The next step is to perform a retrograde urethrogram. Do not insert a Foley urethral catheter before a retrograde urethrogram. Why? A Foley urethral catheter can turn a partial urethral tear into a complete one.

87. How may decompression sickness present in divers?

Decompression sickness occurs when a diver returns to the surface and gas tension in the tissues is greater than

Know the various clinical presentations in decompression sickness.

atmospheric pressure, causing liberation of gas bubbles in the tissues. These gas bubbles cause obstruction of vessels or tissue compression, manifesting as various signs and symptoms such as mild joint pain, pruritic erythematous rash, paresthesia, and paraplegia (spinal cord damage). In addition, air bubbles can cause gas embolism in the pulmonary venous system, producing chest pain, wheezing, and dyspnea ("chokes") or can transverse a patent foramen ovale to cause an arterial gas embolism in the pulmonary artery.

88. What are treatment options for decompression sickness?

Treatment is 100% oxygen with the Trendelenburg position and hyperbaric oxygen therapy to reduce the volume of bubbles.

Chapter 4
Ophthalmology

1. What is the pathogenesis of acute angle closure glaucoma?

Acute angle closure glaucoma is a trabecular meshwork occlusion that is due to persistent bowing of the iris forward, leading to elevated intraocular pressure. The patient presents with red eyes (**ciliary flush**), headache, nausea, vomiting, eye pain, and blurry vision. On examination of the eye, you will see dilated pupils and a cloudy cornea with a steamy appearance (edematous cornea). The first step is to check the intraocular pressure, which is usually elevated. Medical treatment can begin with topical pilocarpine (muscarinic agonist) and topical beta-blockers, followed by systemic medications (acetazolamide) to lower intraocular pressure and definitive therapy with laser surgery.

What is the first step in the evaluation of acute angle glaucoma?

2. What are some precipitants of acute angle closure glaucoma?

Sympathetic agonists, anticholinergic agents, stress, and darkness all lead to a dilated pupil that worsens angle closure.

3. What is the pathogenesis of central retinal artery occlusion?

Central retinal artery occlusion is an atheroembolic or atherosclerotic lesion that causes occlusion of the retinal artery, leading to sudden loss of vision that is painless. On examination of the eye, you will see background whiteness of the retina, an **afferent pupillary defect,** and a cherry-red spot in the macular region because of

Always rule out infraorbital fracture when a patient presents with a punch to the face.

What are the differences between periorbital cellulitis and orbital cellulitis?

What are the differences between hordeolum and chalazion?

the lack of ganglion fibers in the fovea. The first step is ocular massage to dislodge the emboli to the retinal artery branches and systemic or topical medications to lower intraocular pressure.

4. **What is the pathogenesis of infraorbital fracture?**
   Infraorbital fracture occurs when a fist or an object in the shape of the orbit impacts it. The infraorbital location is the most commonly fractured area because the orbital bone is the thinnest there. The patient will present with eye pain and on the physical examination will be unable to gaze upward.

5. **What is the pathogenesis of periorbital cellulitis?**
   Periorbital cellulitis is inflammation of the epidermis and subcutaneous tissues not involving the orbit. The patient will present with swelling, redness, and warmness of the periorbital region.
   Treat with amoxicillin/clavulanate.

6. **What is the pathogenesis of orbital cellulitis?**
   Orbital cellulitis is continuation of periorbital cellulitis that involves the orbit by involving the Tenon capsule (the capsule that separates the eyelid from the orbit). This condition is an emergency; the patient may have eye pain with movement and vision changes.
   Treat with IV penicillin and nafcillin or vancomycin. Why? The most common cause of this condition is Staphylococcus aureus.

7. **What is the pathogenesis of hordeolum (sty)?**
   A hordeolum is an acute staphylococcus infection of the meibomian glands. The patient will present with tender swelling of the eyelid.
   Treat with warm compresses and maintain clean hygiene, with incision and drainage being the last treatment option.

8. **What is the pathogenesis of a chalazion?**
   A chalazion is a chronic lipogranulomatous obstruction of the meibomian gland. The patient may present with nontender swelling of the eyelid. This condition has a high recurrence rate. The patient can first try warm compresses; if this fails, incision and drainage is the last treatment option.

9. What is the pathophysiology of a pterygium?

A connective tissue lesion of the conjunctiva that is common in people from a **warm climate**, a pterygium can cause eye irritation. Emergency ophthalmology referral should be made if it invades the cornea.

10. When a patient presents with "red eye," what is the next step in evaluation?

The most common cause of red eye is conjunctivitis; however, other causes that need to be considered are subconjunctival hemorrhage (trauma associated and unilateral), scleritis, acute angle closure glaucoma, uveitis, and keratitis.

11. Itching, burning, and red eye with follicular conjunctival reaction is usually associated with viral conjunctivitis. True or false?

True. However, itching, tearing eyes and nasal congestion with conjunctival (chemosis) and eyelid edema points more toward allergic conjunctivitis. Crusting with "glued eyes" associated with **purulent discharge** is more likely to be bacterial conjunctivitis.

12. What is the etiology of conjunctivitis in neonates?

Conjunctivitis can be caused by chemicals, viruses or bacteria in neonates.

Bacterial conjunctivitis is either gonococcal or chlamydial. The chlamydial type can cause both conjunctivitis and **pneumonia, with the patient presenting with respiratory distress** and watery (mucopurulent) conjunctivitis in the first 5-14 days after birth.

Treatment of chlamydial conjunctivitis: **Oral erythromycin** will treat both the conjunctivitis and pneumonia.

Gonococcal conjunctivitis is the most severe type and may cause bilateral purulent discharge within the first 2- 5 days after birth and extraocular involvement.

Treatment of gonococcal conjunctivitis: **IV or IM 3rd generation cephalosporin such as ceftriaxone.**

The chemical type of conjunctivitis (occurs within the first 24 hours of birth) is usually due to topical silver nitrate for prophylaxis. It causes mild hyperemia (red eye) with tearing. No treatment is needed but artificial tears can be used.

What is the difference between gonococcal and chlamydial conjunctivitis in neonates?

Fluorescein staining is diagnostic of corneal abrasion.

13. The prevalence of age-related macular degeneration increases in older adults. True or false?

True. Other risk factors are female sex, smoking, and white race. The clinical features are sudden-onset or **gradual unilateral** vision loss, the need for increased lighting, and **facial distortions**.

14. What is the most common cause of glaucoma?

Primary open angle glaucoma is usually due to **age-related optic neuropathy**. Other risk factors are steroid use, diabetic retinopathy, and congenital disorders. Treat with topical beta-blockers, prostaglandin analogs, alpha agonists, and laser trabeculoplasty.

15. What is the diagnostic evaluation of eye pain and foreign body sensation?

This is likely **corneal abrasion**; **fluorescein staining** is diagnostic. Treatment is empirical topical antibiotics (against *Pseudomonas aeruginosa* in those with contact lenses). Another common cause of foreign body sensation is keratoconjunctivitis (dry eyes).

16. What is the differential diagnosis of acute unilateral vision loss?

Consider optic nerve lesion (tumor), inflammation (optic neuritis), retinal artery occlusion, nonarteritic ischemic optic neuropathy (diabetes, hypertension, vascular disease), retinal detachment, temporal arteritis, and amaurosis fugax.

17. What is the differential diagnosis of acute bilateral vision loss?

Consider lesions affecting the **optic tract** or **occipital lobe** causing a posterior circulation stroke, circulatory disturbance (hypotension), or cardiac disease (aortic dissection, MI).

18. A flashing light or a shadow pulled down over the visual field like a curtain suggests what ophthalmologic condition?

This suggests **retinal detachment**. Make sure to differentiate it from **transient unilateral** vision loss (amaurosis fugax), which is usually due to carotid artery disease. In retinal detachment, a funduscopic examination will confirm a tear in the retina, whereas in amaurosis fugax, a **carotid bruit** will be heard.

19. Flare (increased protein content of the aqueous humor) and hypopyon (leukocytes in the anterior chamber) on a slit lamp are clinical features suggestive of what ophthalmologic condition?

Inflammation of the uveal tract (iris, ciliary body, choroid), also known as **uveitis**, can be associated with autoimmune disorders (systemic lupus erythematosus, inflammatory bowel disease, sarcoidosis) and viral and fungal infections.

20. What are the most common causes of uveitis?

Anterior uveitis is usually caused by **herpes simplex 1**; posterior uveitis is usually caused by toxoplasmosis and cytomegalovirus (CMV).

21. What are the most common causes of keratitis (cornea infection)?

The most common cause is **herpes simplex virus** with characteristic **dendritic ulcer** (linear branching ulcer), or bacterial infections (can be associated with ulcerative keratitis with **contact lenses use**).

22. What is the pathophysiology of unilateral eye droop (ptosis)?

The upper eyelid is innervated by the 3rd nerve, which keeps it open, and the 7th nerve, which keeps it closed. Unilateral eyelid droop is usually caused by any lesion affecting the **3rd nerve (oculomotor palsy)** such as transtentorial (uncal) herniation, as well as intracranial aneurysms, cavernous sinus mass, and diabetes (pupillary sparing microvascular palsy). Look for associated symptoms because most patients will also present with pupillary dilation and extraocular muscle weakness in the region of the 3rd nerve. **Oculosympathetic pathway** is also responsible for a minor elevation of the upper eyelid, and any lesion in this pathway can result in ptosis as part of Horner's syndrome (miosis, ptosis, anhidrosis).

Two common causes of ptosis are oculomotor palsy and oculosympathetic pathway lesions.

23. What is the differential diagnosis of ptosis?

In addition to 3rd nerve palsy, and oculosympathetic palsy, consider myasthenia gravis, which may present as ptosis and weakness of multiple extraocular muscles. Severe hyperthyroidism (Graves' disease) can also present in a similar fashion, in addition to ophthalmoplegia.

What is the most common cause of white reflex?

24. What is the definition of strabismus?

Strabismus is the misalignment of the eyes. On examination, the misaligned eye is deviated; in the Hirschberg test, reflected light is seen in a different spot in each eye.

Treatment: Occluding the normal eye, forcing the misaligned eye to realign

Early treatment is crucial; otherwise, a patient may develop amblyopia.

25. What is the definition of amblyopia?

Amblyopia is abnormal vision within a normal eye, most commonly caused by strabismus. In general, it is caused by the repression of images in the misaligned eye by the brain.

26. What is the definition of leukocoria?

Leukocoria is an absent red reflex or the development of a white reflex. The most deadly disease to rule out is retinoblastoma (the most common intraocular childhood tumor), but the most common cause of white reflex is a congenital cataract.

Chapter 5
Ear, Nose, and Throat

1. How do patients present with peritonsillitis?
The patient may present with asymmetric swelling of the tissues around the tonsils (swelling of one tonsil, with the other being normal), erythremia, difficulty swallowing (dysphagia), trismus (pain when attempting to open the mouth), fever, and pain on swallowing (odynophagia). On examination, the uvula may be seen to be deviated to the contra lateral side because of asymmetric swelling of peritonsillar tissue. The first step is to secure the airway if it is compromised. Additional treatment is to administer broad-spectrum IV antibiotics, with possible drainage by an ear, nose, and throat (ENT) specialist.

Always check the airway in patients with peritonsillitis or retropharyngeal abscess.

2. How do patients present with a retropharyngeal abscess?
A retropharyngeal abscess is located between the cervical vertebrae and the posterior pharynx. The patient may present with erythema of the oropharynx, dysphagia, odynophagia, trismus, neck pain, drooling, a hyper-extended neck, and respiratory distress, but absent peritonsillar swelling. The first step is to secure the airway. Additional treatment includes administration of IV antibiotics with possible drainage by an ENT specialist.

3. What are the risk factors for developing otitis media?
Risk factors are age (children are more likely to develop acute otitis media [AOM] and adults are at risk for chronic otitis media), smoking, immunosuppression and Eustachian tube abnormality.

What is the difference between otitis externa and AOM?

Tenderness with tragal pressure suggests otitis externa.

4. What is the pathogenesis of acute otitis media (AOM)?
AOM is common in children because of the small size of the Eustachian tube and its acute angulation.

5. How may a patient present with AOM?
The patient may present with ear pain, fussiness, and fever. Adults can present with unilateral hearing loss, pain, and ear discharge. On examination, the tympanic membrane (TM) is **erythematous with exudates, bulges,** and is **immobile** with insufflation.

6. What are the treatment options for AOM?
The first step is treatment with **high-dose amoxicillin.** If therapy fails, the second line of treatment is **amoxicillin/clavulanate** or **intramuscular ceftriaxone**. Macrolide antibiotic is used if the patient is allergic to penicillin.

7. How do patients with sinusitis present?
The patient presents with purulent nasal drainage, fever, and facial pain. Treatment: **Amoxicillin/clavulanate** is now the first-line treatment against sinusitis.

8. Immunocompromised patients are at risk for what type of sinusitis?
They are at risk for fungal organisms; diabetes patients are predisposed to **mucormycosis**, a deadly sinusitis with a high mortality rate.

9. What complications are patients with sinusitis at risk of developing?
They are at risk for periorbital cellulitis, brain abscess, and meningitis.

10. The most common causative organisms in sinusitis and AOM are *Streptococcus pneumoniae, Haemophilus influenzae,* and *Moraxella catarrhalis*. True or false?
True. Thus, treat with amoxicillin and amoxicillin/clavulanate.

11. What is the most common causative organism in otitis externa?
The most common causative organisms are ***Pseudomonas aeruginosa*** and *Staphylococcus aureus*. The patient presents with severe ear pain, ear discharge, and hearing loss. On examination, the ear canal is erythematous and edematous, and the TM is non-erythematous and mobile with insufflation. Treatment is topical antibiotics or acetic acid plus corticosteroid drops.

12. How is acute serous otitis media treated?
In serous otitis media, on examination, the TM bulges, and is immobile but there is no evidence of inflammation. **Watchful waiting** is advised.

13. List some common complications of otitis media.
- Mastoiditis
- Chronic otitis media
- Cholesteatoma (mass-like excess squamous epithelium causing compressive symptoms resulting from chronic otitis media)
- Malignant otitis (common in diabetes and immunosuppressed patients caused by *Pseudomonas aeruginosa*)

Cholesteatoma should be surgically removed in children to prevent hearing loss, vertigo and infections.

14. List some rare complications of otitis media.
- Brain abscess
- Epidural abscess
- Sinus thrombosis
- Cavernous vein thrombosis
- Carotid artery thrombosis
- Meningitis

15. What are risk factors for external otitis?
Risk factors are water exposure, a foreign body inserted into the ear, and external hearing devices.

16. What are risk factors for upper respiratory infections (URIs)?
Risk factors include age (old or young), overcrowding, immunosuppressed states, and malnutrition.

17. What are clinical features of URI?
Features include runny nose, scratchy throat, and nasal congestion, followed later by cough.

18. What are the most common causative organisms in URI?
Most common are **viral organisms** such as respiratory syncytial virus that are transmitted by aerosol particles or direct contact. Treatment should be symptomatic except if signs/symptoms of bacterial superinfection occur, such as fever, facial/maxillary tooth pain, and symptoms that last >1 week.

19. What is the most common type of epistaxis?
The **anterior type** is most common, occurring when the nasal septum is supplied by Kiesselbach's plexus,

which is usually caused by benign conditions such as trauma, allergic hyperemia, systemic anticoagulation or antiplatelet use, or introduction of a foreign body or intranasal drug (cocaine). Treatment is nasal pressure, intranasal phenylephrine, cotton wool swab insertion, or prophylactic anti-staphylococcal antibiotics.

20. What are rare causes of anterior epistaxis?
Rare causes include Osler Weber-Rendu syndrome, nasal tumor, and aneurysms.

21. What is the differential diagnosis of oral lesions?
- Aphthous ulcers
- Candidiasis (oral white plaques)
- Leukoplakia (white plaque or patch, premalignant lesion)
- Coxsackievirus
- Syphilis
- Human immunodeficiency virus (HIV)
- Neoplasia

22. What is the differential diagnosis of oral white plaque?
Consider **candidiasis** versus leukoplakia, which can be differentiated from risk factors: candidiasis is associated with inhaled steroid use, antibiotic use, having dentures, and immunosuppressed states, whereas leukoplakia is associated with heavy smoking and alcohol.

23. How is sore throat (pharyngitis) evaluated?
The most common cause of pharyngitis is a viral organism or rhinovirus; however, **group A *Streptococcus*** (GAS) infection is associated with some dreaded complications.. The first step in evaluation is to obtain a **rapid antigen assay** test for GAS.

What is the difference between croup and epiglottitis?

24. What is the pathogenesis of croup infection?
Croup is a parainfluenza (RNA virus) infection that causes inflammation of the larynx and tracheal tissues. The patient may present with a hoarse voice, hacking cough with no respiratory distress, and low-grade fever. Diagnosis is clinical, but a chest X-ray (CXR) may show subglottic stenosis (steeple sign) (Figure 5-1).

On examination, the patient has neck lymphadenopathy and inspiratory stridor.

Treatment: Treat mild croup initially with a single dose of oral dexamethasone and cool mist (humidified air); if this fails, or it progresses to respiratory distress, give oxygen and inhaled epinephrine.

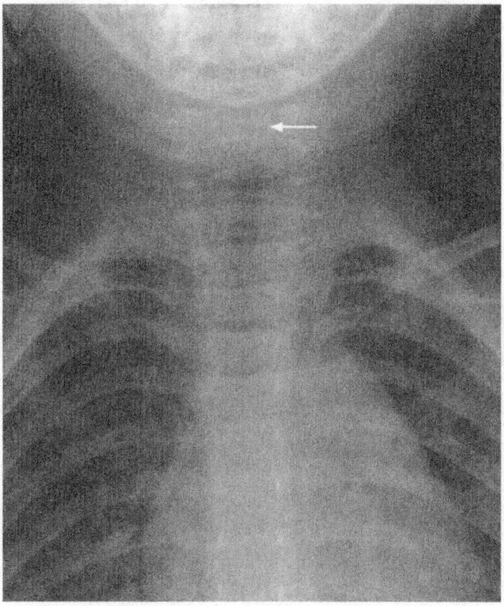

Figure 5-1. *Steeple sign (inverted V shape) of croup from subglottic narrowing (arrow).*

Children not immunized with Hib vaccine are at risk for epiglottitis.

25. What is the pathogenesis of epiglottitis?

Inflammation of the epiglottis and surrounding tissues is caused by Haemophilus influenzae (a gram-negative rod). The patient presents with hoarseness, high fever, sore throat, hyperextended neck, and drooling.

On the physical examination, inspiratory stridor is present, the neck is hyperextended, and the patient is drooling. Lateral X-rays may show the "thumb sign," which is indicative of edematous epiglottis (Figure 5-2).

Treatment: Immediate emergency endotracheal intubation and IV antibiotics. Tracheostomy may be needed if endotracheal intubation fails.

What is the difference between epiglottitis and peritonsillitis or retropharyngeal abscess?

26. How may patients present with Ludwig's angina?

Presentation is similar to that for epiglottitis, typically fever, chills, mouth pain, stiff neck, drooling, and dysphagia. The physical examination may reveal stridor, as in epiglottitis. However, Ludwig's angina is caused by infection of the submandibular space, usually from a

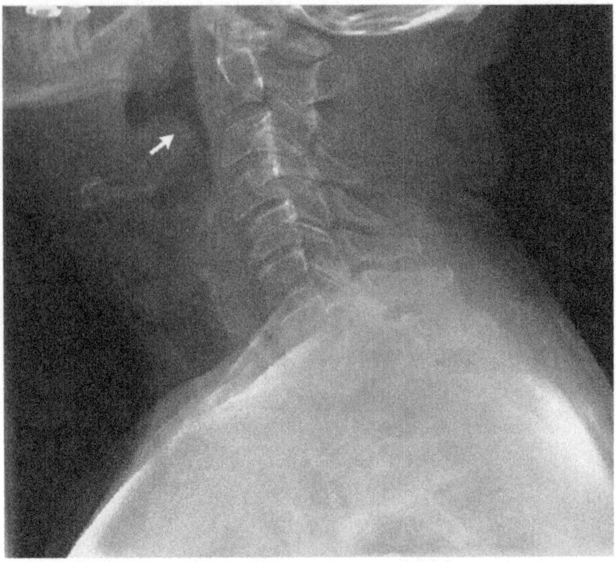

Figure 5-2. *"Thumb sign" of epiglottitis.*

tooth infection. There is cellulitis on floor of the mouth with a "woody" appearance. Treatment is emergency airway maintenance with endotracheal intubation via the nasal route and broad-spectrum IV antibiotics.

Tracheostomy is performed if endotracheal intubation fails.

What is the difference between bronchiolitis and asthma?
Age and upper respiratory tract infection

27. What is the pathogenesis of bronchiolitis?

Bronchiolitis is lower airway inflammation secondary to respiratory syncytial virus. Other causative organisms include adenovirus and parainfluenza virus. The patient may present with symptoms of upper respiratory tract infection (runny nose, nasal congestion),and bronchioles inflammation (tachypnea, respiratory retractions, wheezing), and fever.

Treatment: Oxygen, beta agonists. Patients with bronchiolitis have an increased risk of acquiring asthma. These patients are usually <2 years old and have an associated upper respiratory tract infection.

28. What is the pathogenesis of pertussis?

Pertussis is whooping cough secondary to spasms of the airway due to inflammation caused by Bordetella pertussis (a gram-negative rod). Patients usually present initially with nasal congestion, sneezing, and rhinorrhea, which are similar to symptoms of upper respiratory infections. This is the most infectious stage, known as the catarrhal phase. The second stage of pertussis is characterized by whooping cough.

Treatment: Erythromycin or azithromycin during the catarrhal phase helps limit the course of illness. It is still recommended after cough has appeared because although it does not alter the disease course, it can help limit the secondary spread of the disease.

Prophylaxis: Regardless of their immunization status, individuals in contact with patients who have pertussis require prophylaxis with oral erythromycin for 14 days. Macrolides can be used as an alternative.

What is the prophylaxis for pertussis?

29. List the clinical features of streptococcal pharyngitis.

Streptococcal pharyngitis is caused by *Streptococcus pyogenes* (group A streptococci). The patient will present with sore throat, fever, and absence of cough. Physical examination may reveal swollen, **tender anterior cervical** lymphadenopathy and **tonsillar exudates**.

30. List the clinical features of Epstein-Barr virus (EBV) pharyngitis.

EBV, along with acute retroviral syndrome, is relatively uncommon. The patient will present with sore throat, fever, malaise, and abdominal pain. The patient on examination will have cervical lymphadenopathy. **Splenomegaly** may be present.

Do not forget to advise patients with EBV to abstain from contact sports until their physical examination results are normal.

31. What is the diagnostic evaluation and management of EBV pharyngitis?

The first step is to obtain a **monospot** test to check for **heterophil antibodies**. Laboratory tests may reveal elevated **liver enzyme levels** and **hemolytic anemia. The** patient may develop a **maculopapular rash** after being treated with antibiotics. Advise the patient not to take part in physical activity until the results of the physical examination are normal or for a minimum of 3 weeks to avoid spleen rupture.

32. What are the dreaded complications of streptococcal pharyngitis?

Complications include acute rheumatic fever, acute glomerulonephritis (within 2 weeks of pharyngitis onset), scarlet fever, and retropharyngeal and peritonsillar abscesses.

33. When is primary prophylaxis of rheumatic fever indicated?

In patients with pharyngitis and positive results on the Group A *Streptococcus* rapid test or throat culture, treatment with penicillin reduces the incidence of rheumatic fever.

34. Post-streptococcal glomerulonephritis does not appear to be prevented by antibiotic treatment of pharyngitis. True or false?

True. However, the incidence of acute rheumatic fever and peritonsillar abscess can be reduced after treatment of streptococcal pharyngitis with penicillin.

35. What is the differential diagnosis of acute hearing loss?

Consider drugs (aminoglycosides, cisplatin), infectious labyrinthitis, acoustic neuroma, meningioma, and meningitis.

36. What is the first step in the evaluation of acute hearing loss?

The first step is to perform the Weber and Rinne tests; in Rinne, bone and air conduction are compared by placing the tuning fork on the mastoid and near ear; in Weber, the tuning fork is placed on the forehead.

37. How are the Weber and Rinne tests used for the differential diagnosis of hearing loss?

In the Weber test, the good ear hears the sound better in sensorineural hearing loss and the bad ear hears the sound better in conductive hearing loss. In the Rinne test, if air > bone conduction, it indicates normal hearing; if bone conduction >air conduction, it indicates conductive hearing loss, particularly if the Weber test lateralizes to that side.

Presbycusis causes sensory high frequency hearing loss early on , while meniere disease causes low frequency sensory hearing loss early on.

38. What are causes of sensorineural hearing loss?

Presbycusis due to aging, which is usually bilateral, is the most common cause of chronic sensorineural hearing loss. There can also be inner ear, cochlear, or auditory nerve involvement (acoustic neuroma).

39. What are the causes of conductive hearing loss?

- Cerumen impaction
- External obstruction in the auditory ear canal
- Chronic otitis media
- Cholesteatoma

40. What are the three most common causes of peripheral vertigo?

The most common causes are benign positional vertigo (BPV), labyrinthitis, and Meniere's disease. Peripheral vertigo is usually associated with horizontal or rotatory nystagmus, whereas central vertigo can be associated with vertical or horizontal nystagmus. Neurological symptoms are usually present in central vertigo (e.g., multiple sclerosis, stroke, tumor).

41. Brief episodes (a few seconds) of vertigo worsened by positional changes is usually suggestive of what type of vertigo?

It suggests BPV. Treatment is reassurance and canalith repositioning (Epley's maneuver).

42. Acute vertigo lasting for days occurring after a viral illness is most likely related to what type of vertigo?

It is most likely labyrinthitis. Treat symptomatically, as it usually self-resolves.

The duration of vertigo is usually diagnostic.

43. Chronic or repeated episodes of tinnitus, hearing loss, and severe vertigo are suggestive of what type of vertigo?

They suggest Meniere's disease. Treatment is symptomatic, salt restriction, and diuretics.

44. What is the differential diagnosis of head and neck masses?

Possibilities can be divided into three categories: congenital, inflammatory, and neoplastic.

45. What are some congenital causes of a head and neck mass?

- Brachial cleft cyst (**anterior to the sternocleidomastoid** muscle, not a midline mass)
- Thyroglossal duct (typically a **midline mass**, ectopic thyroid gland can present in the thyroglossal duct)
- Teratoma (consists of all three germ layers)
- Dermoid
- Thymic cyst

46. What are inflammatory causes of a head and neck mass?

Viral infections from upper respiratory infections may produce **reactive** lymphadenopathy in the submandibular region, which is usually tender and mobile and resolves

Viral upper respiratory infections are the most common cause of cervical lymphadenopathy.

in 1-2 weeks. Bacterial infections can cause **suppurative** lymphadenopathy in the submandibular region from infection in the pharynx or skin. Examples of note include *Staphylococcus,* cat scratch disease, toxoplasmosis, tularemia, actinomycosis (associated with dental procedures; biopsy with granulomas and **sulfur granules**), brucellosis (transmitted by **farm animals**), mycobacterial infections, and HIV.

47. What are neoplastic causes of a head and neck mass?

- Metastatic head and neck cancer (usually from squamous cell cancer)
- Thyroid masses
- Salivary gland masses (e.g., parotid gland)
- Schwannoma
- Lymphoma

Chapter 6

Endocrine System

1. What is the pathogenesis of appetite?
Leptin stimulates the appetite when it is released from the hypothalamus. Tumor necrosis factor and interleukin-1 suppress appetite. Loss of appetite can be caused by these mechanisms, leading to weight loss.

2. What is a common cause of weight loss in the elderly?
Inadequate intake due to loss of dentition is a common cause of weight loss in the elderly.

3. List the key features of vitamin deficiencies and excesses.

- Niacin is made from tryptophan; vitamin D is made from cholesterol. Niacin **deficiency causes pellagra (dementia, diarrhea, and dermatitis)**.
- Vitamin D deficiency causes rickets in children (bowing of legs with elevated alkaline phosphatase and parathyroid hormone) and osteomalacia in adults (characteristic symmetrical pseudofractures with elevated alkaline phosphatase and parathyroid hormone).
- Vitamin D deficiency can also be due to renal failure.
- Vitamin A deficiency leads to night blindness and dry skin. Excesses have been associated with benign intracranial hypertension **(pseudotumor cerebri)**.
- Vitamin E deficiency leads to ataxia and telangiectasia.
- Excess vitamin E inhibits vitamin K and leads to easy bruisability.
- Vitamin B6 (pyridoxine) deficiency causes peripheral neuropathy in patients with tuberculosis treated with isoniazid. Why? Isoniazid inhibits vitamin B6.

Excess vitamin A can cause pseudotumor cerebri.

Always rule out vitamin C deficiency in patients presenting with gum bleeding and swelling.

- Vitamin C deficiency causes perifollicular papules and **scurvy (gum swelling and bleeding)**.
- Thiamine deficiency causes Wernicke syndrome (ophthalmoplegia, ataxia, and nystagmus) and Korsakoff syndrome (anterograde amnesia) in alcoholics.
- Folate deficiency and vitamin B12 deficiency both cause pernicious megaloblastic anemia and homocysteine accumulation. Why? Both are responsible for converting homocysteine to methionine. Methylmalonic acid elevation is found only in vitamin B12 deficiency because only vitamin B12 is responsible for the synthesis of succinyl-coenzyme A (CoA) from methylmalonyl-CoA (methylmalonic acid). Accumulation of this intermediate results in neurological problems. Therefore, only vitamin B12 deficiency causes neurological problems.

4. What are the neurological problems found in vitamin B_{12} deficiency?

One neurological problem is subacute combined degeneration of the dorsal (posterior) and lateral spinal (corticospinal tracts) columns. Symptoms are paresthesias and ataxia, due to loss of vibration and position sense. Degeneration can progress to weakness, paraplegia, and fecal and urinary incontinence. Other neurological signs and symptoms are Lhermitte's syndrome (shock-like sensation radiating to feet during neck flexion, optic atrophy and neuropathy, memory loss, and dementia).

5. What are the treatment options for vitamin deficiencies?

Supplemental feeding, especially enteral therapy, is preferred; appetite stimulants, treatment of the underlying causes, and vitamin replacement for deficiencies are other options.

6. Dermatitis, alopecia, and diarrhea are suggestive of what mineral deficiency?

They suggest zinc deficiency. Since animal products represent the primary source of zinc, people with a low intake of protein (alcoholics, vegetarians) can be deficient in zinc. Growth failure, hypogonadism, and impaired immunity are other signs of severe zinc deficiency.

7. What is the pathogenesis of hyperthyroidism?
Hyperthyroidism is the abnormal release of thyroid hormones, leading to excessive sweating, diarrhea, menstrual alteration, and weight loss.

8. How do patients present with Graves' disease?
Graves' disease is the most common type of hyperthyroidism. Antibodies to thyroid-stimulating hormone (TSH) receptors, after binding, cause the release of thyroid hormones. In addition to presenting with hyperthyroid symptoms, patients will present with unique signs, such as proptosis (exophthalmos) and pretibial myxedema.

Graves' disease is the most common cause of primary hyperthyroidism?

9. What antibodies are found in Graves' disease?
Thyroid-stimulating immunoglobulin is diagnostic of Graves' disease; other antibodies that indicate autoimmunity are antithyroid peroxidase (anti-TPO) and antithyroglobulin antibodies.

Secondary hyperthyroidism (High T3 and T4 levels and normal or high TSH) suggests a TSH producing pituitary tumor.

10. What is a life-threatening complication of hyperthyroidism?
A life-threatening complication is thyroid storm, which can be precipitated by radioiodine, sudden cessation of thyroid medications, surgery in those with unrecognized thyrotoxicosis, and acute illness, leading to hypo/hyperthermia, tachycardia, diarrhea, agitation, and seizures or psychosis.

11. What are the treatment options for thyroid storm?
Treatment consists of a combination of propylthiouracil, propranolol, iodine, and hydrocortisone.

12. What is the pathogenesis of subacute thyroiditis (de Quervain thyroiditis), also known as granulomatous thyroiditis?
Subacute thyroiditis is caused by viral infection, which destroys the thyroid gland, leading to the release of thyroid hormones. The patient may present with a painful neck and fever.

13. Most thyroiditis cases have a triphasic pattern? True or false?
True. It usually consists of a thyrotoxic phase, a hypothyroid phase, and finally a euthyroid phase.

14. What is the pathogenesis of postpartum thyroiditis?
Postpartum thyroiditis is an autoimmune reaction that leads to the release of thyroid hormones. It is common

Amiodarone and lithium are common drugs that cause thyroid dysfunction.

If thyroid tests confirm primary hyperthyroidism (low TSH and high free T3 and T4 levels), the next step is to obtain thyroid scintigraphy (radioiodine testing). Scintigraphy is not needed for hypothyroid states.

in pregnancy and typically presents as a **painless** mildly enlarged thyroid gland. **Anti-TPO antibodies** may be present.

15. What is the pathogenesis of multinodular adenoma?

Multinodular adenoma is common in the elderly population. It is the autonomous release of thyroid hormones.

16. What are some causes of elevated TSH and normal free T4 levels?

- Subclinical hypothyroidism
- Sick euthyroid syndrome
- Drugs (amiodarone)
- Transient thyroid states
- TSH-receptor mutation

17. What is the pathogenesis of surreptitious hyperthyroidism?

Surreptitious hyperthyroidism is the ingestion of thyroid hormones. The patient will present with hyperthyroidism symptoms.

18. What drugs are known to cause hyperthyroidism and hypothyroidism?

Amiodarone, lithium, and alpha interferon can cause hyper- and hypothyroidism; interleukin-2 can cause thyroiditis.

19. Excess iodine can cause hyperthyroidism. True or false?

True. Excess iodine can cause increased synthesis of thyroid hormone. Some iodine sources are medications (amiodarone), dietary supplements, iodine-rich water, and topical anesthetics.

20. The first step in diagnosing thyroid conditions is to obtain TSH. True or false?

True. Triiodothyronine (T3) and thyroxine (T4) are subsequently ordered.

21. The test that is usually used for differential diagnosis in primary hyperthyroidism is iodine-131. True or false?

False. Radioiodine-123 (in capsule or liquid form) is usually used for diagnosis and radioiodine-131 (also in capsule or liquid form, given orally as a single dose, is usually used for therapeutic purposes.

22. Radioiodine treatment can worsen Graves' ophthalmopathy. True or false?

True. Graves' ophthalmopathy is less likely to be worsened in those treated with surgery or thyroid medications.

23. What types of hyperthyroidism show increased uptake of iodine-123 in the affected gland?

Types of hyperthyroidism that show increased uptake are those that actively produce thyroid hormones:

- Graves' disease: Diffuse uptake **(>30% uptake)**
- Multinodal adenoma: Multiple nodular uptake **(>30% uptake)**
- Single adenoma: Single uptake, with normal surroundings (>30% uptake)

Know the specific types of uptake (diffuse vs. nodular) in different types of hyperactive glands.

24. What types of hyperthyroidism show lack of uptake of iodine-123 contrast?

Types of hyperthyroidism that show lack of uptake are those that involve destruction of the thyroid glands or no active thyroid production:

- Surreptitious intake/euthyroid (10-30% uptake)
- Thyroiditis (low uptake, <10%)
- Thyroid malignancy (uptake less than surrounding thyroid tissue [cold nodules])

All solid hypoechoic thyroid nodules >1cm should be biopsied with fine needle aspiration (FNA).

25. Hyperfunctioning thyroid nodules (increased uptake) detected via radionuclide scanning suggest what?

They suggest an autonomously secreting thyroid nodule; this is seen in various causes of hyperthyroidism. Hyperfunctioning nodules are almost never malignant, and fine needle aspiration is not needed.

26. What are the therapies of choice in hyperthyroidism?

Therapies of choice are antithyroid medications (methimazole or propylthiouracil), radiation ablation, and surgery (thyroidectomy).

Beta-blockers are used for acute episodes.

Note: Treatment of hyperthyroidism will not cause regression or ameliorate progression of **Graves' ophthalmopathy or** myxedema.

The first steps in evaluating incidentally discovered thyroid nodule (palpated or located radiographically) are to perform history, physical, obtain neck ultrasound and measure serum TSH.

27. What are the complications of hyperthyroidism treatment?

The most common surgical complication is hypothyroidism; others are hoarseness from recurrent laryngeal nerve transaction and hypoparathyroidism. Medical

Central hypothyroidism (Low TSH and low T4 and T3 levels) suggests a pituitary mass.

The most common cause of primary hypothyroidism (High TSH and low T3 and T4 levels) is Hashimoto's thyroiditis.

Which antibodies are found in Hashimoto thyroiditis?

therapies for hyperthyroidism, such as methimazole, can cause neutropenia.

28. What is the definition of hypothyroidism?
Hypothyroidism is low levels of thyroid hormones because of the destruction of the gland or inadequate iodine intake, leading to fatigue, cold intolerance, constipation, weight gain, facial puffiness, myxedema coma, and carpel tunnel syndrome.

29. What is a life-threatening complication of hypothyroidism?
A life-threatening complication is **myxedema coma**, which can be precipitated by infection, sedatives, or cold exposure, leading to hypothermia and coma. Treatment is intravenous levothyroxine and corticosteroids.

30. What are the types of hypothyroidism?
- Hashimoto: Antibodies to thyroglobulin and peroxidase, leading to damage of the thyroid gland
- Surgery: Surgery indicated for hyperthyroidism
- Drugs: amiodarone, lithium
- Hypopituitarism (secondary hypothyroidism)

Treatment of hypothyroidism: Levothyroxine

31. What is a long-term complication of Hashimoto thyroiditis?
Monitor patients with Hashimoto thyroiditis carefully for the potential development of lymphoma.

32. What is the most common type of thyroid cancer?
The most common is **papillary cancer**; other types are follicular (the only thyroid cancer that spreads hematogenously; therefore, there is no lymph node involvement), medullary (elevated calcitonin levels), and anaplastic cancer (very rare).

33. Medullary thyroid cancer (MTC) is associated with what proto-oncogene?
It is associated with the RET-proto-oncogene.

34. Radioiodine is not taken up by C-cells, and so MTC can only be treated with total resection, in contrast to papillary and follicular cancers, which are treated with radiation and total resection. True or false?
True.

35. How do patients present with hypercalcemia?
The patient can present with polyuria, polydipsia, and bone and abdominal pain.

Hypercalcemia may present with diabetes-like symptoms.

36. What are the causes of hypercalcemia?
- Hyperparathyroidism: The most common cause of hyperparathyroidism is primary hyperparathyroidism. Patients are usually older.
- Malignancy: This occurs either by secretion of a parathyroid-like peptide or by lysis of the bone (multiple myeloma).
- Multiple endocrine neoplasia (MEN) 1 and IIa syndrome.
- Chronic diseases (sarcoidosis, excess vitamin D or vitamin A, granulomatous diseases)
- Tertiary hyperparathyroidism or Drugs (thiazide)
- Acidosis
- Familial hypocalciuric hypercalcemia (calcium sensing receptor defect)

37. How does acidosis cause hypercalcemia?
Acidosis leaves fewer binding sites for calcium on albumin, increasing the level of free calcium.

38. How is familial hypercalcemia distinguished from primary hyperparathyroidism?
Both have elevated calcium and parathyroid hormone levels, but familial hypercalcemia has a low **urinary calcium/creatinine ratio** (<0.01) and would be found in **first-degree relatives** since it is an autosomal dominant condition.

39. What is the only cause of tertiary hyperparathyroidism?
The only cause is **chronic renal failure**, leading to parathyroid hyperplasia and causing autonomously functioning parathyroid glands.

40. What is the first step in assessing patients with acute hypercalcemia?
Administer intravenous (IV) saline to replenish lost fluids in severe and symptomatic hypercalcemia. The next step is to order a parathyroid hormone (PTH) test. Why? It allows you to look for the underlying cause of hypercalcemia.

41. If testing reveals elevated PTH and low phosphate levels, what is the most likely cause of hypercalcemia?
The most likely cause is primary hyperparathyroidism, for which parathyroidectomy is the definitive

Markedly elevated calcium levels usually indicates malignancy.

treatment. The other possible causes are Familial hypercalcemia, MEN I and IIa syndrome and tertiary hyperparathyroidism.

42. If testing reveals a low or normal PTH level, what is the most likely cause of hypercalcemia?

The most likely cause is malignancy especially if serum calcium level is severely elevated (>12 mg/dl). Obtain a chest X-ray to look for primary cancer. The other possible causes are non-PTH mediated causes of hypercalcemia (Vitamin D intoxication, drugs, chronic granulomatous diseases, acidosis).

43. When is asymptomatic primary hyperparathyroidism treated with surgery (hyperparathyroidectomy)?

It is treated when calcium is >1.0 mg/dl above the baseline normal reference range, the bone mineral density (BMD) T score is below −2.5 at any site, age is younger than 50, and there is a 30% reduction in creatinine clearance or <60 ml/min.

44. What are some pharmacological therapies for primary hyperparathyroidism?

Estrogen therapy in postmenopausal women can reduce calcium levels and has a beneficial effect on BMD. Bisphosphonates have been shown to improve BMD, and calcimimetic drugs (e.g., cinacalcet) increase the sensitivity of calcium-sensing receptors on parathyroid cells, inhibiting parathyroid cell function. They have also been shown to reduce PTH levels and normalize serum calcium levels. Practically, bisphosphonate is used in those with low bone density and a calcimimetic drug is used in those with normal bone density.

45. All postmenopausal women and men ≥50 years of age with vertebral or hip fracture automatically have a diagnosis of osteoporosis and should be treated as such. True or false?

True.

46. Bisphosphonates should be used to prevent bone loss if prednisone >5 mg/day is planned to be used >3 months. True or false?

True. A complication of bisphosphonate is **osteonecrosis of the jaw**, and so a dental evaluation is required prior to using it.

47. Osteomalacia can present with bone pain, fatigue, and malaise in adults. True or false?

True. Because it can lead to fractures, look for low calcium and phosphate levels, which are both required for mineralization, and radiograph evidence of symmetric pseudofractures.

48. How may patients present with hypocalcemia?

Patients may present with tremors, muscle spasm, **Trousseau sign**, **Chvostek's sign**, tetany, and seizures. EKG may show a **prolonged QT** interval.

49. What are some causes of low calcium levels?

- Hypoparathyroidism
- Pseudohypoparathyroidism
- Hypomagnesemia
- Hungry bone syndrome
- Large blood transfusions
- Renal failure (secondary hyperparathyroidism)
- Vitamin D deficiency
- Osteoblastic metastasis (prostate, breast cancer)
- Alkalosis

50. How does hypomagnesemia cause low calcium?

It inhibits the action of PTH and its release.

How does low magnesium cause hypocalcemia?

51. How does hungry bone syndrome cause low calcium?

In those with hungry bone syndrome, surgical resection of the parathyroid glands leads to inhibition of bone resorption, which results in large amounts of calcium and phosphate **uptake into the bone**, causing low serum calcium and phosphate levels.

52. What are some clinical features and laboratory findings in pseudohypoparathyroidism?

Clinical features include congenital disorder (maternally transmitted mutation in cyclase-stimulating G alpha protein) and dysmorphic features, and laboratory findings are **low calcium level** and **resistance to PTH** (**high PTH level**). Differentiate this from **Albright osteodystrophy** (AKA pseudopseudohypoparathyroidism), which is a paternally transmitted mutation in the same protein resulting in **osteodystrophy,** but normal renal response to PTH. Patients with Albright osteodystrophy present with a **missing fourth knuckle**. X-ray shows a short fourth metacarpal and metatarsal with osteodystrophic

Why is the phosphate level elevated in secondary hyperparathyroidism?

features, but no cognitive deficits or dysmorphic faces. Usually the calcium, phosphorus, and PTH levels are normal and no treatment is needed.

53. What is the pathogenesis and workup for secondary hyperparathyroidism?

Secondary hyperparathyroidism is mostly due to chronic renal failure. It manifests as a low serum calcium level. The next step is to look for elevated serum PTH and phosphate levels. Why is the phosphate level elevated? Renal function is compromised, thus altering phosphate secretion. Secondary hyperparathyroidism can also occur in vitamin D deficiency, as it can occur from gastrointestinal diseases or malabsorption. In this case, secondary hyperparathyroidism will manifest as elevated PTH and a low-to-normal calcium level.

54. What is the pathogenesis of elevated cortisol?

Excess cortisol production by the pituitary gland (Cushing disease) or the adrenal gland (Cushing syndrome) or cortisol intake can lead to buffalo hump, facial puffiness, central obesity, and abdominal striae. Cortisol can also stimulate the mineral corticoid receptor (MCR) and cause increased sodium reabsorption in the distal tubule and secretion of potassium and hydrogen ions, causing **hypertension**, **hypokalemia**, and **metabolic alkalosis**.

55. The initial preferred test for evaluation of elevated cortisol level is a 24-hour urine free cortisol test. True or false?

True. This is because it provides measurement over 24 hours. A dexamethasone suppression test is an alternative and confirmatory test for the diagnosis of Cushing syndrome or disease, but it is not the initial preferred test.

56. How is a dexamethasone test performed?

Obtain baseline adrenocorticotropic hormone (ACTH) and cortisol levels. If, after an overnight dexamethasone test, cortisol remains >20 mcg/dl, this means that the portal axis is not suppressed and cortisol excess is confirmed.

57. How is the cause of elevated cortisol evaluated during a dexamethasone suppression test?

Use the baseline ACTH obtained at the beginning of the dexamethasone suppression test. If ACTH at baseline is elevated, the differential diagnosis is **pituitary mass** versus **ectopic mass**; if ACTH at baseline is low, consider **adrenal tumor** as the cause.

58. How is an ectopic mass differentiated from a pituitary mass as the cause of excess cortisol?

High-dose dexamethasone will suppress a pituitary tumor, but not an ectopic mass.

59. What is the pathogenesis of hyperaldosteronism?

Hyperaldosteronism is excess aldosterone production, which leads to hypertension, polyuria, polydipsia, muscle pain, and other nonspecific symptoms. The first step is to obtain an aldosterone/renin ratio test. If the ratio is >20-25 ng/d, then the result is positive for hyperaldosteronism. A high aldosterone level suppresses renin activity via a feedback mechanism. Aldosterone stimulates MCR and causes sodium reabsorption in the distal tubule and secretion of potassium and hydrogen ions at the corticomedullary collecting ducts, causing **hypertension, hypokalemia, and metabolic alkalosis.**

60. What is the pathogenesis of virilism?

Virilism is excess androgen production that leads to hoarseness, ambiguous genitalia, clitoromegaly, and hirsutism. The first step is to obtain the serum dehydroepiandrosterone (DHEA) sulfate and DHEA levels. Markedly elevated DHEA and DHEA sulfate levels point to the adrenal cortex (e.g., adrenal tumors, premature adrenache) as the cause of virilism rather than the gonads (e.g., PCOS) or ACTH mediation (e.g., congenital adrenal hyperplasia [CAH], Cushing syndrome). Why? These enzymes are made mainly in the adrenal cortex.

What is the difference between virilism originating from the gonads and that from the adrenal cortex?

61. List endocrine syndromes that may present with secondary hypertension.

- Hyperaldosteronism (Conn syndrome)
- Cushing syndrome/disease
- Pheochromocytoma

62. What is the pathogenesis of pheochromocytoma?

Pheochromocytoma is excess adrenal medulla enzyme (catecholamine) production, leading to a triad of palpitations, perspiration, and pounding headache. If suspicion is low, the first step is to obtain a fractionated urine catecholamine level. If suspicion is high, obtain **fractionated plasma metanephrine, fractionated urine**

catecholamine, and fractionated urine metanephrine levels. Pheochromocytoma is associated with MEN 2a syndrome (pheochromocytoma, medullary carcinoma, and parathyroid adenoma) and MEN 2b syndrome (pheochromocytoma, medullary carcinoma, and mucosal neuromas).

63. What are the treatment options for pheochromocytoma?

Treat preoperative patients with alpha blockers, phenoxybenzamine, and volume repletion, and then proceed with surgical resection.

64. What is the rule of 10s in pheochromocytoma?

The rule is that 10% are bilateral, 10% are malignant, 10% are extra-adrenal, and 10% are familial.

65. How are low serum cortisol levels approached?

Consider primary, secondary or tertiary adrenal insufficiency. Addison disease (primary adrenal insufficiency) is the loss of adrenal cortex cells, leading patients to report nonspecific symptoms such as nausea, vomiting, and hypotension. The diagnosis is confirmed by high potassium and low sodium serum levels. Diminished cortisol leads to low serum glucose levels. The first step in diagnosis is to perform baseline serum ACTH and cortisol and ACTH stimulation test. Why? These tests help us to learn whether adrenal insufficiency is due to Addison disease (primary adrenal insufficiency) or pituitary/hypothalamus dysfunction (secondary and tertiary adrenal insufficiency).

High ACTH and low cortisol suggest primary adrenal insufficiency.

Low ACTH and low cortisol suggest secondary and tertiary adrenal insufficiency.

66. Which clinical and chemical findings differentiate adrenal insufficiency from pituitary dysfunction in patients with a low cortisol level?

Hyperpigmentation does not occur in pituitary dysfunction (no melanocyte-stimulating hormone); hypoglycemia is more common in pituitary dysfunction (ACTH and GH dysfunction) and electrolyte abnormalities are less common in pituitary dysfunction (aldosterone still works in pituitary dysfunction).

67. Autoimmune adrenal dysfunction is the most common cause of Addison disease in the young adult population. True or false?

True. Patients may present with hyperpigmentation in addition to nausea, vomiting, and hypotension.

68. Sudden stoppage in the intake of extrinsic steroids is the most common cause of Addison disease. True or false?

True. Always check for the history of steroid usage in patients with a low cortisol level and a high suspicion for Addison disease. Exogenous steroids can suppress the adrenals after 3 weeks of use.

Remember that cortisol is low in patients with extrinsic steroid intake.

69. What is the most common symptom of Paget's disease of the bone?

The most common symptom is osteolytic disease, which causes dull, aching bone or joint pain, most commonly in the pelvis; in addition, there can be high output failure plus compression neuropathies. Radiographs may reveal focal osteolysis, bone expansion, and cortical thickening (**"cotton wool"** appearance), and an **elevated serum alkaline phosphatase** level may be seen (Figure 6-1). Treatment is bisphosphonates.

Obtain a CT scan of the abdomen to evaluate the adrenal glands after diagnosis of primary adrenal insufficiency.

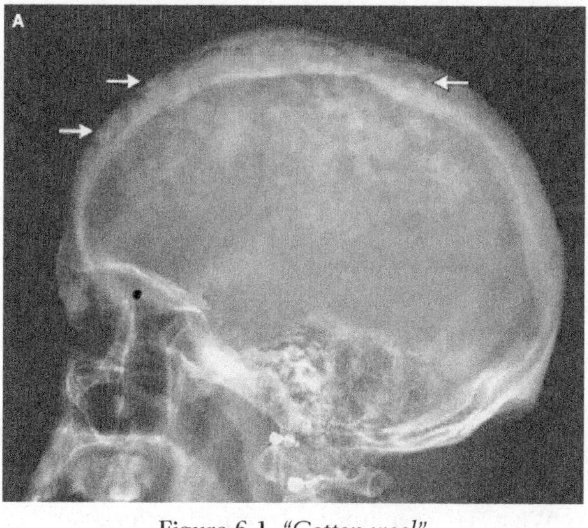

Figure 6-1. *"Cotton wool" appearance of Paget's disease of the bone.*

70. What comprises polyglandular endocrine syndrome type II?

This is the most common endocrinopathy syndrome. Polyglandular endocrine syndrome type II consists of **Addison's disease** in combination with **thyroid autoimmune disease** and/or type 1 diabetes. Hypogonadism, celiac disease, and myasthenia gravis can also be observed in this syndrome.

Differentiate the initial test and confirmatory test for the diagnosis of acromegaly.

71. What are treatment options for adrenal disorders?

- Cushing disease (adrenal mass): Surgery to remove the mass
- Hyperaldosteronism due to hyperplasia: Spironolactone or amiloride
- Virilism: Cortisol, which will inhibit ACTH and stop production of androgens in CAH. Surgery is used to remove adrenal tumors.
- Addison disease: Cortisol and fludrocortisone

72. What is the pathogenesis of hyperprolactinemia?

Hyperprolactinemia is excess prolactin production due to a tumor of the pituitary gland. The patient may present with galactorrhea/ gynecomastia, amenorrhea/ erectile dysfunction, and infertility. Visual field defects can occur from mass effects. The first step is to order a serum prolactin test, which is usually >200 ng/ml.

Treatment of microadenoma is with bromocriptine.

73. What is the pathogenesis of acromegaly?

Acromegaly is production of excess growth hormone (GH) from a pituitary tumor. The patient may present with hoarseness, sweaty palms, skin tags, and polyps. Hyperprolactinemia, hypogonadism, and visual field defects can also occur. The first step is to order a serum insulin-like growth factor-1 (IGF-1) test. An elevated serum IGF-1 level confirms the diagnosis of acromegaly.

74. How do patients with a nonfunctional pituitary mass present?

A nonfunctional pituitary mass can cause headache, nausea, and bitemporal hemianopsia by compressing the crossing fibers of the optic nerve.

75. What is the confirmatory test used to diagnose acromegaly?

The confirmatory test is **oral glucose load** with failure to suppress GH. It is the most specific test used to confirm diagnosis.

76. What is the pathogenesis of hypopituitarism?

Hypopituitarism is the loss of hormones from the anterior and posterior pituitary gland, leading to low levels of cortisol, androgens and aldosterone, thyroid hormones, antidiuretic hormone (ADH), and oxytocin.

The first step is to obtain the serum levels of follicle-stimulating hormone (FSH), luteinizing hormone (LH), GH, ACTH, and TSH.

77. How do patients with hypopituitarism present?
Hypopituitarism can lead to hypotension, hypothyroidism, hypogonadism (e.g., loss of axillary hair, lack of lactation after childbirth), and diabetes insipidus.

78. How may patients present with pituitary apoplexy?
Patients may present with acute hemorrhage into the pituitary gland (**pituitary apoplexy**), which can cause sudden headache, visual changes, and ophthalmoplegia.

79. What are the causes of hypopituitarism?
- Vascular causes (infarction, postpartum infarction [Sheehan syndrome: occurs in the postpartum period secondary to loss of blood], diabetes, temporal arteritis, acute coronary syndrome)
- Pituitary adenoma apoplexy: Bleeding into the tumor
- Nonpituitary masses
- Autoimmune diseases
- Infiltrative diseases (amyloidosis, hemochromatosis, tuberculosis)
- Infection (bacterial, tuberculosis, sarcoidosis, meningitis)

Infectious diseases (e.g., tuberculosis), hemorrhage, drugs (ketoconazole) can also cause Addison disease.

80. What is the pathogenesis of the syndrome of inappropriate ADH (SIADH)?
SIADH is excess ADH production from a tumor or drug reaction, leading to low serum osmolality (low sodium), lethargy, and eventually neurological signs such as coma. The first step is to obtain the urine osmolality level, which is usually >100 mOsm/kg in SIADH in the setting of low serum osmolality of <275 mOsm/kg. Although nonspecific, urine sodium is generally >20 mmol/L.

What is the difference between SIADH and primary polydipsia?

81. What are the laboratory abnormalities in primary polydipsia (excessive water drinking)?
The patient has low urine osmolality because the body compensates for excessive water by ridding itself of the excess. Urine osmolality is usually <100 mOsm/kg in the setting of low serum osmolality of <275 mOsm/kg. Urine osmolality >100 mOsm/kg in the context of increased total body water (low serum osmolality)

indicates impaired ability of the kidneys to dilute urine. Primary polydipsia is usually present in psychiatric patients.

What is the difference between DI and primary polydipsia.

82. What is the treatment for SIADH?

The treatment is fluid restriction for mild cases. If the patient has neurological signs, 3% saline should be given.

83. What is the pathogenesis of diabetes insipidus (DI)?

Diabetes insipidus is lack of response to ADH or the lack of ADH production due to hypopituitarism/tumor, sellar surgery, trauma, or infiltrative disease.

84. How may patients present with DI?

The patient may present with polydipsia and polyuria. The first step is to obtain a water deprivation test. Water intake is withheld the night before to allow maximal concentration of urine. If urine is still not concentrated, then the diagnosis is confirmed. In patients with diabetes insipidus, urine osmolality is usually ≤200 mOsm/kg, urine specific gravity <1.005, and random serum osmolality >287 mOsm/kg.

85. How is central diabetes insipidus differentiated from nephrogenic diabetes insipidus?

ADH is administered after an **overnight water deprivation test**. A response of urinary osmolality by≥50% is suggestive of central diabetes insipidus, whereas a lack of response is suggestive of nephrogenic diabetes insipidus. In healthy individuals, urine osmolality is usually 2-4 times greater than plasma osmolality at the end of this test.

The treatment is to administer amiloride to conserve potassium. Patients who are hypotensive or severely dehydrated can be treated with IV normal saline. Those with central DI can receive desmopressin (synthetic ADH).

86. What are some causes of nephrogenic diabetes insipidus?

This is due to resistance to ADH activity in the kidneys caused by drugs (e.g., lithium, demeclocycline, cisplatin, methoxyflurane), hypercalcemia, hypokalemia, chronic renal insufficiency, tubulointerstitial disease, and, rarely, heredity. Other causes are due to lack of a receptor for antidiuretic hormone (ADH), and a mutation in the vasopressin receptor aquaporin-2 water channel.

Treatment of nephrogenic diabetes insipidus: Renal response to ADH can be promoted by chlorpropamide or thiazide diuretics. Nonsteroidal anti-inflammatory drugs (NSAIDs) can also be used as treatment.

87. What are the causes of low testosterone in men?
There are two major causes: primary hypogonadism (affecting the gonads) and secondary hypogonadism (affecting the hypothalamus or pituitary glands).

88. What is the differential diagnosis of primary hypogonadism in men?
Consider chromosomal/congenital causes, toxins, trauma, and infiltrative disorders.

Primary hypogonadism is disease of the testes, while secondary hypogonadism is disease of the pituitary or hypothalamus.

89. Most men born with cryptorchidism go through puberty and are fertile early in life. True or false?
True. However, they become infertile later in life and have a low testosterone level.

90. What is the most common cause of secondary hypogonadism in men?
The most common cause is a tumor; other causes are congenital/infiltrative, trauma, toxins, and drug (steroids) use.

91. What is the next step after finding a low testosterone level?
Obtain FSH, LH, and prolactin levels. High FSH and LH levels suggest gonadal failure, whereas low FSH and LH levels, along with a high prolactin level, suggest pituitary disease.

92. What is the definition of metabolic syndrome?
Metabolic syndrome consists of insulin resistance, hyperlipidemia, obesity, and hypertension. The criteria are the presence of any three of the following:

- Fasting glucose ≥100 md/dl
- Serum HDL <40 mg/dl
- Triglycerides ≥150 mg/dl
- Blood pressure ≥130/85
- Obesity: men (waist) ≥40 in; women ≥35 in

Metabolic syndrome is an important risk factor for the development of type 2 diabetes and/or cardiovascular disease. Thus, aggressive lifestyle modification is required after it is identified.

Measuring FSH and LH, distinguishes between primary and secondary hypogonadism.

93. List the types of treatment and goal LDL recommended for patients with the following risk factors and low-density lipoprotein (LDL) levels (ml/dl):

- Risk factor: 0-1: LDL≥190, start pharmacological therapy with a goal of LDL <160.
- Two or more risk factors: LDL ≥160, start pharmacological therapy with a goal of LDL <130.
- CAD or CAD equivalent: LDL ≥130, start pharmacological therapy with a goal of LDL <100 (<70 is an optional goal).

Special situations: When patients have two or more risk factors and a Framingham risk score between 10% and 20%, the LDL goal should be <130, with <100 as an optional goal; if there are more than two CAD risk factors and a Framingham risk score of≥20%, then the LDL goal should be <100, with an optional goal of <70.

Understand that lifestyle modifications are started in addition to pharmacological therapy for all of these patients. In those with risk factors but without CAD or its equivalent, always try lifestyle modifications first. For example, in a patient with two or more risk factors presenting with LDL ≥160 for the first time, you should encourage lifestyle modifications for 3-6 months, and then if that makes no difference, begin pharmacological therapy. Why? Patients with CAD or its equivalent have been shown to benefit from a reduction in LDL levels by preventing future ischemic heart events.

Pancreatitis does not occur until triglycerides are >1000mg/dl.

94. When are elevated triglycerides treated?

In mild to moderately elevated triglycerides of 150 mg/dl-500 mg/dl, the aim of treatment is to reduce cardiovascular risk; therefore, treatment should be targeted against LDL with statin therapy. In severe pancreatitis with triglycerides of ≥500 to 1000 mg/dl, the aim is to prevent pancreatitis; therefore, initiate a fibrate, nicotinic acid, or fish oil to reduce triglycerides. However, pancreatitis does not occur until triglycerides are >1000 mg/dl.

95. What are the risk factors for hyperlipidemia?

The risk factors include smoking, hypertension, diabetes, family history, and a low high-density lipoprotein (HDL) level. Hypothyroidism should be ruled out in these patients. The LDL values determine when to start treating hyperlipidemia. Why? LDL (not HDL) is the most important determinant of atherosclerosis.

96. What are the pharmacological therapies for hyperlipidemia?

The first line of treatment is HMG-CoA reductase inhibitors, called statins, which reduces LDL by 60%. The main adverse effects are muscle injury and elevated transaminases. Other treatments are as follows:

- Fibrates: Fibric acid (gemfibrozil) increases the metabolism of very low-density lipoproteins, reducing triglyceride levels as a result. It is the first line of treatment for triglyceridemia. Fibrates reduce triglyceride levels and increase HDL levels, but may cause muscle injury when combined with statins.
- Nicotinic acid: This significantly increases the HDL level more than any other drug and can modestly reduce LDL and triglyceride levels. Adverse effects include flushing and diarrhea.
- Ezetimibe: This can reduce LDL when used alone or combined with statins.
- Fish oil and omega 3 acids: These can reduce triglycerides, but they also increase LDL levels.
- Bile acid sequestrants (cholestyramine): These can lower LDL levels by binding LDL in the gut, but their use is limited by gastrointestinal side effects.

What is the number one drug used to reduce high triglycerides?

What is the number one drug used to reduce high LDL?

97. What is the progression of diabetes mellitus (DM) type 2?

DM is a metabolic disease that eventually leads to insulin deficiency. Patients with DM may present with polyuria, polydipsia, or blurry vision, or they may be asymptomatic.

DM causes insulin resistance early on.

98. What is the pathogenesis of type 1 DM?

Type 1 DM is an autoimmune destruction of the pancreatic islet cells, leading to insulin deficiency. This results in fatty acid accumulation that is converted to ketones. The patient can develop diabetic ketoacidosis (DKA) as a result of infection or dehydration.

99. How do patients with DKA present?

Patients are young and have abdominal pain, nausea, and vomiting. Serum ketones are high and metabolic acidosis (anion gap) is present. Potassium can be depleted from osmotic diuresis and acidosis.

The treatment is to replace fluids and administer IV insulin. The blood sugar is usually between 400 and 500

Remember to replace potassium in patients with DKA even if potassium is initially normal.

How are patients with DKA monitored?

What is the difference between DKA and hyperosmolar coma?

Tight glucose control is the number one prevention of microvascular complications.

mg/dl. Remember that you may need to replace potassium, but the trick here is that it may be falsely elevated because of insulin deficiency and hyperosmolarity.

100. How are patients with DKA monitored?

Monitor metabolic acidosis by watching the anion gap.

101. What is the pathogenesis of type 2 DM?

Type 2 DM is the most common type of diabetes. It is due to altered insulin receptor sensitivity, eventually leading to diminished insulin production.

Complication: The patient can present with hyperosmolar coma (similar to DKA, but the blood sugar is much higher [1000 mg/dl]). Treatment is IV fluids and insulin.

102. How is DM usually diagnosed?

Obtaining two episodes of fasting glucose ≥126 mg/dl is the best diagnostic test, or one episode of fasting glucose ≥126 mg/dl and symptoms of hyperglycemia. A random blood glucose level of ≥200 mg/dl and hemoglobin A1C ≥6.5% are alternative criteria for the diagnosis of diabetes.

103. What are the most common treatment options for type 2 DM?

Metformin: This is first-line therapy. Its mechanism of action is by decreasing hepatic glucose output and increasing glucose utilization. Adverse effects include lactic acidosis; therefore, do not give this to patients with renal failure (elevated creatinine) and liver failure (elevated results of liver function tests).

Sulfonylurea: This is second-line therapy to metformin. Its mechanism of action is to act as a secretagogue by stimulating the secretion of insulin. Side effects include allergies to sulfur, hypoglycemia, and weight gain.

Nephropathy: Patients with nephropathy should be checked for retinopathy. Why? Retinopathy precedes nephropathy.

104. What are the long-term complications of DM?

Complications are microvascular (nephropathy, retinopathy) and macrovascular disease (atherosclerotic disease; e.g., peripheral artery disease, coronary heart disease).

105. How are complications of DM prevented?

Low blood glucose or tight glucose control has been shown to reduce the incidence of microvascular disease (nephropathy and retinopathy) better than any other method. Other methods include diabetic shoes, angiotensin-converting enzyme inhibitors, and control of blood pressure below 130/80.

106. What is the pathogenesis of diabetic nephropathy and treatment?

Diabetic nephropathy begins with the proliferation of the renal glomerulus basement membrane, which eventually leads to microalbuminuria. The patient can be treated for microalbuminuria with angiotensin-converting enzyme inhibitors. Keeping tight control of blood pressure <130/80 is ideal.

107. Tight glucose control reduces the progression of diabetic nephropathy. True or false?

False. Tight glucose control only reduces the **incidence of diabetic nephropathy**. However ACE inhibitors and angiotensin receptor blockers both decrease the incidence and progression of diabetic nephropathy.

108. Tight glucose control reduces the incidence and progression of diabetic retinopathy. True or false?

True. In addition to reducing the incidence of diabetic retinopathy, tight glucose control also reduces the progression of diabetic retinopathy.

109. In type 1 diabetics, renin-angiotensin system inhibitors reduce the incidence and progression of diabetic retinopathy. True or false?

True. This is now standard therapy in this patient population.

110. List the stages of diabetic retinopathy.

Microaneurysms (normal vision) progress to exudative changes, causing hemorrhages that lead to macular edema, ischemic infarcts (**cotton wool spots**), and proliferative changes (**neovascularization**). Then newly formed vessels are prone to **hemorrhage**.

111. Which medications have been shown to lower the mortality rate from cardiovascular events in patients with diabetes?

- Metformin
- ACE inhibitor
- Statins
- Aspirin

What is the difference between diabetic retinopathy and hypertensive retinopathy?

C-peptide level can be used to differentiate various causes of hypoglycemia.

Tight glucose control can prevent incidence and the progression of diabetic neuropathy.

Foot care can prevent complications of diabetic neuropathy.

112. List other types of diabetes.

Secondary diabetes can be caused by pancreatitis, cystic fibrosis, hemochromatosis, endocrine disease (hyperthyroidism, Cushing disease, acromegaly, pheochromocytoma), genetic disease (Klinefelter syndrome, Prader-Willi syndrome, and maturity-onset diabetes).

113. What is maturity-onset diabetes of the young?

Genetic defects of beta-cell function cause diabetes at an early age (teens to early 20s). Diabetes can be found in family members, and hyperglycemia can be severe, but can be treated with oral agents.

114. What are the causes of hypoglycemia?

- Exogenous insulin: Low C-peptide level
- Secretagogue: Elevated C-peptide level
- Insulinoma: High insulin and C-peptide levels
- Insulin-like growth factor: Increased glucose use by tumors, low insulin level
- Decrease in glucose supply
- Severe starvation
- Alcohol intake
- Sepsis
- Liver dysfunction
- Nutritional deficiency
- Endocrine diseases (Addison's, hypopituitarism, growth hormone deficiency)

115. Diabetic neuropathy may present as great toe sole ulcer. True or false?

True. Always do a foot X-ray of patients with diabetes who present with great toe sole ulcer to rule out orthopedic involvement. It is common in patients with diabetes.

116. **Necrobiosis lipoidica is an inflammatory skin disorder commonly found on the shin and frequently associated with diabetes. True or false?**

True. It consists of oval, yellow-red plaques with telangiectasia and atrophy. Topical steroids are used to treat it.

Chapter 7

Gastrointestinal System

1. **What are the types of diarrhea?**
   - Osmotic
   - Secretory
   - Inflammatory
   - Alteration of intestinal motility
   - Malabsorptive

2. **What is the pathogenesis of osmotic diarrhea?**
   Osmotic diarrhea is the accumulation of indigestible contents in the intestine due to enzyme deficiency or intestinal dysfunction (lactose intolerance, celiac disease). Fasting halts diarrhea.

3. **What is the pathogenesis of secretory diarrhea?**
   Secretory diarrhea is caused by an organism that releases toxins or chemicals, leading to secretion of fluid into the intestine (Escherichia coli enterotoxin, cholera). Fasting does not halt diarrhea. In peptide-secreting tumors (carcinoid, VIPoma, gastrinoma), 5-hydroxyindoleacetic acid, vasoactive intestinal polypeptide, and a high volume of gastric acid cause secretory diarrhea. Other causes are structural diseases (intestinal tumors) and endocrinopathy (e.g., diabetes, hyperthyroidism, adrenal insufficiency, systemic mastocytosis).

Fasting halts osmotic diarrhea but does not halt secretory diarrhea.

4. **What are some diagnostic studies for acute diarrhea?**
   Diagnostic tests include stool leukocytes, *Clostridium difficile* Ag, stool culture, and stool ova and parasites.

5. **What is the pathogenesis of inflammatory diarrhea?**
   Inflammatory diarrhea is the destruction of the mucosa

of the intestine. Examples are bacterial inflammation (Shigella, Salmonella, hemorrhagic E. coli) and inflammatory bowel disease (IBD).

6. **What is the pathogenesis of malabsorptive diarrhea?**
The villi of the intestine are altered. Examples are celiac disease, Whipple disease, post-bowel resection syndrome, and **pancreatic insufficiency**. Most patients present with iron-deficiency anemia and fat-soluble vitamin deficiency (vitamins A, K, E, and D).

7. **What is the pathogenesis of altered intestinal motility?**
Secretion of hormones or bowel resection causes increased intestinal motility. Hyperthyroidism, short bowel syndrome, and small bowel resection are examples in which this occurs.

8. **What are two classifications of diarrhea?**
   - Mild benign diarrhea: The passage of watery stools with no blood or fever
   - Severe diarrhea: The passage of stools >4 times a day, bloody stools (invasive enteropathy), fever, antibiotic usage, and history of foreign travel

9. **How do patients with diarrhea generally present?**
The patient may present with fever and have diarrhea that may be foul smelling, watery, and bloody.

10. **What are some diagnostic studies in chronic diarrhea (>4 weeks)?**
These include fecal studies, fecal leukocytes, and osmotic gap (the difference in stool osmolality in milliosmoles per kilogram of water, and twice the sum of stool sodium and potassium in milliosmoles per liter). An osmotic gap <50 is suggestive of secretory diarrhea and ≥125 is suggestive of an osmotic process.

11. **What are the laboratory findings in malabsorptive diarrhea?**
   - Chronic anemia with thrombocytosis suggests iron-deficiency anemia
   - Elevated fecal fat
   - Elevated prothrombin time suggests vitamin K deficiency
   - Macrocytosis suggests vitamin B12 deficiency

Low serum calcium, phosphate, and serum albumin levels can also occur.

Anemia may be suggestive of chronic malabsorptive diarrhea.

12. What are the treatment options in diarrhea?

Administer supportive therapy with intravenous fluids or oral rehydration therapy.

Treat Clostridium difficile with metronidazole or vancomycin (alternative). Treat patients with Giardia or amebiasis with metronidazole.

13. What are some empiric pharmacological therapies for diarrhea?

Do not treat diarrhea with antibiotics except if the patient has persistent symptoms with volume depletion, invasive enteropathy (presenting as bloody diarrhea), and immunosuppression. Treat empirically with oral fluoroquinolone. Azithromycin and erythromycin are other options.

14. Antibiotics should be avoided in suspected enterohemorrhagic E. coli (EHEC). True or false?

True. Suspected EHEC presents as bloody diarrhea with abdominal pain and little or no fever. Antibiotics can lead to hemolytic uremic syndrome, which results from an increase in the release of Shiga toxin when antibiotics are given.

Why are antibiotics avoided in EHEC?

15. What is the pathogenesis of irritable bowel syndrome?

Irritable bowel syndrome is altered bowel motility that can result in **alternating constipation and diarrhea** and abdominal pain relieved with defecation, but a **lack of alarming symptoms** (weight loss, fever, and rectal bleed). The patient may present with loose stools with no blood or with constipation and relief of abdominal pain on defecation, which has been going on for 12 weeks. Irritable bowel syndrome is a diagnosis of exclusion.

The first step is to do a stool test and culture of stool to rule out other serious conditions; consider colonoscopy to rule out colitis. Treat with antispasmodic and antidiarrhea agents and recommend ingestion of highly fibrous foods if the patient is constipated.

16. What is the pathogenesis of Whipple disease?

Whipple disease is the destruction of the intestinal villi (villous atrophy as seen on PAS positive staining of duodenal biopsies) due to Tropheryma whipplei, a rod shaped bacteria, leading to malabsorptive, foul-smelling diarrhea. The patient will also present with a systemic

PAS positive staining of duodenal biopsies is suggestive of Whipple disease.

manifestation of **joint and lymph node involvement**, as well as hyperpigmentation.

17. What is the pathogenesis of carcinoid syndrome?
Carcinoid syndrome is secondary to a carcinoid tumor, which releases serotonin (5-hydroxyindoleacetic acid), leading to diarrhea and flushing (carcinoid syndrome). The most common type of carcinoid tumor that causes this syndrome is found in the ileum.

18. What is the pathogenesis of tropical sprue?
Tropical sprue is the blunting of the small intestine's villi, leading to foul-smelling diarrhea (malabsorptive diarrhea) that occurs in residents of or visitors to the tropics. Mononuclear infiltrates, enlarged nuclei, and epithelial cells are found in the intestinal biopsy sample.

19. What is the pathogenesis of celiac disease?
This disease involves a T-cell mediated immune response. Celiac disease is the blunting of the small intestine's villi, leading to malabsorption. It is associated with dermatitis herpetiformis (pruritic rash). Patients present with chronic diarrhea, malabsorption features (e.g., iron deficiency), and extraintestinal features (e.g., atrophic glossitis).

20. What is the serological test for celiac disease?
Anti-tissue transglutaminase is the most reliable test, but a confirmatory small bowel biopsy is needed. Treatment is a **gluten-free diet**.

21. What laboratory tests may suggest small bowel overgrowth syndrome?
Low B12 and high folate levels due to production of folate by bacteria may suggest this syndrome. Causes are hypochlorhydria, blind loop syndrome, diabetes, and scleroderma. Treatment is empiric antibiotics.

22. What is the pathogenesis of gastric esophageal reflux disease (GERD)?
GERD is the reflux of the contents of the stomach because of an incompetent lower esophageal sphincter (LES). The patient may present with heartburn that becomes worse when certain foods are ingested and a bitter taste in the mouth. Risk factors are smoking, ingesting chocolate and coffee, and use of choline agonists.

The first step is to empirically treat with antacids and eliminate risk factors.

Where is the most common type of carcinoid tumor that triggers carcinoid syndrome found?

Why are mononuclear infiltrates and enlarged nuclei cells found in an intestinal biopsy sample from patients with tropical sprue? ***Folate, vitamin B12 deficiency***

What is dermatitis herpetiformis?

What is the difference among GERD, achalasia, and scleroderma?

23. What are the indications for endoscopy (EGD) in patients with GERD?

Candidates for upper endoscopy are those with a complication such as a stricture that can present clinically **as dysphagia and vomiting, long-standing disease of >5 years, age ≥50, or who have red flags such as weight loss or anemia.**

When is endoscopy indicated for patients with GERD?

24. How do patients present with dysphagia?

Patients present with the inability to swallow liquids, solids, or both. Oropharyngeal dysphagia due to hypopharynx can cause drooling and chronic cough. Barium swallow is the first test of choice.

25. How do patients present with achalasia?

Patients may present with an inability to swallow both liquids and solids and chest pain because of the denervation of the LES. The definitive test is manometry. Why? It demonstrates increased LES tone. There is a **bird's beak appearance** on the esophagram (barium swallow).

Why is there elevated LES pressure by manometry in achalasia?

What is the test of choice for achalasia and why?

26. What are some causes of oropharyngeal dysphagia?

- Cervical osteophytes
- Cricoid webs
- Zenker's diverticulum
- Myasthenia gravis
- Parkinson's disease
- Stroke
- Thyroid goiter
- Amyotrophic lateral sclerosis

27. What are some causes of esophageal dysphagia?

- Achalasia
- Esophageal spasm
- Muscular dystrophy
- Scleroderma
- Esophageal strictures
- Malignancy
- Esophageal web and rings (Schatzki)

28. The intermittent inability to swallow solid foods (meat impaction) in the setting of alcohol abuse, which has been present in the past months to years, is suggestive of what type of dysphagia?

This is suggestive of esophageal webs or rings.

Barium swallow study (esophagram) is the initial test in patients with dysphagia.

29. How do patients present with esophageal cancer?

With esophageal cancer, the patient is unable first to swallow solids and then liquids, associated with **weight loss**. The risk factors are smoking, chronic GERD, and Barrett esophagus. Esophagoscopy (endoscopy) is the test of choice if esophageal cancer is highly suspected.

30. How may patients present with esophageal spasms?

Patients may present with nonspecific symptoms such as GERD, chest pain, and dysphagia. Barium swallow may show "**rosary bead**" or "corkscrew" esophagus. Esophageal spasms should be confirmed with **manometry** testing. Treatment is a calcium channel blocker for dysphagia, and tricyclic antidepressants for pain.

31. How do patients with scleroderma present?

The patient presents with heartburn in addition to dysphagia associated with **Raynaud's phenomenon** and periungual telangiectasia. LES tone is low on manometry.

32. What does the manometry test show in esophageal spasm?

The manometry test will show intermittent exaggerated contraction of the esophageal muscle and normal peristalsis.

33. Which esophageal dysmotility disease will show very high amplitude peristaltic contractions on manometry?

Nutcracker esophagus will show this. Patients can present with symptoms that are similar to esophageal spasm and the treatment is similar.

34. List some causes of odynophagia (painful swallowing).

- *Candida* infection
- Cytomegalovirus infection
- Herpes infection
- HIV
- Drugs such as aspirin
- NSAIDs
- Bisphosphonates
- Iron
- Radiation
- Peptic ulcer disease (PUD)

35. *Candida albicans* is the most common cause of infectious esophagitis. True or false?

True. Patients may present with odynophagia and **oral**

thrush. Viral infection (cytomegalovirus [CMV]) is the most common cause of esophagitis in immunosuppressed patients. Treat *Candida* with nystatin solution or fluconazole and CMV with ganciclovir (after confirmation with endoscopic biopsy).

36. What is the pathogenesis of gastritis?

Gastritis is inflammation of the gastric mucosa, which can be due to systemic diseases that reduce the blood supply, extreme stress reactions, drugs, or hypersensitivity reactions. However, the most common causes are infectious or autoimmune diseases. It may present asymptomatically or as blood in the stool. Gastritis is common in postoperative surgical patients.

37. What are types of Helicobacter pylori infections?

- Chronic atrophic gastritis
- Type B gastritis
- Duodenal ulcer
- Gastric ulcer
- Nonulcer dyspepsia
- GERD
- Mucosa-associated lymphoid tissue (MALT)

Atrophic gastritis and gastric ulcer predisposes individuals to gastric cancer, especially gastric lymphoma (**MALT**). Gastric lymphoma is treated with a combination of amoxicillin, clarithromycin, and a PPI against H. pylori.

38. How do patients present with gastric ulcer?

The patient may present with epigastric abdominal pain that varies with intake of food. Approximately 60-70% of gastric ulcer cases are associated with H. pylori. If H. pylori are detected, treat with a combination of amoxicillin, clarithromycin, and a PPI.

39. How do patients with duodenal ulcer present?

Patients present with epigastric pain that feels better after food, but worsens 2-3 hours later. About 90% of duodenal ulcer cases are associated with H. pylori. If H. pylori are found, treat with proton pump inhibitors and antibiotics against H. pylori (amoxicillin and clarithromycin) for 10-14 days.

The first step in the definitive diagnosis of duodenal or gastric ulcer is to perform an endoscopy or barium swallow test. Endoscopy is much more specific.

What is the treatment of gastric lymphoma?

Gastric and duodenal ulcers are referred to as peptic ulcer disease (PUD).

PUD can be aggravated by NSAIDs use.

Nitrate is a risk factor for what type of cancer?

40. What is the best test for eradication of *H. pylori* after treatment?

This is done 4 weeks after treatment if symptoms recur. A stool antigen test or urea breath test is more specific than serological tests for eradication testing.

41. What are complications of PUD (duodenal and gastric ulcers)?

- Obstruction (least common complication)
- Perforation (2nd most common complication)
- Bleeding (most common complication)

42. List the risk factors associated with gastric cancer.

- Nitrates (found in **smoked meats** commonly found in Japan and Korea)
- Chronic atrophic gastritis
- Pernicious anemia
- *H. pylori*
- Gastric adenomatous polyps
- Gastrectomy
- Hereditary nonpolyposis colon cancer
- Familial adenomatous polyposis (BRCA-2 mutation)

43. Left supraclavicular adenopathy can be an indicator for metastatic abdominal cancer. True or false?

True. However, this is most commonly found in metastatic gastric cancer. This is referred to as **Virchow's node** and is due to supraclavicular node involvement with cancer. Nodal enlargement is caused by metastatic gastric cancer via the thoracic duct. Other physical findings suggestive of metastatic gastric cancer are periumbilical nodule (**Sister Mary Joseph's node**), axillary node (Irish node), peritoneal spread causing enlarged ovary (**Krukenberg's tumor**), and **ascites** indicating peritoneal carcinomatosis. Sister Mary Joseph's node can also be found in metastatic ovarian cancer.

44. What is the pathogenesis of IBD?

IBD is a chronic idiopathic inflammation of the bowel, a multifactorial disease. The two most common types are Crohn's disease (CD) and ulcerative colitis (UC). Microscopic colitis is less common and can cause chronic diarrhea and mild weight loss.

45. What is the pathogenesis of CD?

CD is a transmural granulomatous disease that affects the patient anywhere from the mouth to the anus, but most commonly involves the ileum. The patient may present acutely with abdominal pain, diarrhea, low-grade fever, and sometimes blood in the stool.

The first step is to look for WBCs, ova, and parasites in the stool and to perform a stool culture to rule out infectious causes of diarrhea. The next steps are to do a colonoscopy to look for gross changes and then to perform a biopsy.

46. What is the pathogenesis of UC?

UC is a multifactorial inflammatory disease characterized by gastrointestinal mucosal inflammation and pseudopolyps that almost always involves the colon. The patient may present acutely with abdominal pain, blood in the stool, and fever. Look for WBCs in the stool and perform a colonoscopy to confirm the diagnosis.

47. Tobacco use is protective of ulcerative colitis. True or false?

True. However, it is harmful to those with CD.

48. What are the complications of IBD?

- Obstruction
- Perforation
- Toxic megacolon in UC
- Fistulas in CD

49. What are extraintestinal manifestations in IBD?

- Liver disease: Sclerosing cholangitis in UC
- Nephrolithiasis in CD
- Uveitis
- Oral ulcers (aphthous ulcer)
- Arthritis
- Pyoderma gangrenosum
- Gallstones
- Ankylosing spondylitis
- Erythema nodosum
- Metabolic bone disease

50. Are transmural inflammation, skip lesions, and rectal sparing, perianal abscess and fistulas more likely to develop in CD or ulcerative colitis?

These are more likely to develop in CD.

What is the histological difference between Crohn disease and ulcerative colitis?

What is the most common cause of hepatitis in the United States?

Most patients with PSC will have associated ulcerative colitis.

51. What are treatment options in IBD?

5-Amino-salicylic acid can be used to treat both CD and UC. Metronidazole can be used for perianal disease in CD. Surgery is indicated for obstruction, perforation, or excessive use of steroids.

Patients with long-term IBD need to undergo screening for malignancy by means of a colonoscopy at 2-year intervals.

52. How do patients present with toxic megacolon?

The patient presents with underlying UC and fever, abdominal pain, and abdominal distention. Treat with nothing by mouth, nasogastric suction, and bed rest. If this fails, perform surgery.

53. What is the definition of hepatitis?

Hepatitis is inflammation of the liver secondary to the body's response to infection. Viruses are the most common cause of hepatitis in the United States.

54. What are other causes of hepatitis?

- Drugs (isoniazid, halothane, azoles, HMG-CoA dehydrogenase inhibitors)
- Cytomegalovirus
- Alcohol
- Hereditary (hemochromatosis, Wilson disease, alpha 1-antitrypsin deficiency)
- Autoimmune hepatitis
- Nonalcoholic steatohepatitis
- Primary sclerosing cholangitis (PSC)
- Primary biliary cirrhosis (PBC)

55. How do patients present with primary sclerosing cholangitis?

The patient may present with cholestasis. The pathogenesis is intrahepatic and extrahepatic biliary duct stenosis. Elevation of the serum alkaline phosphatase level dominates the picture, along with elevated autoimmune antibodies and immunoglobulins and mildly elevated bilirubin. Endoscopic retrograde cholangiopancreatography (ERCP) is standard for diagnosis and may show multiple strictures and dilations of intrahepatic and extrahepatic ducts. Approximately 75-90% of patients with primary sclerosing cholangitis have associated IBD. Treatment is palliative, with cholestyramine or ursodiol.

Liver failure is treated with a liver transplant.

56. What is the pathogenesis of primary biliary cirrhosis?

The pathogenesis is autoimmune small to medium bile duct destruction. Primary biliary cirrhosis is the destruction of the intrahepatic bile ducts. The patient may present with fatigue and pruritus. Aspartate aminotransferase and alanine aminotransferase levels are mildly elevated, alkaline phosphatase levels are much more elevated than in primary sclerosing cholangitis, and y-glutamyl transpeptidase (GGTP) and immunoglobulin levels are also very prominent. Bilirubin becomes elevated as the disease progresses. Serum antimitochondrial antibody is diagnostic. Treatment is the alleviation of symptoms by cholestyramine or ursodiol. Liver failure is treated with a liver transplant.

57. How may patients present with acute hepatitis?

The patient may present with abdominal (right upper quadrant) pain, fever, jaundice, and hepatosplenomegaly.

Know the presentation of patients with acute hepatitis.

58. How is hepatitis A infection evaluated?

Risk factors are fecal oral transmission and breakouts with diarrhea.

The first step in diagnosis is to obtain serum anti-hepatitis A from the patient. You can treat the immunosuppressed patient with immunoglobulin at postexposure. Positive anti-IgM indicates an acute infection and +IgG to hepatitis A indicates a previous infection.

59. How is hepatitis B evaluated?

The risk factors for hepatitis B are multiple sexual partners and use of serum and blood products. Perinatal transmission is common in developing countries. Most people who recover from an acute infection develop immunity against it; only a small minority of patients develops chronic infection.

The first step is to obtain the serum hepatitis B surface antigen (HBsAg) level, which is the first to show up in acute infection; hepatitis B core antibody, IgM subtype, is the first antibody to show up in the serum.

What is the first thing to show up in the serum in hepatitis B infection?

What is the first antibody to show up in hepatitis B infection?

60. What does the presence of HBsAg for more than 6 months suggest?

The presence of HBsAg for more than 6 months is indicative of chronic **hepatitis B** infection.

What serological test suggests hepatitis B clearance?

61. What does the presence of anti-HBsAg suggest?
The presence of anti-HBsAg (HBsAb) is indicative of immunity against hepatitis B.

62. What does the presence of hepatitis B e antigen (HBeAg) indicate?
HBeAg indicates high infectivity.

63. What does seroconversion of HBeAg to anti-HBe mean?
It indicates clearance of hepatitis B infection.

64. What is the treatment for hepatitis B infection?
Because immunity is altered, interferon can be used to treat chronic severe (elevated transaminases) hepatitis. How does it work? It boosts the immune system. Treatment is indicated when hepatitis B viral DNA is elevated, transaminases are elevated, and liver biopsy results show active disease.

65. What is the recommended screening after exposure (e.g., needle stick) to a patient with hepatitis C virus (HCV) infection or a patient with an unknown status of hepatitis C virus infection?
Screen with initial baseline HCV testing, and then HCV RNA 4 weeks after the incident, if baseline HCV testing is negative.

66. What is the recommended evaluation after exposure (e.g., needle stick or sexual intercourse) to a contact with a known hepatitis B status or a patient with an unknown hepatitis B status?
If the contact hepatitis B status is positive, assess for hepatitis B vaccine immunity in the victim; if immune, hepatitis B immunoglobulin is given. If the victim is not immune, give the hepatitis B vaccine series plus immunoglobulin. On the other hand, if the contact hepatitis B status is unknown and the victim is immune, no further treatment is needed. If the victim is not immune, give the hepatitis B vaccine series.

67. How are patients with hepatitis C evaluated?
Patients are usually asymptomatic and are usually found from test results showing elevated serum transaminases. The most common form of transmission is **intravenous drug use**. Multiple sexual partners as a risk factor is rare.

The first step is to obtain anti-hepatitis C antibody. This antibody does not mean that there is protection against the virus. Serum hepatitis C RNA is the best test for diagnosis.

Treatment for severe (elevated transaminases) chronic disease is interferon and ribavirin.

68. Intravenous drug users are at risk for hepatitis D viral infection. True or false?

True. However, the presence of hepatitis B is usually needed for hepatitis D infection.

69. What is the transmission route for hepatitis E?

The transmission route is fecal-oral, but hepatitis E is most commonly found in pregnant women.

70. Hepatitis B and C are the only viruses that can lead to the development of liver cirrhosis and hepatocellular carcinoma. True or false?

True.

71. Which causes of acute hepatitis can cause markedly elevated transaminases (≥1000 u/L)?

Viruses and drugs (acetaminophen) cause such markedly elevated transaminases in acute hepatitis. Ischemic hepatitis (hypotension) can also cause such markedly elevated transaminases, which can be transient, returning to normal in 48 hours.

72. What is the pathogenesis of hemochromatosis?

Hemochromatosis is an autosomal recessive disorder that causes iron absorption to be altered, leading to the accumulation of iron in the liver (hepatitis, hepatomegaly), brain (lenticular lesions), testes (enlargement, impotence), heart (restrictive disease), skin (hyperpigmentation), joints (arthritis), and pancreas (diabetes). Laboratory tests will show an increased ferritin level and an elevated percentage of saturation (≥55%). Liver biopsy is used to confirm diagnosis.

Treat with an iron binder (e.g., deferoxamine) and liver transplant for liver failure.

73. A young adult found to have mildly elevated indirect bilirubin during an acute illness should be ruled out for what congenital syndrome?

Gilbert's syndrome, a syndrome of abnormal conjugation of bilirubin, should be ruled out.

The classic triad of skin hyperpigmentation, liver cirrhosis and diabetes mellitus ("bronze diabetes"), occur late in hemochromatosis.

No specific therapy is needed in patients with Gibert's syndrome as it is a self resolving condition.

The predominant symptoms in Wilson disease are hepatic, neurologic and psychiatric.

74. What is the pathogenesis of Wilson disease?

Autosomal recessive disorder is usually present in those <40 years. Wilson disease involves a dysfunctional copper transporter, leading to copper accumulation in the liver (hepatitis, hepatomegaly), brain (lenticular lesions), and eyes (Kayser-Fleischer rings). Laboratory tests reveal low-serum ceruloplasmin and elevated urine copper levels. A liver biopsy confirms diagnosis.

Treat with penicillamine (binds copper) and liver transplant for end-stage disease.

75. How do patients present with alpha 1-antitrypsin deficiency?

Patients are young and those with no risk factors usually present with emphysema and liver failure due to alpha 1-antitrypsin inactivity in the lungs and liver. Treat with intravenous (IV) antitrypsin.

76. How do patients with autoimmune hepatitis present?

Autoimmune hepatitis is usually present in women with elevated transaminases in the absence of viral serological markers. It presents as insidious fatigue and mild **hyperbilirubinemia** of <3 mg/dl (jaundice). Antinuclear antibodies, anti-smooth antibodies, and antimicrosomal antibodies may be present. Treatment is prednisone.

Fatigue and pruritus are the most common presenting symptoms of PBC but half are asymptomatic.

77. What are characteristic liver function test (LFT) results for alcohol hepatitis?

An aspartate aminotransferase to alanine aminotransferase ratio of 2:1 is diagnostic.

78. What is the alkaline phosphatase level in autoimmune hepatitis versus PBC or PSC?

It is mildly elevated in autoimmune hepatitis, but markedly elevated in PBC or PSC.

PSC is often found as part of IBD, and those that have symptoms will present with fatigue and pruritus.

79. How do patients with nonalcoholic steatohepatitis present?

A patient will present with obesity and abdominal pain, or asymptomatically with elevated serum transaminases, but will be a nondrinker. Liver ultrasound may reveal fatty liver infiltration. A liver biopsy will reveal elevated fatty acids in liver cells. LFT results may be elevated. Treatment is weight loss, but a small number of patients may develop cirrhosis.

80. What are some ominous complications of hepatitis?

- Cirrhosis
- Hepatocellular carcinoma

81. How is chronic liver disease and cirrhosis monitored?

Liver disease is monitored by obtaining serum prothrombin time (PT), ammonia, albumin, bilirubin, and vitamin K levels. Severe liver disease may show elevated PT, bilirubin, and ammonia levels and low albumin (low serum urea nitrogen) and vitamin K levels.

82. In alcoholic hepatitis, discriminant factor (PT and bilirubin level) is used to estimate liver disease severity. True or false?

True. Steroids are given to those with a score ≥32.

83. How do patients with chronic liver disease present?

Patients may present with signs of portal hypertension such as encephalopathy, ascites, palmar erythema, bleeding, esophageal varices, gastric varices, hypoglycemia, testicular atrophy, dilation of umbilical veins and superficial abdominal veins (caput medusa), splenomegaly from venous congestion, and internal hemorrhoids. Portal hypertension develops from increased pressure of the portal system due to obstruction of portal venous flow. Obstruction can be presinusoidal (portal vein thrombosis, portal fibrosis, or infiltrative diseases), sinusoidal (liver cirrhosis), or postsinusoidal (Budd-Chiari syndrome, hepatic venous disease).

84. Liver cirrhosis is the most common cause of portal hypertension. True or false?

True. In these patients, portal pressure is enhanced by arterial vasodilation.

85. How do patients present with ascites?

Ascites may present as abdominal protrusion, as well as abdominal pain and shifting dullness, during the physical examination. The first step is to obtain abdominal fluid for analysis (paracentesis). The serum ascitic albumin gradient (SAAG) is calculated by subtracting the albumin concentration of the ascitic fluid from the albumin concentration of the serum.

What is SAAG?

If SAAG is ≥1.1 g/dl, high portal pressure is present; consider any disorder leading to portal hypertension such as liver cirrhosis. Non-cirrhotic causes of portal hypertension such as heart failure, liver metastasis, and Budd-Chiari syndrome may also be considered.

If SAAG is <1.1 g/dl, portal hypertension is absent; consider malignancy of the peritoneum, nephrotic syndrome, ischemic or obstructed bowel, pancreatitis, and peritonitis as possible causes.

Since ascites in cirrhosis is caused by increased hydrostatic pressure, sodium accumulation, and low serum albumin levels, it can be treated with a potassium-sparing diuretic and albumin.

What is the most common infective organism in SBP?

86. What is an ominous complication of ascites?

An ominous complication of ascites is spontaneous bacterial peritonitis (SBP). The patient may present with abdominal pain and fever. Differentiate SBP from other types of peritonitis. Paracentesis, with a single type of gram-negative organism, is diagnostic. The most common organism causing it is the Enterobacteriacae group (E. coli, Klebsiella). A **neutrophil or PMN count ≥250 cells/mm^3** in the ascitic fluid is diagnostic.

Treat SBP with broad-spectrum drugs such as cefotaxime that cover gram-negative enteric organisms.

Why is a beta-blocker effective in the prevention of esophageal varices?

Child-Pugh classification is used to estimate the severity of liver cirrhosis according to ascites, albumin, prothrombin time, bilirubin and encephalopathy, with class C indicating decompensated liver disease.

87. How are patients with esophageal varices evaluated?

The patient may present with hematemesis. Varices develop from attempted decompression of portal hypertension. The first step is to administer IV normal saline. The next step is to use an alternative treatment of octreotide/somatostatin if there is **active bleeding**. Why? It constricts the involved vessels. The third step is to perform endoscopic sclerotherapy or band ligation.

If all treatments fail, the last step is an emergency transjugular intrahepatic portosystemic shunt (TIPS), a shunt between the hepatic vein and the portal system, to relieve portal hypertension, or surgery

The first step in prevention is with beta-blockers, which reduce portal hypertension.

88. How do patients with hepatic encephalopathy present?

Patients may present nonspecifically with lethargy and drowsiness. The physical examination may reveal a flapping tremor on extension of the arms. The cause is nitrogenous compounds that bypass the diseased liver and enter the brain.

The treatment goal is to reduce ammonia because it is thought to be the culprit; therefore, administer lactulose, neomycin, or rifaximin and reduce risk factors such as a high-protein diet and infection, bleeding, use of sedatives, and constipation.

89. What is the pathogenesis of palmer erythema, testicular atrophy, and spider telangiectasia (angioma)?

These symptoms are mostly caused by excess estrogen due to inadequate metabolism in the diseased liver. Palmer erythema and spider angioma can also be found in pregnancy.

90. When is a liver transplant indicated?

A liver transplant is indicated when there are recalcitrant liver complications (encephalopathy, esophageal varices, or ascites).

91. What are contraindications to a liver transplant?

A liver transplant is contraindicated with metastatic liver disease, infection (AIDS), and alcohol abuse.

92. A model for end-stage liver disease (MELD) is used to determine who gets a liver, allowing the sickest person to receive a liver first. True or false?

True. INR, bilirubin, and serum creatinine are used to calculate the MELD score.

93. How do patients present with cholestasis?

The patient may present with jaundice, clay-colored stool, dark yellow urine, and pruritus because of obstruction of the common bile duct (CBD). The first step in the evaluation of jaundice is to obtain serum direct and indirect bilirubin levels. Conjugated bilirubin ≥20% of the total suggests cholestasis (hepatobiliary causes), while elevated indirect bilirubin suggests increased bilirubin production (hemolysis), reduced clearance (Gilbert or Crigler Najjar syndrome), or impaired hepatic uptake(congestive heart failure, portosystemic shunts).

What is the first step in the evaluation of jaundice?

94. In patients with jaundice, what does the presence of bilirubin in the urine suggest?

It suggests hepatobiliary causes of jaundice. In contrast unconjugated bilirubin is bound to albumin and so unable to be filtrated across the glomerulus into the urine.

When is ERCP useful?

What is the Courvoisier sign?

95. What is the evaluation of patients presenting with cholestasis?

Once cholestasis is confirmed by elevated serum direct bilirubin level, the first step is to obtain an ultrasound. Why? Ultrasound differentiates between extrinsic and intrinsic causes of cholestasis.

96. If ultrasound shows thickening of the gallbladder and dilation of the CBD, what does this mean?

It means that a stone is obstructing the CBD (choledocholithiasis). The next step would be to obtain endoscopic retrograde cholangiopancreatography (ERCP or cholangiogram) to characterize the stone and its location. Laboratory results will show an elevated alkaline phosphatase level more than an elevated transaminase level in choledocholithiasis.

97. If ultrasound shows dilation of the CBD, but absence of gallbladder thickening, what does this mean?

This result may indicate a mass that is obstructing the CBD. The next step in this case will be a computed tomography (CT) scan (not ERCP). Why? An extrinsic factor (e.g., tumor) is responsible for CBD dilatation.

98. List the risk factors for pancreatic cancer.

- Smoking
- Chronic pancreatitis
- Familial adenomatous polyposis
- Peutz-Jeghers syndrome
- Von Hippel-Lindau syndrome
- Advanced age (most common)
- High-fat diet
- Partial gastrectomy

99. What are other factors that will cause one to obtain a CT scan instead of ERCP in the evaluation of patients with cholestasis?

A CT scan should be obtained if the Courvoisier sign is present, a nontender right upper quadrant on palpation, with ultrasound evidence of **CBD dilation** and significant weight loss, all suggesting possible pancreatic cancer.

100. List the triad of cholangitis.

The triad is fever, right upper quadrant tenderness, and jaundice. The first step is to initiate broad-spectrum antibiotics empirically and then proceed to ERCP sphincterotomy or stent placement.

101. What are other causes of cholestasis?
- Nonalcoholic hepatic steatosis
- Drugs (penicillin, sulfur, antipsychotics)
- Pregnancy
- Primary biliary cirrhosis (PBC)
- Primary sclerosing cholangitis (PSC)

102. What is the definition of pancreatitis?
Pancreatitis is an inflammation of the pancreas due to premature activation of its enzymes.

103. How may patients with acute pancreatitis present?
The patient may present with epigastric, severe dull pain radiating to the back that is associated with nausea and vomiting.

The most common causes in the United States are gallstones and alcohol abuse. Other causes are viruses (mumps), hyperlipidemia, hypercalcemia, scorpion bites, trauma (post-ERCP), and drugs (diuretics).

The first step is to obtain an ultrasound if the vignette suggests gallstone pancreatitis. Once a diagnosis is made, a CT scan can be used to evaluate the extent of pancreatitis.

104. What are the complications of acute pancreatitis?
- Pancreatic abscess
- Pancreatic pseudocysts
- Chronic pancreatitis
- Acute respiratory distress syndrome
- Pleural effusion
- Adynamic ileus
- Portal vein thrombosis and gastric varices
- Fistulas after percutaneous drainage
- Pancreatic pseudoaneurysm

105. What criteria are used for prognosis of acute pancreatitis?
Ranson's criteria are used. The mnemonic is GA LAW in the first 24 hours: glucose ≥200 mg/dl; age ≥55; lactate dehydrogenase (LDH) ≥350; aspartate transaminase (AST) ≥250; WBC ≥16000/mm3.

The mnemonic is C-Hobbs in the next 48 hours: calcium ≤8 mEq/L, hematocrit decrease ≥10%; PO2 ≤60 mm Hg; BUN increase ≥5 mg/dl; base deficit ≥4 mEq/L; fluid sequestration ≥6 L.

Know the criteria for the prognosis of patients with pancreatitis.

Severe pancreatitis indicates a high mortality rate.

Each is assigned 1 point; if the score is ≥3, pancreatitis is considered severe.

An alternative scoring system is **APACHE II**, which assigns points for age, previous health, temperature, heart rate, respiratory rate, PaO2, pH, K, Na, MAP, creatinine, Hct, WBC, and GCS. A score of ≥8 indicates severe pancreatitis.

106. What are the treatment options for acute pancreatitis?

With aggressive intravenous **hydration**, the stone will usually pass in gallstone pancreatitis, but consider **ERCP** for stone removal if CBD dilation is present. Give nothing by mouth to reduce stimulation of the inflammation. Give medications for pain (meperidine, not morphine). Why meperidine? Morphine will stimulate the sphincter of Oddi and aggravate pancreatitis. Consider **elective cholecystectomy** in the presence of gallstone pancreatitis.

107. What is the pathogenesis of pancreatic pseudocyst?

A pancreatic pseudocyst occurs when pancreatic enzymes have been walled off, resembling a cyst. The patient presents with dull epigastric pain, early satiety, and a history of pancreatitis. The next step is to watch a patient with an acute pseudocyst that is smaller than 5 cm for 4-6 weeks because most of these pseudocysts self-resolve. If it is larger than 5 cm, wait 4-6 weeks for the pseudocyst wall to mature before drainage. Other indications for surgical or endoscopic drainage are infections, pain, and concern for malignancy.

Up to half of all pseudocysts will self resolve without any intervention.

108. How do patients with pancreatic abscess present?

Patients may present with fever, abdominal pain, and a history of pancreatitis. This usually results from **necrotizing pancreatitis**. The risk of infection can be reduced if broad-spectrum antibiotics are given in patients with necrotizing pancreatitis. Treat with surgical drainage.

109. How do patients present with chronic pancreatitis?

Chronic pancreatitis is usually due to alcohol abuse. Patients may present with nonspecific, chronic abdominal pain, or classically with chronic upper abdominal pain radiating to the back associated with steatorrhea (with only an elevation of amylase and lipase on screening), or they may present with hyperglycemia, diabetes, vitamin deficiency, and malabsorption. A secretin stimulation test, CT scan, and endoscopic ultrasound can help confirm the diagnosis. Treat pain with analgesics, nerve blocks, ductal stenting, or pseudocyst drainage. Treat vitamin deficiency with replacement and pancreatic enzymes with lipase replacement.

110. What is the workup for diverticulitis?

Diverticulitis is common in the elderly population. Patients can present with left lower quadrant pain, fever, nausea, and vomiting. If diverticulitis is mild and stable, a CT scan is the first step in diagnosis. If diverticulitis is severe, an abdominal X-ray will rule out perforation.

111. Patients with diverticulosis may present with a nonpainful rectal bleed. True or false?

True. Sigmoidoscopy may reveal multiple diverticula.

112. What is the pathogenesis of angiodysplasia (vascular ectasia)?

Angiodysplasia involves abnormal, malformed vessels in the colon. Rule out other causes of nonpainful rectal bleeding; sigmoidoscopy may reveal no abnormalities. Angiodysplasia is mostly found in the colon with colonoscopy.

Differentiate angiodysplasia from diverticulitis.

113. Recurrent nausea or vomiting in a patient with early satiety, bloating, and abdominal pain, plus a history of diabetes, suggests what diagnosis?

Consider diabetic gastroparesis, diagnosed with a gastric emptying study, after ruling out acute causes of nausea or vomiting.

114. List some causes of constipation.

Causes include drugs (anticholinergics, iron supplements, calcium-containing medications, opiates), low-fiber diet, rectocele, autonomic neuropathy, spinal cord lesions, and scleroderma.

115. Angiodysplasia may be associated with what heart murmur?

It may be associated with aortic stenosis.

116. What is the workup for an acute upper gastrointestinal (GI) bleed?

The patient presents with persistent hematemesis or melena.

The first step is to check the airway, breathing, and circulation and to administer IV fluids. Next, obtain

The most common cause of upper GI bleeding is due to peptic ulcer disease.

Other common causes of upper GI bleed are esophageal/gastric varices, Mallory-Weiss tears, and esophagitis/gastritis and dieulafoy's lesion.

Know the most common cause of a lower GI bleed in adults.

Other common causes of lower GI bleed are vascular (angiodysplasia, ischemic, radiation induced); inflammatory (IBD, infectious); and neoplastic.

a gastric lavage to determine whether it is an upper GI bleed or a lower GI bleed if you are unsure of the source or it is a recalcitrant bleed. An upper endoscopy should be done in 24 hours to identify the source of the bleed. After the source of bleeding is found, initiate intravenous **proton pump inhibitors** and perform **endoscopy** therapy to stabilize the bleed (epinephrine, sclerosing agents, balloon tamponade). If this fails, **surgery** may be needed.

117. Most episodes of upper GI bleed due to peptic ulcer disease will self-resolve. True or false?

True.

118. An upper GI bleed can present with hematochezia. True or false?

True. This signifies that there is a significant amount of blood in the upper GI tract.

119. What is the workup of an acute lower GI bleed?

The patient presents with hematochezia.

The first step is to check airway, breathing, and circulation, and to administer IV fluids. Rectal heme occult blood testing should be done if melena is present; anoscopy should be performed if hematochezia is present to rule out hemorrhoids. The most common cause of a lower GI bleed is diverticulosis. A colonoscopy should be performed first; however, if upper GI symptoms such as hematemesis or a bloody aspirate from gastric lavage are present, an upper endoscopy should be done first.

120. When is angiography performed in rectal bleeding?

It is performed in patients when endoscopy is not able to locate the source of bleed and there is refractory bleeding. A **radionuclide scan** can be performed before angiography because it is more sensitive for diagnosis but less specific. If angiography fails to locate the source of the bleed, imaging of the small bowel by **push or capsule enteroscopy** is the next step. Consider a **Meckel** scan in younger patients.

121. List some congenital syndromes that can cause occult GI bleeding in young adolescents.

- Peutz-Jeghers syndrome (**perioral pigmentation**, intestinal obstruction from multiple hamartomatous polyps)
- Meckel's diverticulum

- Arterial venous malformation
- Dieulafoy's lesion (large superficial artery usually in the proximal stomach not associated with an ulcer)
- Hemangiomas

122. List some causes of occult GI bleed in adults.

- Radiation
- Drugs (NSAIDs)
- Tumors
- Angiectasis
- Hereditary hemorrhagic telangiectasia
- Gastric antral vascular ectasia (**watermelon stomach**)
- Aortoenteric fistula
- Crohn's disease

123. What are the gastrointestinal manifestations of Chagas disease?

Chagas disease is an esophagus and colon disease manifesting as **megaesophagus** and **megacolon**. *Trypanosoma cruzi* is carried in the gut of reduviid bugs and transmitted by inoculation of their feces into humans. Treatment is largely supportive.

Mallory Weiss tears are mucosal lacerations in the distal esophagus/ proximal stomach due to forceful vomiting. It is associated with alcoholism and hiatal hernia.

Gastrointestinal Chagas is common in the southernmost areas of South America (Brazil, Bolivia, Argentina, Paraguay, Chile)

Chapter 8

Male Genitourinary Disorders

1. Erectile dysfunction evaluation should include in its first step nocturnal penile tumescence or history of morning erection. True or false?

True. If it is positive, this suggests a psychological cause of erectile dysfunction. Other tests of utility are testosterone, TSH, and prolactin.

2. List the causes of erectile dysfunction in men.

- Psychogenic disorder
- Obesity, smoking, alcohol abuse
- Vascular disorders
- Drugs (antihypertensives, narcotics, antidepressants)

3. Selective serotonin reuptake inhibitors (SSRIs) can delay ejaculation and thus can be used to treat premature ejaculation. True or false?

True.

4. DIAPPERS is a mnemonic for causes of urinary incontinence. True or false?

True. **DIAPPERS**: delirium, infection (urinary tract infection [UTI]), atrophic vaginitis/urethritis, pharmacologic therapy, psychogenic disorder, excessive urine (CHF, hyperglycemia), restricted mobility, stool impaction

5. What is the first step in the evaluation of patients with suspected benign prostatic hyperplasia (BPH)?

Patients usually present with frequency, urgency, nocturia, hesitancy, straining, and incomplete emptying. Urinalysis

There's an association between ED and bicycling and this has been thought to be a potential problem for serious cyclists.

Always rule out genitourinary infections in patients presenting with BPH.

is obtained first to rule out UTI. PSA can be offered. Treatment is alpha antagonists, with 5-alpha reductase inhibitors as second-line therapy. Surgical therapy with transurethral resection of the prostate (TURP) is the gold standard treatment for refractory cases.

6. What is the differential diagnosis of acute testicular pain?

Testicular pain is classified according to age:

Age: Adolescence to 20s

Consider testicular torsion.

Age: 30s

Consider epididymitis; it can present similarly to torsion, but is associated with UTI symptoms and gradual onset of scrotal pain. It can be caused by mumps, *E. coli,* and gonococcal and tuberculosis infections. If the patient is **younger than 35**, treat epididymitis with antibiotics that are similar to those for urethritis. If the patient is **older than 35** or has receptive anal intercourse, add ofloxacin to target coliform bacteria.

7. What is the differential diagnosis of testicular mass?

- Cyst
- Hydrocele
- Varicocele (bag of worms)
- Inguinal hernia
- Testicular cancer (age 20-35)

8. Describe the physical examination in patients presenting with physical testicular torsion.

Patients can present with acute nausea and vomiting. The physical examination shows testicular pain and swelling, with **elevation of the testes**, **horizontal orientation**, and an **absent cremasteric reflex**.

What type of hydrocele should be treated?

9. What is the definition of a hydrocele?

A hydrocele is a fluid-filled sac caused by a **patent processus vaginalis**. The patient presents with an enlarged scrotum.

Do not treat in children if it is a **non-communicating** processus vaginalis, because this type self-resolves at 12 months of age. A **communicating type** (usually associated with a hernia) should be repaired surgically. Hydrocele can also be associated with local infection (epididymitis) or testicular mass.

10. How does an adult patient present when a urinary tract infection (UTI) is present?

The patient presents with dysuria, frequency, and urgency. **The first step is** to obtain urinalysis (UA) to look for **pyuria** (leukocytes), leukocyte esterase, and nitrites; sometimes hematuria is present. Culture is indicated for complicated UTI, pyelonephritis and in men. Why? Culture and sensitivity is used to narrow the coverage of antibiotics.

Treatment: Nitrofurantoin or trimethoprim/sulfamethoxazole or fluoroquinolone, or beta lactams for uncomplicated cystitis. Empiric nitrofurantoin and beta lactams not as effective in prostatitis, so avoid in men with UTI.

If fever and flank pain (**pyelonephritis**) or complicated cystitis (associated with renal failure, BPH, and altered mental status) are present, admit the patient to hospital or treat longer (10-14 days) with fluoroquinolone or 3rd generation cephalosporin.

11. What are the risk factors for uncomplicated cystitis and pyelonephritis in adults?

Risk factors for women include sexual intercourse, use of spermicides, a previous UTI, and a new sexual partner. Risk factors for men are similar including BPH.

12. How do patients present with prostatitis?

The patient can present with back pain, urinary frequency, and urgency. The prostate examination will reveal a tender prostate.

The first step is to obtain a UA and culture. **Why? The causative organism is usually *E. coli*.** In sexually active young men, *Neisseria gonorrhoeae* and *Chlamydia trachomatis* are possible causes.

Treatment: The first step in treatment is to treat empirically against gram-negative organisms with trimethoprim/sulfamethoxazole or a fluoroquinolone. If prostatitis is present in a **sexually active young man** with concomitant urethritis or epididymitis, treat it empirically as an **STD**.

Know the different organisms in prostatitis in elderly and young patients.

Chapter 9

Gynecology

1. What is the most commonly found vaginal cyst?
The Bartholin cyst is the most common. It is found on the labia inferiorly. If it is infected, treat it with incision and drainage and with antibiotics.

2. How do patients with lichen sclerosis present?
Lichen sclerosis is most commonly found in postmenopausal women. The patient will present with itching and pain during sexual intercourse (dyspareunia). On examination of the patient, you will see labial fusion and atrophic labia. Rule out squamous carcinoma by doing a biopsy.

Treatment: Administer high-potency topical steroids.

3. What is the definition of vaginismus?
Vaginismus is the tensing or contraction of the perineal musculature, making sexual intercourse painful (dyspareunia). The treatment is dilatation techniques.

4. What is the definition of recurrent UTI in women?
≥2 UTI within 6 months or three or more within the previous 12 months.

Treatment is initial behavioral modification including postcoital voiding, and avoiding spermicides. Antibiotics prophylaxis (either postcoital or intermittent) is effective for those refractory or unable tolerate behavioral changes. Topical estrogen for postmenopausal women.

Know the various approaches to recurrent UTI in women.

5. What is the most commonly found ovarian cyst?
The corpus luteum cyst is most common.

Treatment: Observe or treat with oral contraceptives.

What is the difference between leiomyoma and adenomyosis?

6. How do oral contraceptives work against ovarian cysts?

Oral contraceptives prevent the stimulation of gonadotropin-releasing hormone (GnRH) to prevent the maturation of follicles and thus cyst formation.

Simple and complex cysts ≥5-10 cm by ultrasound should be considered for surgical removal to confirm diagnosis of the cyst.

7. In anovulatory vaginal bleeding, the menstrual cycle falls out of the normal range of the cycle. True or false?

True. It usually falls 10 days out of the normal menses cycle. Treatment is oral contraceptives.

8. What is the pathogenesis of uterine fibroids (leiomyoma)?

Uterine fibroids are abnormal growths in the smooth muscle of the uterus. The patient can present with heavy or prolonged bleeding, abdominal swelling, and pain, or can be asymptomatic. On examination, the mass is bumpy and nodular. Abdominal ultrasound should be performed to rule out adenomyoma.

Treatment: Myomectomy or hysterectomy

9. What is an indication for myomectomy in leiomyoma?

Myomectomy is indicated when the patient desires to be pregnant.

10. What is an indication for hysterectomy in leiomyoma?

Hysterectomy is indicated when the patient does not desire to be pregnant.

11. What is the pathogenesis of endometriosis?

Endometriosis is invasion of the various extrauterine tissues by the endometrium of the uterus. The patient presents with heavy or prolonged bleeding, dysmenorrhea, abdominal pain, painful defecation, and pain during sexual intercourse (dyspareunia).

The diagnosis is clinical, but a definitive diagnosis is by laparoscopy for direct visualization.

Complication: Scars in the fallopian tubes cause infertility.

Treatment is the administration of oral contraceptives to control heavy menstrual bleeding and NSAIDs for pain. **Gonadotropin-releasing hormone agonists** are the second-line agent for treatment. Surgery is the treatment for lysis of fibrotic lesions and hysterectomy is for refractory cases.

12. What is the difference between primary dysmenorrhea and endometriosis?

Abdominal pain due to endometriosis stops prior to menses, whereas that due to primary dysmenorrhea continues throughout menses. In the first 1-3 days of menses, elevated prostaglandins from low levels of estrogen and progesterone in the luteal phase cause abdominal pain in primary dysmenorrhea; treatment is thus NSAIDs or oral contraceptives.

13. What is the pathogenesis of adenomyosis?

Adenomyosis is the invasion of the myometrium by the endometrium. The patient may present with heavy or prolonged bleeding (menorrhagia) and dysmenorrhea. On examination, the mass is diffuse or symmetric.

Treatment is oral contraceptives and NSAIDs. Refractory medical cases are treated with hysterectomy.

14. What is the pathogenesis of pelvic organ prolapse (cystocele, rectocele, urethrocele)?

The pelvic floor muscles and fascia are loose as a result of childbirth, obesity, menopause, and increased intra-abdominal pressure, causing herniation of the genitourinary organs or the rectum into the vagina wall.

What is the difference among cystocele, urethrocele, and rectocele?

15. How do patients generally present with cystocele/ urethrocele?

The patient will present with urgency, frequency, lower abdominal fullness, and stress urinary incontinence. On the pelvic examination, a cystocele (herniated bladder) and urethrocele (herniated urethra) present as a protrusion of the anterior vaginal wall.

16. How do patients with a rectocele present?

Patients may have problems with incomplete evacuation and difficulty in defecating. On the physical examination, the rectum is seen protruding into the posterior vaginal wall.

17. What are the treatment options for cystocele, rectocele, or urethrocele?

Treatment is hormonal therapy for postmenopausal patients and Kegel exercises for others. For patients who do not desire surgery, but do not respond to the preceding treatment, treat with pessaries (cone-like structures inserted into the vagina to act as a pelvic support).

18. What are types of urinary incontinence?

- Stress
- Urge
- Overflow
- Continuous

Workup for urinary incontinence should include a urinalysis.

19. What is the pathogenesis of stress incontinence?

Stress incontinence is caused by pelvic floor relaxation, which leads to a slanting down of the urethrovesical junction, causing a nonequal distribution of intra-abdominal pressure between the bladder and the urethral sphincter. Risk factors are the same as for pelvic organ prolapse.

20. How do patients present with stress incontinence?

Incontinence is due to increased intra-abdominal pressure (cough, Valsalva maneuver, obesity, lifting), sometimes with concurring prolapse such as a cystocele and a urethrocele. Treatment is the same as for cystocele with **Kegel exercises**.

Pharmacological treatment is an alpha agonist to increase internal sphincter resistance. However this is no longer recommended due to the high rate of adverse effects. Surgery can help those without improvement from Kegel exercises.

21. What is the pathogenesis of urge incontinence (urinary frequency > 8 times in 24 hours)?

The bladder muscle (detrusor) repeatedly contracts. Risk factors are diabetes, neuropathy, and neurological disorders.

The patient may present with urgency, frequency, and nocturia. Conservative treatment is to reduce caffeine and treatment is weight loss in obese patients. Pharmacologic treatment is a muscarinic antagonist, such as tolterodine (Detrol), solifenacin (Vesicare), or oxybutynin.

22. What are the risk factors for overflow incontinence, also known as atonic bladder?

The risk factors for overflow incontinence are spinal cord paralysis, diabetes, urethral stenosis, **enlarged prostate**, and **postsurgical** use of an epidural anesthesia, all of which cause atonic bladder. The patient will present with urinary retention, overdistention, incomplete voiding, and dribbling, or mixed symptoms of urge and stress incontinence. Post-void residual (PVR) should be >100 ml to cause urinary retention. Normal PVR is <45 ml. This is the only type of incontinence that has elevated PVR. The treatment is urinary catheterization and use of an alpha 1 antagonist such as tamsulosin (Flomax).

What is the criterion needed to have overflow incontinence?

23. What are the characteristics of human papillomavirus lesions (condyloma acuminata)?

Human papillomavirus lesions are cauliflower-like, flesh-colored lesions that are nonpainful and seen during the physical examination. Differentiate from **angiofibromas** (pearly penile papules on the corona of the penis) in men and **papillomatosis** of the vulva in women (multiple papules that arise from a single base), which are similar in shape to condyloma acuminata, but are benign lesions. Treatment is Condylox ointment or trichloroacetic acid, cryotherapy, or excision.

24. How do patients with Gardnerella vaginalis *(bacteria vaginitis)* present?

The patient presents with white vaginal discharge that has a **fishy odor**. Microscopic examination of the discharge reveals clue cells (epithelial cells covered with bacteria). Treatment is metronidazole.

25. How do patients with Candidiasis vaginitis present?

The patient presents with a cottage cheese-like discharge and itching, and an erythematous vulvar is seen on examination. Microscopic examination reveals pseudohyphae and spores after application of potassium hydroxide. Treatment is Diflucan or topical azoles.

26. How do patients present with Trichomoniasis (caused by Trichomonas vaginalis)?

The patient presents with a colored (grey, yellow, green), foul-smelling discharge. An erythematous vulva and cervix (strawberry cervix) are seen on examination. Microscopic examination of the wet preparation shows a motile, flagellated organism.

Treat the patient and her sexual partner with metronidazole. All metronidazole users need to avoid the use of alcohol to prevent a disulfiram reaction.

Trichomoniasis is considered a sexually transmitted infection.

27. How do patients present with pelvic inflammatory disease (PID)?

The patient may present with lower abdominal pain and discharge, intermenstrual bleed, dysuria, and frequent urination, with a history of sexually transmitted disease (STD) (remember that fever is rare). Vaginal examination reveals uterine or cervical motion tenderness.

Treatment: If PID is severe, admit the patient to hospital and treat with broad-spectrum antibiotics. Cefotetan or cefoxitin IV plus doxycycline IV for 14 days. Gentamycin IV and clindamycin IV is an alternative regimen for inpatients. For outpatients, a single intramuscular dose of ceftriaxone and oral doxycycline for 14 days is recommended.

28. In a sexually active woman presenting with right upper quadrant abdominal pain with a pleuritic component that is sometimes referred to the right shoulder, who has with normal liver test results, what diagnosis should be considered?

Consider perihepatitis (Fitz-Hugh-Curtis syndrome) associated with PID caused by exudates coating the surface of the liver.

Staphylococcus aureus can produce exotoxin that can lead to three syndromes: food poisoning, scalded skin syndrome and toxic shock syndrome.

29. What is the most common risk factor for toxic shock syndrome?

The most common risk factor is use of highly absorptive tampons. Toxic shock syndrome is caused by Staphylococcus aureus and Group A streptococci. The syndrome is due to an exotoxin, a bacterial superantigen causing extensive activation of inflammatory cells. The patient presents with fever, a desquamative rash on the palms and soles, and hypotension. Thrombotic complications and multiple organ involvement can occur. Treatment is IV fluids and broad-spectrum antibiotics. Early treatment with **clindamycin** reduces the production and release of exotoxins.

30. What is the pathogenesis of menopause?

Atrophy of oocytes leads to lack of estrogen, which results in elevated follicle-stimulating hormone (FSH) and luteinizing hormone (LH) levels.

The patient may present with hot flushes, night sweats, bone fractures, vaginal dryness, vaginal atrophy, and pain during sexual intercourse. The atrophic vagina is susceptible to *E. coli* infection, which can present as multiple UTIs.

Treatment is hormonal replacement therapy (estrogen and progesterone) for a limited period (6 months to a year) to prevent osteoporosis and alleviate other symptoms. Treat with topical vaginal estrogen for vaginal symptoms. Alternatives to hormonal therapy are clonidine, **SSRIs**, and gabapentin.

Why are postmenopausal women susceptible to UTIs?

31. What are complications of estrogen therapy?

- Endometrial hyperplasia and endometrial cancer
- Withdrawal bleeding

32. Estrogen replacement is associated with cardiovascular disease, thromboembolism, and breast and endometrial cancers. True or false?

True.

33. How do patients with amenorrhea present?

The patient with no menses by age 16 has primary amenorrhea. Patients with no menses for three consecutive cycles (those with regular menses) or who have not had menses for 6 months (those with irregular menses) have secondary amenorrhea.

34. What are the causes of primary amenorrhea?

- Ovarian failure (Turner syndrome, autoimmune ovarian failure, polycystic ovarian syndrome)
- Androgen hyperplasia (21-hydroxylase deficiency): Chronic anovulation with estrogen
- Testicular feminization: Chronic anovulation with estrogen present
- Kallmann syndrome: Absent estrogen
- Anatomical defects (imperforate hymen)
- Anorexia nervosa

35. How do patients with Turner syndrome present?

Turner syndrome is the most common cause of primary amenorrhea. As a result of a 45,XO karyotype and consequent ovarian failure, the patient presents with a webbed neck, broad chest, and lymphedema in the neck and extremities. An elevated FSH level is present because of ovarian failure.

A definitive diagnosis can be obtained with karyotype analysis.

Treatment: Estrogen replacement therapy

What is the difference between CAH and Sertoli-Leydig cell tumors?

What are similarities between CAH and Addison disease?

36. What are the classic features of 21-hydroxylase deficiency?

Classic features are adrenal insufficiency (shock or hypotension, hyponatremia, hyperkalemia) virilization, and salt wasting; however, mild forms may present with virilization only.

37. What is the pathogenesis of testicular feminization (androgen insensitivity)?

Testicular feminization is the lack of receptor sensitivity to testosterone, leading to conversion of testosterone to estrogen and an elevated serum testosterone level. Müllerian inhibiting factor is persistent, responsible for the lack of uterus and fallopian tubes. The testes are retained in the inguinal canal.

Treatment: Remove testes to prevent cancer and hormonal replacement.

38. What is the pathogenesis of Kallmann syndrome?

Kallmann syndrome is anosmia and the congenital absence of GnRH and, as a result, FSH levels are diminished.

39. What is the pathogenesis of congenital adrenal hyperplasia (CAH)?

CAH is caused by excess androgens as a result of a deficiency of **21-alpha dehydroxylase (classic CAH)**. The patient will present with **virilization** (hoarse voice, hirsutism, ambiguous genitalia, clitoromegaly) and **amenorrhea** over an **extended time**. The levels of **androgen precursors**, urine **17-alpha dihydroxyprogesterone (this enzyme elevation is diagnostic of classic CAH)**, serum dehydroepiandrosterone (DHEA), and its sulfate (DHEAS) are elevated. The first step is to rule out **ovarian/adrenal tumors,** which can cause hirsutism and virilization, but usually **occur rapidly**. Since aldosterone and cortisol are both diminished in CAH, patients can also present with nausea, vomiting, hypotension and salt wasting, and skin hyperpigmentation (Addison-like symptoms).

40. What is the first step in the diagnosis of primary amenorrhea?

To diagnose primary amenorrhea, determine whether the breast or uterus is present

41. What would the presence of a breast and uterus indicate on a physical examination?

The presence of a breast indicates the presence of estrogen, and the presence of a uterus indicates normal female development.

Understand the workup for primary and secondary amenorrhea.

42. What would the presence of breasts but an absent uterus on the physical examination indicate in patients with primary amenorrhea?

The absence of uterus suggests abnormal mullerian development (46, XX karyotype with normal female testosterone), androgen insensitivity syndrome (46, XY karyotype) or 5-alpha-reductase deficiency (46, XY with increased testosterone but male phenotype unlike androgen insensitivity). Obtain serum testosterone level and karyotype analysis for diagnosis..

43. What would the presence of a uterus but absent breasts on the physical examination indicate in patients with primary amenorrhea?

After checking for absence of imperforate hymen, vaginal septum, or congenital absence of vagina, the first thing to consider is gonadal failure (e.g., Turner syndrome) or hypothalamic failure (Kallmann syndrome), which can both cause a diminished estrogen level. Hypothalamic failure may lead to low FSH levels, whereas ovarian failure may lead to elevated FSH levels. Therefore, the next step would be to order serum FSH levels, then serum beta human chorionic gonadotropin, to rule out pregnancy.

44. List other causes of primary amenorrhea.

- Prolactinoma-prolactin suppresses GnRH
- Aromatase deficiency
- Gonadal dysgenesis
- LH, FSH resistance
- Hypothyroidism, hyperthyroidism, sarcoidosis, galactosemia

45. What are the causes of secondary amenorrhea?

- Polycystic ovarian syndrome (PCOS)
- Premature ovarian failure
- Pregnancy
- Hypothalamic-pituitary axis dysfunction (anovulation)

- Outflow tract obstruction
- Prolactinoma
- Hypothyroidism
- Congenital adrenal hyperplasia (late onset)
- Sarcoidosis
- Anorexia nervosa

46. What is the most common cause of secondary amenorrhea?

The most common cause is chronic anovulation with estrogen, such as **PCOS**, Cushing syndrome, 21-hydroxylase deficiency, and luteal phase defects.

47. What is the pathogenesis of PCOS?

PCOS is caused by elevated androgen levels, leading to oligo-anovulation, obesity, insulin insensitivity, hirsutism, and an LH/FSH ratio >2:1. Treatment is metformin exercise, weight loss, and oral contraceptives. **Clomiphene citrate** can be used to induce ovulation for those who desire to be pregnant.

Two out of three of Rotterdam criteria are needed to diagnosis PCOS and they are oligo-and/or anovulation, clinical or biochemical signs of hyperandrogenism, polycystic ovaries by ultrasound.

48. What are the causes of hypothalamic-pituitary axis dysfunction (anovulation)?

One of the most common causes of secondary amenorrhea is functional hypothalamic amenorrhea which is usually secondary to stress, exercise, and low body fat (anorexia). Patients can present with decrease in GnRH secretion, and consequent anovulation. This is ultimately a diagnosis of exclusion after work-up for organic causes of secondary amenorrhea. Treatment is to reduce exercise, consult a nutritionist, and reduce stress.

49. How do patients present with prolactinoma?

Patients can present with galactorrhea, headaches, and vision changes.

50. What is the pathogenesis of outflow tract obstruction (Asherman syndrome)?

Asherman syndrome is caused by adhesions in the uterine canal secondary to previous uterine surgeries, PID, and procedures (cesarean section, dilation and curettage).

51. The first step in the diagnosis of secondary amenorrhea is to obtain a pregnancy test (beta human chorionic gonadotropin [B-HCG] test). True or false?

True. Next, obtain prolactin, thyroid-stimulating hormone (TSH), and FSH levels. Why TSH and FSH?

Elevated TSH, FSH, or thyrotropin-releasing hormone levels can cause hyperprolactinemia and amenorrhea. Obtain serum total testosterone level if there is evidence of hyperandrogenism.

If the above tests are normal, perform a progesterone challenge test.

Why is the TSH level obtained in the evaluation of secondary amenorrhea?

52. What is the progesterone challenge test?

Administer progesterone for 7 days; if the patient has a withdrawal bleed, then the test result is positive. This means that estrogen is adequate (Figure 9-1).

If the test result is negative, this usually means that the estrogen level is low; therefore, administer estrogen and progesterone. If the test result is still negative, consider Asherman syndrome (Figure 9-1).

Treatment: Progesterone or combination oral contraceptives if the progesterone challenge test is positive.

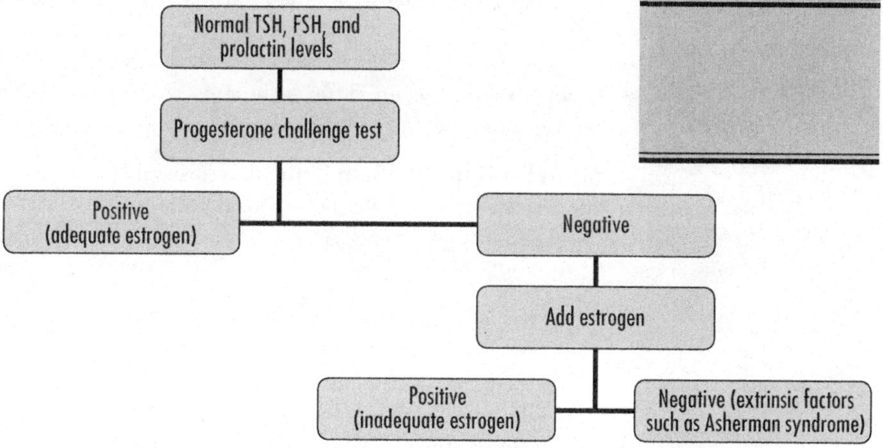

Figure 9-1. *Workup of secondary amenorrhea. TSH, thyroid-stimulating hormone.*

53. What is the pathogenesis of dysfunctional uterine bleed (DUB)?

DUB is the most common cause of abnormal vaginal bleeding in adolescents. In the first decade after menarche, the hypothalamic portal axis is immature, leading to anovulation (periods of amenorrhea alternating with polymenorrhea). Anovulation is also common in the transition period to menopause; these are periods when ovarian function begins and declines.

What is the most common cause of abnormal uterine bleeding in postmenopausal women?

54. What is the approach to diagnosis of abnormal vaginal bleeding?

Evaluate according to age, as follows:

Adolescents

Consider anovulation, pregnancy, infection, and bleeding disorders.

20s-40s

Consider pregnancy, endometriosis, infection, fibroids, cervical/endometrial polyps, adenomyosis, ovarian tumors, and endocrine disorders.

50s

Consider anovulation, endometrial hyperplasia, and malignancy.

Postmenopause

Consider malignancy, endometrial hyperplasia, vaginal atrophy, and hormonal replacement therapy.

55. How do patients with endometrial or vaginal atrophy present?

Patients with endometrial or vaginal atrophy present with vaginal bleed. This is the most common cause of abnormal uterine bleeding in postmenopausal women.

56. What is the first step in the diagnosis of abnormal uterine bleeding in postmenopausal patients?

The first step is to perform an endometrial biopsy to rule out endometrial cancer.

57. What is the treatment for abnormal uterine bleeding?

If bleeding is continuous or active when the patient is seen, IV estrogen is given. When the patient becomes stable, or if the patient is stable on arrival or has been previously diagnosed with DUB, she can be treated with oral contraceptives, or a progesterone-only contraceptive if she is a smoker and ≥35 years old.

58. How is chronic abdominal pain (≥6 months' duration) approached in women?

It should be evaluated according to age.

20s: Consider primary dysmenorrhea and endometriosis.

30s-40s: Consider leiomyoma (fibroids).

40s and older: Consider ovarian cancer.

59. How do patients with premenstrual dysphoric disorder present?

The patient presents with mood symptoms such as difficulty concentrating, loss of interest in activities, lethargy, depressed mood, and irritability, as well as physical symptoms, including headache, abdominal bloating, and cramps a few days before menses. Symptoms must be severe enough to interfere with work or school.

Treatment: Hormones (oral contraceptives) or anxiolytics (selective serotonin reuptake inhibitors). Other treatment options: diuretics, vitamin B6, beta-blockers, NSAIDs, and cognitive-behavioral treatment.

60. What is the pathogenesis of Sertoli-Leydig cell tumors?

A Sertoli-Leydig cell tumor of the ovary produces elevated androgen levels. The patient presents with rapid onset of hirsutism and virilization (weeks to months) and a very high level of testosterone. DHEA and DHEAS levels are absent.

Why are DHEA and DHEAS absent in patients with Sertoli-Leydig cell tumors?

61. Women presenting with a markedly elevated testosterone level ≥150 ng/dl should be checked for ovarian or adrenal tumors. True or false?

True. The most common cause of elevated testosterone in women is PCOS, but it rarely exceeds 150 ng/dl; a higher value should be an alert to check for an ovarian or adrenal tumor.

62. How do patients with a granulosa-theca ovarian tumor (a sex cord stromal tumor) present?

The patient will present with abnormal uterine bleeding and underlying endometrial hyperplasia, and breast tenderness due to increased estrogen production. In patients with endometrial cancer, always search for a granulosa-theca tumor. They are the most common malignant potential ovarian sex cord stromal tumor, however fibromas (associated with Meig's syndrome) are the most common sex cord stromal tumors.

Treatment: Total abdominal hysterectomy and bilateral oophorectomy.

63. What is the pathogenesis of endometrial hyperplasia?

Endometrial hyperplasia is caused by an elevated estrogen level. The patient may present with postcoital bleeding.

Why are certain types of endometrial hyperplasia treated with progestin?

Why are patients who are smokers and older than 35 years treated with a progesterone-only pill? ***Higher risk of coagulation***

Treatment: If it is an atypical complex endometrial hyperplasia, the treatment is a hysterectomy. If it is a complex endometrial hyperplasia without atypia, treat it with progestin to oppose excess estrogen.

64. What are some contraceptive methods?

- Barrier method (condoms)
- Hormonal (oral contraceptives)
- Intrauterine device (IUD)
- Emergency contraception
- Sterilization

65. What are the advantages of oral contraceptives?

Oral contraceptives prevent ovarian and endometrial cancer, and menses are less frequent.

66. What are the disadvantages of oral contraceptives?

Oral contraceptives are contraindicated in smokers ≥35 years old and in patients with coagulopathy, an estrogen responsive tumor, hypertension, and migraine headaches.

67. What are the advantages of an IUD?

An IUD is one of the most effective, long-term contraceptives (lasts 5-10 years).

68. What are the disadvantages of an IUD?

IUDs are contraindicated in patients with PID, who have had recent STDs or multiple sexual partners, or who have never been pregnant. They are associated with vaginal bleeding and cramping (copper form).

69. How is emergency contraception (levonorgestrel) used?

Emergency contraception is effective up to 120 hours after unprotected sexual intercourse to prevent possible pregnancy. The patient is usually given high-dose progestin, levonorgestrel.

70. Sterilization is the most effective form of contraception. True or false?

True. However, it is a permanent method of contraception.

71. What form of prophylaxis is recommended for victims of sexual abuse?

Recommended are a progestin-only pill and treatment with antibiotics against gonorrhea, *Chlamydia*, bacterial vaginosis, *Trichomonas vaginalis*, and hepatitis B. Test for syphilis and HIV. Treat for HIV if the assailant is HIV positive; if assailant's HIV status is unknown, do repeat testing for HIV at 6 weeks, 3 months, and 6 months (this is the same recommendation as for needle-stick injuries).

72. What is the first approach to couples presenting with infertility?

The first step is to ask about the frequency of sexual activity and interest and the duration of sexual intercourse. Why? Because infertility is defined as failure to conceive 1 year after unprotected intercourse.

73. The most common cause of infertility in women is ovarian and fallopian tube disorders (e.g., PID, adhesions). True or false?

True. Other causes of infertility in women are peritoneal (endometriosis), cervical defects, uterine abnormalities, and ovarian abnormalities.

74. The most common cause of infertility in men is a low number of functional sperm in the ejaculate. True or false?

True.

75. The first step in the work-up of infertility in men is to obtain a serum analysis. True or false?

True. If the results are abnormal, obtain serum hormone levels (FSH, LH, testosterone) to look for the underlying cause. In women, the initial evaluation is documentation of ovulation, and then imaging to evaluate the uterine cavity and tubal patency (hysterosalpingography).

76. What is one infertility treatment option?

Ovarian stimulation: Clomiphene citrate can stimulate follicles to mature for artificial uterine insemination via in vitro fertilization or other methods.

77. What is a serious complication of uterine insemination?

One serious complication is ovarian torsion due to enlarged cysts as a consequence of follicular stimulation.

The most common complication, however, is multiple gestations due to implantation of several follicles.

What is a common complication of artificial uterine insemination?

Chapter 10

Hematology/Oncology

1. What are three major factors causing anemia?
Anemia is caused by destruction of red blood cells (RBCs), reduced production of RBCs, and blood loss.

2. What is the definition of anemia?
Anemia is considered to be hemoglobin (Hb) <12 g/dl in women and Hb <14 g/dl in men.
The patient may present with fatigue and depression-like symptoms.

3. What are types of microcytic anemia (mean corpuscular volume <80 fl, low reticulocyte count <1%)?

- Iron deficiency
- Sideroblastic
- Thalassemia
- Anemia of chronic disease

4. What are the causes of iron-deficiency anemia?
The most common cause of iron-deficiency anemia in men is fecal occult blood loss (malignancy sign). The most common cause in infants is reduced iron intake. Laboratory tests may reveal an elevated red cell distribution width and hypochromic microcytic anemia (Figure 10-1).

The major cause of iron deficiency in developed countries is blood loss. Thus, always search for the presence of blood loss.

5. List some causes of sideroblastic anemia.
Sideroblastic anemia is caused by lack of incorporation of iron into heme. It can be caused by myelodysplastic syndrome, lead poisoning, nutritional deficiencies (vitamin B6, copper), alcohol, drugs (anti-tuberculosis drugs), and hypothermia. It can also be idiopathic or

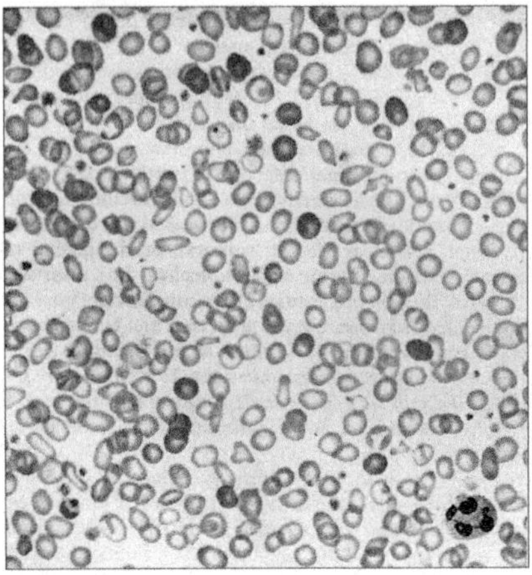

Figure 10-1. *Hypochromic microcytic anemia. Note the central pallor of the small red blood cells. Courtesy of Robert W. McKenna, MD, University of Minnesota and Elsevier Saunders.*

have congenital causes (mitochondrial disorders). Ringed sideroblasts (with nuclear ring of iron deposits) are found in the bone marrow smear.

Treatment: Pyridoxine (vitamin B6) should be tried in all cases of sideroblastic anemia.

The peripheral smear in thalassemia can differentiate it from the anemia of iron deficiency anemia.

6. **What is the pathogenesis of alpha thalassemia major?**
Alpha thalassemia major is the deletion of three or more alpha genes. Deletion of all four alpha genes causes the remaining gamma chains to form high-affinity Hb Bart. This causes lack of oxygen delivery to the tissues (anoxia) and eventually hydrops fetalis at birth. Inheriting only one functional alpha gene (deletion of three alpha genes) results in hemoglobin H with neonatal jaundice at birth and lifelong hemolytic anemia.

Why are patients with beta thalassemia asymptomatic until they are 6 months old?

7. **What is the pathogenesis of beta thalassemia major?**
Beta thalassemia major is the alteration of beta gene transcription and translation from no production or severely limited production of beta globin. Since the infant's hemoglobin consists of two alpha and two gamma chains, beta thalassemia is not symptomatic until the age of 6 months to a year, when the infant develops neonatal jaundice. The adult patient may have hemolytic anemia, which will lead to extramedullary hyperplasia as a compensatory response, causing the patient to have an

enlarged skull and prominent cheek bones. Pulmonary arterial hypertension is due to chronic anemia, hemolysis, and microscopic thrombi.

Treatment: Scheduled blood transfusions

Treatment of complications: Administer blood transfusions and an iron chelator to avoid iron overload.

8. How do patients with alpha and beta thalassemia trait (thalassemia minor) present?

The most important thing about beta thalassemia minor (reduced beta globin production) is to differentiate it from iron-deficiency anemia. How? The patient may present with microcytic anemia and you may be asked to interpret the smear (which will probably show target cells). A patient who is continuously being treated for microcytic anemia with an iron supplement but does not improve could also present with beta thalassemia minor. Hemoglobin electrophoresis usually reveals an elevated **HbA2 level**, and target cells, tear drop red cells on the peripheral smear, normal to increased serum iron and ferritin. Patients with alpha thalassemia trait may have mild anemia and present similarly to those with beta thalassemia trait, but their HbA2 level is not elevated and their HbF level may be elevated.

Treatment: No treatment is needed.

9. How is thalassemia minor differentiated from other causes of microcytosis on peripheral smear?

Patients with thalassemia minor have an extremely low mean corpuscular volume (<70 fl) that is not compatible with the degree of anemia (RBC >4 million, Hct >30).

10. What is the cause of anemia of chronic disease?

Anemia of chronic disease is caused by inflammatory diseases (e.g., rheumatoid arthritis) and infectious diseases.

11. How is microcytic anemia worked up?

Obtain the total iron-binding capacity, percent saturation, ferritin level, and iron level (Table 10-1).

TIBC, total iron-binding capacity.

Anemia of chronic disease involves high levels of ferritin (intracellular iron-storage protein) because the iron transporter is inactivated by a C-reactive protein.

Memorize Table 10-1. The normal serum iron level is 50-150 μg. Normal TIBC is 300-360 μg.

What is the difference between beta thalassemia minor and iron-deficiency anemia?

Why is the ferritin level elevated in patients with anemia of chronic disease?

Table 10-1. *Microcytic Anemia Workup*

Microcytic Workup	Iron-Deficiency Anemia	Chronic Disease Anemia	Sideroblastic Anemia
TIBC	Increased	Decreased	Decreased
Percent saturation	Decreased	Decreased (<20%)	Unknown
Ferritin	Decreased	Increased	Unknown
Iron	Decreased	Decreased	Increased or normal

Iron deficiency anemia may present with pica for ice, clay, or starch. Pica for ice is very specific for iron deficiency anemia.

12. What is the definition of chronic iron-deficiency anemia?

Chronic iron-deficiency anemia is compensated iron-deficiency anemia. Examples are fecal occult blood loss or nutritional deficiency.

13. How do patients with mild chronic iron deficiency present on physical examination?

On physical examination, the patient will have pale mucous membranes, angular stomatitis, koilonychia (spoon nails), and glossitis. The laboratory results show a hemoglobin level of between 6 and 8 g/dl.

14. How do patients with severe chronic iron deficiency present?

The patient may present with signs and symptoms of heart failure, especially in children. Laboratory results show a hemoglobin of <3 g/dl.

15. What is the treatment for chronic iron-deficiency anemia?

Give oral iron to patients with mild anemia, and transfuse blood to those with severe anemia. Vitamin C also increases the absorption of iron.

16. What are types of macrocytic anemia (mean corpuscular volume >100 fl, low reticulocytes)?

- Vitamin B12/folate deficiency
- Myelodysplasia
- Alcohol abuse
- Liver disease
- Hypothyroidism

17. How do patients present with vitamin B_{12} deficiency?

The patient will present with megaloblastic anemia, atrophic glossitis (shiny tongue), angular cheilitis, and neurological problems (see chapter 6). Laboratory tests will reveal large polymorphonuclear neutrophils with multiple nuclei and increased methylmalonic acid and homocysteine levels (Figure 10-2).

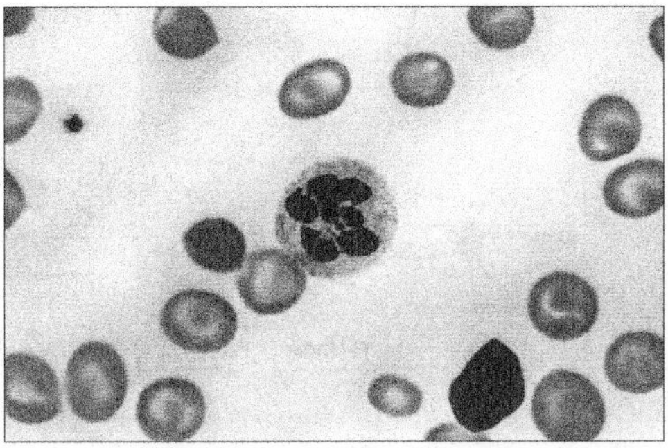

Figure 10-2. *Hypersegmented neutrophil. Note the hypersegmented multilobed nucleus of the neutrophil, characteristic of megaloblastic anemia. Courtesy of Robert W. McKenna, MD, University of Minnesota and Elsevier Saunders.*

18. What is the Schilling test?

It is a test used to diagnose causes of vitamin B12 deficiency. Intravenous (IV) cobalamin and oral labeled cobalamin are administered. If the labeled cobalamin is seen in the urine, the patient's deficiency is nutritional. Add intrinsic factor to the oral labeled cobalamin if the labeled cobalamin is not seen in the urine. If cobalamin is seen in the urine, intrinsic factor is deficient (e.g., pernicious anemia). If cobalamin is not seen in the urine, add antibiotics. If cobalamin is seen, blind loop syndrome (or bacterial overgrowth syndrome) is the diagnosis. If labeled cobalamin is still not seen, the diagnosis is atrophy of villi (e.g., celiac or Whipple disease) or resection of intestinal ileum (Figure 10-3).

19. How do patients present with folate deficiency?

Patients present with pernicious anemia with no neurological deficits. Laboratory test results will show an elevated homocysteine level only.

What is the difference between folate and vitamin B_{12} deficiency?

Pancreatic insufficiency can be diagnosed with schilling test by adding oral labeled vitamin B12 to pancreatic enzymes and checking for oral labeled B12 in the urine.

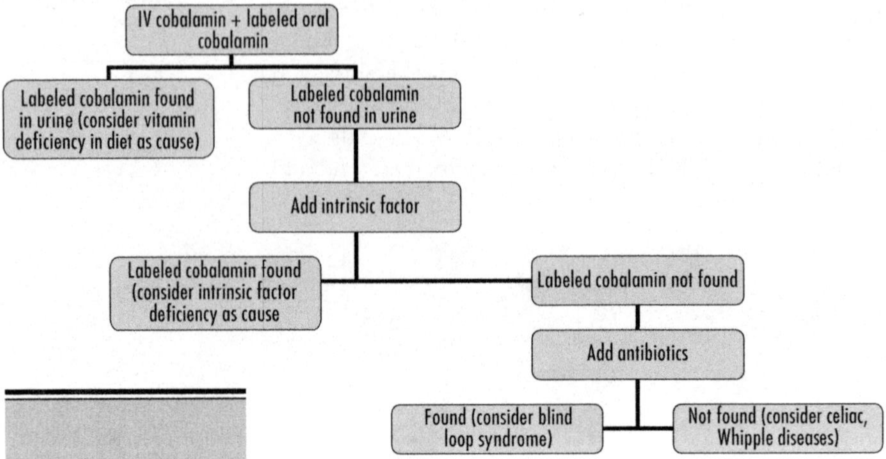

Figure 10-3. *Schilling test. IV, intravenous.*

Copper deficiency and zinc excess can also cause neutropenia or cytopenias.

20. What are some common causes of a low neutrophil count or cytopenias?
- Vitamin deficiency (B12, folate)
- Infections (hepatitis virus, HIV, malaria, ehrlichiosis)
- Drugs (NSAIDs, antibiotics, clozapine)
- Congenital

21. List some causes of aplastic anemia (hypoplastic hematopoietic stem cells in the bone marrow).
- Fanconi anemia (pancytopenia, urogenital disorders, and myeloid cancers)
- Chronic red cell aplasia (severe anemia)
- Paroxysmal nocturnal hemoglobinuria

22. Myelodysplasia is inefficient hematopoiesis leading to low cell counts in all cell lines (pancytopenia). True or false?

True.

23. **What is the most common finding in myelodysplasia?**

Anemia is the most common finding, followed by leukopenia and thrombocytopenia. The median age of diagnosis is 70 years old. Acute myelogenous leukemia develops in a subset of patients with primary myelodysplastic syndrome.

24. What are the causes of hemolytic anemia?
- Autoimmune hemolytic anemia

- Hereditary (sickle cell anemia, hereditary spherocytosis, beta thalassemia, glucose 6-phosphate dehydrogenase)
- Microangiopathic (thrombocytopenic thrombotic purpura [TTP], hemolytic uremic syndrome [HUS], disseminated intravascular coagulopathy [DIC]) (Figure 10-4)

The reticulocyte count is usually elevated (reticulocytosis) in hemolytic anemia as a compensatory response to RBC destruction. Elevated lactate dehydrogenase (LDH) and bilirubin levels (indirect) may also be seen.

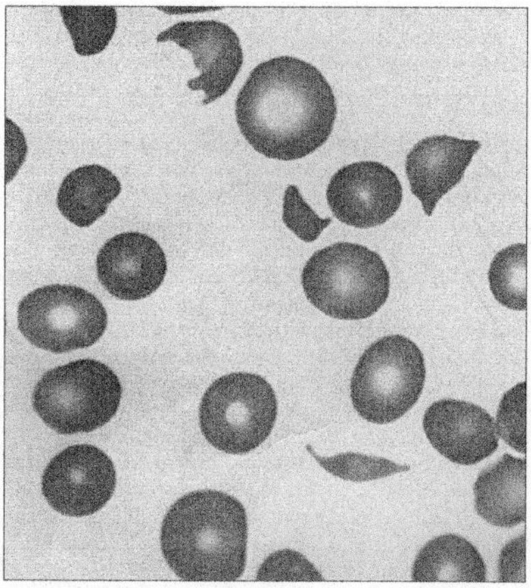

Figure 10-4. *Schistocytes. Note the fragmented red blood cells. Courtesy of Robert W. McKenna, MD, University of Minnesota and Elsevier Saunders.*

25. What is the pathogenesis of cold and warm hemolytic anemia?

Cold: Immunoglobulin M (IgM) binds to RBCs and C3 and lyses RBCs in cold conditions. It is a type of autoimmune hemolytic anemia. Results of the direct antiglobulin test (Coombs test) will be positive. Examples of conditions in which cold hemolytic anemia may occur are lymphoma, Epstein-Barr virus (EBV) (mononucleosis), and Mycoplasma infection.

Warm: Immunoglobulin G (IgG) binds C3 at all times and does not complete lysis. IgG bound to C3 is found on RBCs and phagocytosed in the spleen. It is also a type of autoimmune hemolytic anemia and the results of the direct Coombs test will be positive. Warm hemolytic

What are examples of cold and warm hemolytic anemia?

What is the difference between cold and warm hemolytic anemia?

Mycoplasma pneumonia is an example of cold hemolytic anemia.

Why is the reticulocyte count high in patients with hemolytic anemia?

The acidified glycerol lysis and the eosin-5-maleimide binding tests are more sensitive and specific than the osmotic fragility test, in diagnosing spherocytosis.

anemia can be induced by drugs such as methyldopa, penicillin, and quinine.

26. What is the pathogenesis of hereditary spherocytosis?

Hereditary spherocytosis is an autosomal dominant disease consisting of microspherocytes (small RBCs) that result from a red cell membrane defect (Figure 10-5). The patient can present with anemia and an elevated unconjugated hyperbilirubinemia level after birth or later in life.

Laboratory tests will reveal an elevated mean cell hemoglobin concentration (MCHC) and hemolysis (osmotic fragility test).

Complication: Parvo virus infection can cause aplastic anemia and cholelithiasis can result from hemolysis.

Treatment: Administer folic acid to replenish RBCs; if spherocytosis is severe, a splenectomy may be done. Why? Destruction of RBCs occurs in the spleen.

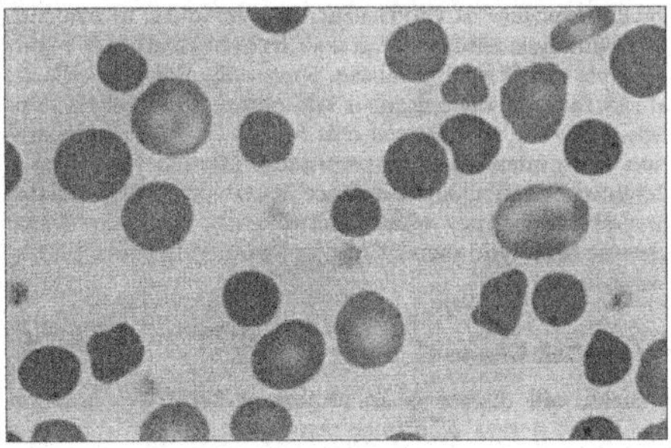

Figure 10-5. *Hereditary spherocytosis. Note the small red blood cells (RBCs) and lack of central pallor in some RBCs. Courtesy of Robert W. McKenna, MD, University of Minnesota and Elsevier Saunders.*

27. What is the pathogenesis of sickle cell anemia?

Switching of valine for glutamate at the sixth position of the beta globin gene on chromosome 11 causes sickled RBCs, especially when the oxygen level is low. The patient presents with a multiple pain syndrome worsened by dehydration. Chest syndrome, splenomegaly, and eventually autosplenectomy are other complications. Laboratory tests show hyperbilirubinemia and reticulocytosis. An RBC smear shows sickled cells. Electrophoresis shows 80-90% of HbSS, 2-4% of HbA2 and 2-20% of HbF (Figure 10-6).

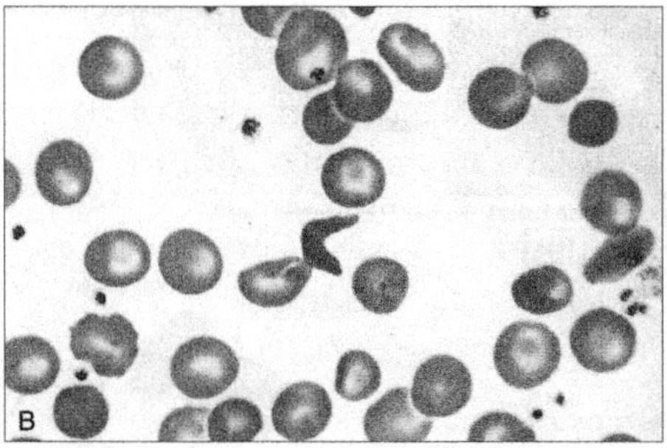

Figure 10-6. *Note the sickle cell in the center of the figure. Courtesy of Robert W. McKenna, MD, University of Minnesota and Elsevier Saunders.*

28. How do patients with sickle cell trait present?

The patient can present with isosthenuria (diluted urine) or hematuria at high altitude.

29. What are the complications of sickle cell anemia?

Complications include parvovirus aplastic anemia, acute chest syndrome, cholelithiasis, dactylitis (swollen and painful hand and foot due to occlusive vessel disease), avascular necrosis of the femoral head, and iron overload.

Treatment: Folic acid supplement and hydroxyurea (to prevent frequency of pain syndrome by replenishing Hb F) and iron binders for iron overload

30. Recommended immunizations for autosplenectomy are pneumococcal, meningococcal, and Haemophilus influenzae vaccinations. Why?

These immunizations are recommended because one of the functions of the spleen is to synthesize IgG, and a component of the complement pathway, properdin, needed for opsonization of bacteria. Since the job of the spleen is also to remove old RBCs, defective cells, and nuclear remnants of RBCs, the peripheral smear after splenectomy would show Howell-Jolly bodies (presents as a single inclusion body inside RBCs).

31. What is the treatment for complications of sickle cell anemia?

Treatment of parvovirus aplastic crisis or chest or lung syndrome consists of exchange transfusion.

What is dactylitis?

Parvovirus infections and cholelithiasis are complications of sickle cell anemia.

What are Heinz bodies?

What is a Bite cell?

32. What are porphyrias?

Porphyrias are disorders in which there is a deficiency of enzymes in the heme synthetic pathway that leads to accumulation of intermediates, such as porphobilinogen, causing a variety of symptoms that are either neurologic or cutaneous. The three most common types are acute intermittent porphyria (AIP), cutaneous porphyria, and erythropoietic protoporphyria.

33. How may patients with AIP present?

Patients present with acute intermittent abdominal pain with neurological and psychiatric symptoms that are mostly precipitated by drugs (P-450 inducers), progesterone, and dietary restrictions. Urine is red due to urinary porphobilinogen. Treatment is hemin or glucose.

34. What is the pathogenesis of glucose-6-phosphate dehydrogenase (G-6-PD)?

Lack of G-6-PD leads to the inability to form nicotinamide adenine dinucleotide phosphate, which is needed to form glutathione, an antioxidant of RBCs. The patient presents with hemolytic anemia after ingestion of drugs that precipitate RBC oxidation. Examples of such drugs are sulfa/nitrofurantoin and Primaquine (antimalaria). On RBC smear, bite cells are seen (Heinz bodies that have been phagocytosed). On laboratory tests, the LDH level is elevated and the haptoglobin level is low. Immediate evaluation may show normal RBCs because young RBCs are normal and are the only RBCs left (Figure 10-7).

Treatment: Discontinue drugs or precipitants.

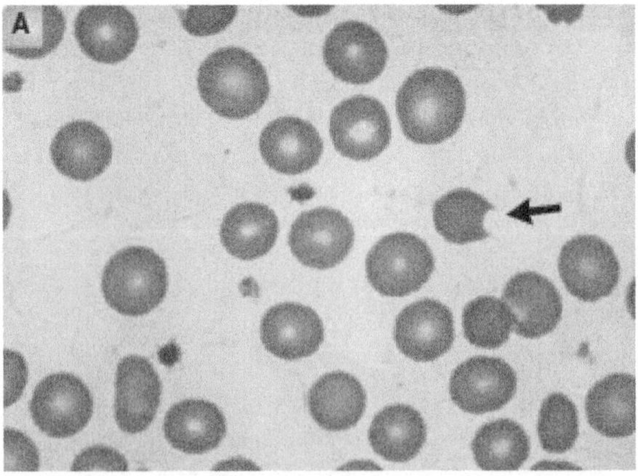

Figure 10-7. *Bite cell*

35. What is the pathogenesis of paroxysmal nocturnal hemoglobinuria?

Paroxysmal nocturnal hemoglobinuria is an RBC membrane defect, where hemolysis occurs at night, leading to presentation of dark urine in the morning. Laboratory tests show pancytopenia from hypocellular bone marrow. The RBC defect may lead to **venous thrombosis.**

36. List the key findings in a blood smear diagnosis.

- Schistocytes: Consider microangiopathic hemolytic anemia.
- Teardrop: Consider myelofibrosis.
- Howell-Jolly bodies: Consider splenectomy.
- Heinz bodies (bite cells): Consider G-6-PD disorder.
- Basophilic stippling (inclusion bodies characterized by multiple small purple granules inside RBCs): Consider sideroblastic anemia.
- Reticulocytes: Hemolytic anemia
- Hypersegmented polymorphonuclear neutrophils: Vitamin B12 and folate deficiency
- Target cells: Consider thalassemia and liver disease.

37. What are indications for a bone marrow biopsy?

- Pancytopenia
- Myelodysplasia
- Myelophthisis: The infiltration of bone marrow with cancer
- Leukemia/lymphoma

38. What is the treatment for uremia-associated anemia?

If the patient is actively bleeding, desmopressin (a vasopressin analogue) is recommended as immediate treatment. Why? It is thought that platelet dysfunction is caused by uremia-secreting, platelet-inhibiting factors. Long-term treatment is dialysis, which removes these platelet-inhibiting factors.

39. What is the pathogenesis of splenectomy?

Splenectomy can occur spontaneously due to splenic infarcts in sickle cell anemia or in a variety of settings. It can be indicated in various hematologic disorders.

The patient's peripheral blood smear will reveal Howell-Jolly bodies (nuclear remnant RBCs) and Heinz

The central pallor of a normal RBC should equal 1/3rd of its diameter.

Howell-Jolly body is a round, single, purple inclusion body to the side of a central pallor in a RBC.

Target lesion is a red dot in the center of a central pallor in a RBC.

How do patients with microangiopathic hemolytic anemia present?

bodies (precipitated hemoglobin). Pretreat with pneumococcal, meningococcal, and haemophilus vaccines. Treat immunocompromised patients with antibiotics against encapsulated organisms such as Streptococcus pneumoniae, Haemophilus influenzae, and Neisseria meningitidis.

40. List the causes of thrombocytopenia.

- Immune-mediated platelet destruction: **immune** thrombocytopenic purpura (ITP), TTP, and drugs (heparin-induced thrombocytopenia)
- Nonimmune destruction: DIC, HUS, vasculitis, vitamin B12, folate deficiency, viral infections, and other drugs (chemotherapy, alcohol)
- Inherited disorders of platelet production: Wiskott Aldrich and Bernard-Soulier syndromes.

41. What are the causes of microangiopathic hemolytic anemia?

Microangiopathic hemolytic anemia is caused by thrombocytopenic thrombotic purpura (TTP), hemolytic uremic syndrome (HUS), disseminated intravascular coagulopathy (DIC), and defective valves (aortic stenosis and other valvular defects).

The first step is to obtain a peripheral smear to check for schistocytes (fragmented RBCs). See Figure 10-4.

Most patients present with bleeding disorders and thrombocytopenia (low platelet count).

42. How do patients present with TTP?

The patient may present with thrombocytopenia, hemolysis, and encephalopathy.

Treatment is exchange transfusion (plasma-pheresis).

43. How do patients present with HUS?

The patient presents with thrombocytopenia, hemolysis, and kidney failure.

Treatment is plasmapheresis.

44. How do patients present with DIC?

The patient presents with thrombocytopenia, decreased fibrinogen, and decreased clotting factors. The patient can also present with diffuse bleeding from IV sites, skin, the gastrointestinal (GI) tract, and other organs. Laboratory tests may reveal a low serum fibrinogen level, but both prothrombin time (PT) and activated partial thromboplastin time (aPTT) are usually elevated. Common causes are sepsis, trauma and obstetric procedures, and malignancy.

Treatment is fresh frozen plasma (FFP) and rarely with heparin if there is thrombosis.

Never transfuse with platelets in patients who have ITP, TTP, HUS and DIC.

45. How do patients with valve defects (e.g., aortic stenosis) present with microangiopathic anemia?

The patient may present with signs and symptoms of anemia; the physical examination may reveal heart murmur and the peripheral smear will show schistocytes. See Figure 10-4.

46. What is the definition of immune thrombocytopenic purpura (ITP)?

Antibodies against platelets cause thrombocytopenia. A blood smear will show megakaryoblasts. The patient will present with nosebleeds and heavy menses, usually following a viral illness. The cause is unknown. ITP is associated with systemic lupus erythematosus, infection, and human immunodeficiency virus (HIV) (immunosuppressive diseases).

Treatment: Administer steroids. Why not plasmapheresis? This is not a microangiopathic hemolytic anemia.

Never transfuse with platelets in patients who have ITP, TTP, HUS, and DIC. Why? These conditions will cause further consumption of platelets.

If the platelet count is >30,000, ITP can self-resolve.

47. What is the definition of Wiskott-Aldrich syndrome?

Wiskott-Aldrich syndrome: X-linked recessive condition affecting actin filaments and hematopoietic cells, causing **eczema**, **immunodeficiency**, and **thrombocytopenia** (bleeding). There is a predisposition to malignancy.

48. What are platelet abnormalities that do not involve destruction of platelets?

- Leukemia (look for associated multiple lymph nodes and organomegaly)
- Infiltrative bone marrow disorders
- Myelodysplasia

49. How do patients present with hemorrhagic disease of the newborn?

The patient may present with ecchymosis due to lack of administration of vitamin K to neonates at birth.

Why does liver disease predispose an individual to hemorrhagic disorder?

50. How does liver disease predispose to hemorrhagic disorder?

Cirrhosis can predispose the patient to having vitamin K deficiency. Why? Coagulation factors are made in the liver with vitamin K. Always consider giving these patients vitamin K, even if they are asymptomatic.

51. What is the first step in the evaluation of clotting factor disorders?

The first step is to obtain a peripheral smear, PT, and aPTT.

52. What is the pathogenesis of von Willebrand disease?

Von Willebrand factor (VWF) attaches factor VIII to the endothelium. VWF is altered in this disease. The patient will present with easy bruising, skin bleeding, minor excessive bleeding (e.g., nosebleed) and prolonged bleeding in mucosal surfaces (e.g., after dental surgery). Sometimes, depending on the severity of the disease, the patient may present with joint hemarthrosis because of the qualitative defect in factor VIII.

Laboratory tests show that aPTT and bleeding time are increased. Treat with desmopressin. Why? It stimulates the release of VWF from endothelial cells.

53. What is the pathogenesis of hemophilia A?

Hemophilia A is an X-linked recessive disorder that causes factor VIII deficiency. The patient will present with hemarthrosis from birth. The bleeding can be spontaneous or occur with minor bruises depending on severity of the disease.

Treat with factor VIII.

54. What is the pathogenesis of warfarin toxicity?

PT is elevated. Warfarin inhibits vitamin K and causes bleeding.

Treatment: Oral or subcutaneous vitamin K. Fresh frozen plasma is given if urgent treatment is needed.

55. What is the pathogenesis of heparin toxicity?

aPTT is elevated. Heparin activates antithrombin III, which in turn inactivates thrombin and other clotting factors.

Treatment: Protamine sulfate

56. What are some complications of blood transfusions?

- ABO hemolytic reaction

- Febrile, nonhemolytic reaction
- Transfusion-related acute lung injury (TRALI)
- Volume overload
- Anaphylaxis (e.g., IGA deficiency)
- Iron overload
- Sepsis

57. What is the pathogenesis of heparin-induced thrombocytopenia?

Antibodies to heparin develop and activate platelets, and the tendency for thrombosis is increased.

Treatment: Stop heparin and treat with antithrombin.

58. Why does stored blood have low calcium?

The citrate that is used to store blood binds to calcium, which can lead to hypocalcemia. Stored blood also has low platelets, elevated CO2, elevated lactate (from citrate), and low pH.

59. What is the pathogenesis of hemolytic ABO incompatibility?

ABO incompatibility causes hemolysis due to preformed antibodies against RBCs. The patient presents with fever, hematuria, unconjugated **hyperbilirubinemia**, hypotension, and back pain after transfusion. Stop transfusion and perform an indirect Coombs test.

60. What is the pathogenesis of febrile reactions?

A rise in temperature occurs after a blood transfusion. Patients may present with fever, chills, and back pain due to preformed antibodies against white blood cells (WBCs). Prevent ABO febrile reaction by washing blood (deplete WBCs) prior to transfusion. Stop transfusion and obtain laboratory results of blood work to rule out an acute hemolytic reaction. Give antipyretics, steroids, or both.

What is the cause of febrile reactions of ABO incompatibility?

61. What is the pathogenesis of allergic reactions of rash (urticaria) in selective immunoglobulin A (IgA) deficiency?

Urticaria can occur after transfusion because of IgA antibodies in the recipient.

62. What is the most common hereditary hypercoagulability disorder?

Factor V Leiden mutation is the most common. Factor V is present but cannot be inactivated by anti-thrombin III.

VDRL may be falsely positive in patients with antiphospholipid syndrome.

63. What is the pathogenesis of antiphospholipid syndrome?

In antiphospholipid syndrome, aPTT is increased, but the tendency for thrombosis is increased. Look for multiple pregnancy loss and recurrent deep vein thrombosis in the patient's history.

The results of the Venereal Disease Research Laboratory (VDRL) test may be positive.

Treatment: Anticoagulants

64. What is the pathogenesis of polycythemia?

Polycythemia can be primary or secondary. Erythropoietin is usually low in most patients with **primary polycythemia**, also known as **polycythemia vera** (PCV). The patient may present with a ruddy skin complexion. Laboratory findings for primary polycythemia will show **elevation in all blood cell lines**, including elevated hemoglobin and hematocrit levels; elevated white blood cells, platelets, and leukocyte alkaline phosphatase levels; and the presence of hypercellularity and hyperplasia in erythroid, granulocytic, and megakaryocytic cell lines in bone marrow studies.

65. What may peripheral smear cytogenetics show in polycythemia vera?

Peripheral smear polymerase chain reaction reverse transcriptase may be positive for JAK2 mutations.

66. What are some causes of secondary polycythemia?

Secondary polycythemia is due to hypoxia (e.g., sleep apnea, chronic lung diseases, or any other cause of hypoxia for long periods) or ectopic production of erythropoietin (e.g., renal cell carcinoma and steroid use). In secondary polycythemia, the erythropoietin level is elevated.

67. What are some complications of hyperproliferative syndromes (e.g., polycythemia vera)?

Hyperviscosity syndrome (blood thickening) in the brain vessels and peripheral blood vessels can lead to headache, dizziness, peripheral neuropathy, and hypertension. **Venous and arterial thrombosis** and bleeding can also occur.

68. What are treatment options for PCV?

Current treatments for PCV are **phlebotomy and aspirin**. Hydroxyurea can be used if phlebotomy is refractory, cannot be tolerated, or thrombocytosis is very high.

69. What is the definition of myeloproliferative syndrome?

This syndrome involves proliferation of **myeloid cell lines** (erythrocytes, leukocytes, and platelets). **Polycythemia vera, essential thrombocytosis** (the most common myeloproliferative syndrome), myelofibrosis, and chronic myelogenous leukemia are all myeloproliferative syndromes.

70. How may hereditary telangiectasia (Osler-Weber-Rendu syndrome) produce polycythemia?

Arterial venous malformations in the lungs may lead to shunting from right to left, leading to hypoxemia and secondary polycythemia.

71. What is the definition of Waldenström macroglobulinemia?

Waldenström macroglobulinemia is a hyperviscosity syndrome and organomegaly caused by monoclonal hyper-IgM (elevated IgM level). Treatment is **plasma exchange for acute** management of symptoms and rituximab **and** fludarabine for Waldenström macroglobulinemia.

72. What is the pathogenesis of multiple myeloma?

Multiple myeloma produces monoclonal immunoglobulin, which is a hyperproliferation of one type of plasma cell in the bone marrow, especially the IgG type, leading to ineffective immunoglobulins. The patient will present predominantly with bone pain and infections. Patients may also present with **hypercalcemia**, **anemia**, **renal failure**, and **lytic bone lesions**.

73. What is the pathogenesis of leukemia?

In leukemia, abnormal hematopoietic cells in the bone marrow proliferate and spread to the peripheral blood organs (spleen, liver, and lymph nodes).

74. What is the pathogenesis of lymphoma?

In lymphoma, abnormal hematopoietic cells in the lymph nodes proliferate and spread to the peripheral blood cells and bone marrow.

75. How are types of leukemia/lymphoma evaluated?

Leukemia/lymphoma can be acute (fast growing) or chronic (slow growing). Acute leukemia/lymphoma patients may present with B symptoms (night sweats and

What is the difference between Waldenström macroglobulinemia and multiple myeloma?

What is the difference between EBV infection and leukemia?

What is the difference between lymphoma or leukemia and EBV mononucleosis?

weight loss). Chronic leukemia/lymphoma may present as bone pain or infection (fever, cough, and dyspnea).

The first step is to obtain a peripheral blood smear and a complete blood cell (CBC) count. **Why? To** look for **blast cells.** A serum **lactate dehydrogenase** level can also be obtained.

Definitive diagnosis: A bone marrow biopsy, CT scan, and PET scan are other studies used for staging.

76. What is prototypical slow-growing (indolent) lymphoma/leukemia?

Chronic lymphocytic leukemia (CLL)/small B-cell lymphocytic lymphoma, and follicular lymphoma are the most common examples.

77. What are the three classifications of lymphoid malignancies?

- B cell
- T cell/NK
- Hodgkin lymphoma

78. What is the prototypical aggressive lymphoma?

Diffuse large B-cell lymphoma is the most common example. Aggressive lymphoma has an excellent prognosis with combination chemotherapy. Autologous stem cell transplantation can be considered for younger patients.

79. What is seen in the evaluation of acute promyelocytic leukemia (APL)?

APL is a subset of acute myelocytic leukemia and most patients present with coagulopathy in the form of disseminated intravascular coagulopathy (DIC).

Why are there numerous blast cells in acute promyelocytic leukemia?

Why? There is an increased expression of a receptor for plasminogen and plasminogen activating factor on the surface of promyelocytic cells. Other laboratory tests may show Auer rods (blue rods in blast cells) and promyeloblast cells in the peripheral or bone marrow smear. The CBC count may show an elevated, normal, or reduced WBC count. The bone marrow biopsy sample may show >20% blast cells. Why? One mechanism is fusion of trans-retinoic acid via a balanced translocation between chromosome 17q21 and chromosome 15q22.

Treatment: DIC is an emergency. APL is treated with all trans-retinoic acid, which causes apoptosis.

80. How do patients with chronic myelogenous leukemia (CML) present?

The patient usually presents asymptomatically, an incidental finding of an elevated WBC count often being found during a routine checkup. Basophilia and an elevated alkaline phosphatase level may be seen.

On the boards, watch out for a patient presenting for a routine checkup who has an elevated WBC count, specifically a granulocyte count. Diagnosis is confirmed by **the presence of t(9;22), the Philadelphia chromosome,** a fusion tyrosine kinase, by PCR of the bone marrow aspirate.

Treatment is imatinib, a tyrosine kinase inhibitor that inhibits the aberrant fusion tyrosine kinase.

81. How do patients with acute lymphoblastic leukemia present (ALL)?

ALL presents in young children. ALL is a **highly aggressive** disease, usually involving the blood, bone marrow, and mediastinum and frequently metastasizing to the **testes** and CNS. Laboratory tests reveal blast cells in the peripheral smear, similar to acute myelogenous leukemia, which is present in adults. Treatment is a combination chemotherapy regimen.

82. How do patients with chronic lymphocytic leukemia present?

Chronic lymphocytic leukemia presents **insidiously**, similarly to CML. The patient usually presents for a routine checkup and routine blood work reveals **lymphocytosis**. Laboratory tests will show numerous matured lymphocytes and fragile lymphocytes (smudge cells). Immunologic findings include hemolytic anemia and immune **thrombocytopenia.** Peripheral flow cytometry analysis is diagnostic.

Treatment: Excision of the lymph node to confirm diagnosis and then chemotherapy

83. What is seen in a bone marrow smear in patients with hairy cell leukemia?

Spiny projections of lymphocytes, tartrate-resistant acid phosphatase-positive cells, are seen in the bone marrow smear (Figure 10-8).

Diagnosis: The bone marrow tap is dry because of fibrosis.

What malignancy is characteristic of smudge cells?

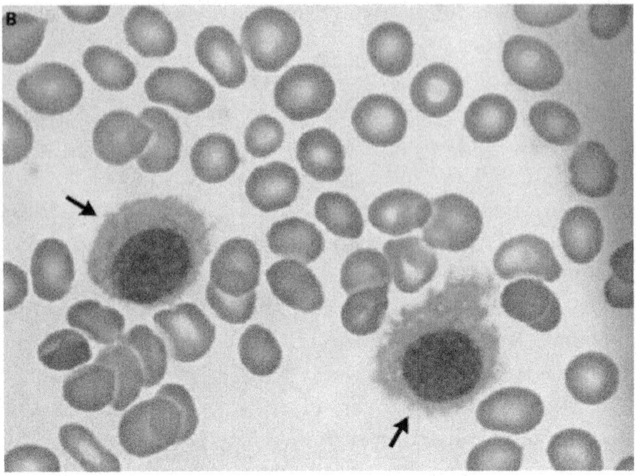

Figure 10-8. *Hairy Cell Leukemia lymphocytes with irregular projections (arrows)*

84. Human T-lymphotropic virus can be associated with leukemia, especially in the tropics. True or false?
True.

85. List some infectious causes of lymphoma.

- EBV
- HIV
- Human T-cell lymphotropic virus 1 (HTLV1)
- Human herpes 8 with HIV
- Hepatitis C
- *H. pylori*
- *Campylobacter jejuni*

86. What is the pathogenesis of Burkitt lymphoma?
This is an **aggressive lymphoma** associated with EBV, presenting with B symptoms. If the tumor is associated with EBV, the patient may present with a **tumor in the jaw if in Africa** or a **tumor in the GI tract** in developed Western nations.

What is the difference between Hodgkin and non-Hodgkin lymphoma?

87. What is the pathogenesis of Hodgkin lymphoma?
The tumor usually migrates through contiguous lymph nodes. Some types are associated with EBV. Children may present with cervical, supraclavicular, axilla, or inguinal **lymphadenopathy** or with a **mediastinal mass** on chest X-ray (CXR). Adults may present with lymphadenopathy or a mass on CXR. The presence of **Reed-Sternberg** cells (bilobed or multinucleated cell

nucleus) in a biopsy sample is pathognomonic.
Treatment: Combination chemotherapy

88. What is the pathogenesis of non-Hodgkin lymphoma?

This tumor easily migrates to the peripheral blood cells (noncontiguous spread); therefore, the patient can present with organomegaly in addition to adenopathy.

89. What is the current recommendation for screening of prostate cancer?

The USPTF recommends against screening in those who are 75 or older. The evidence is inconclusive in those that are younger.

90. How do patients with lymphoma generally present?

Patients with lymphoma generally present with single or multiple lymphadenopathy (painless, rubbery, nonmobile). The patient may also present with organomegaly (splenomegaly and hepatomegaly).

91. In any patient with suspicious cervical, supraclavicular, axillary, or inguinal adenopathy, the first step is to obtain a CXR. True or false?

True. Why? A CXR will help rule out mediastinal lymphadenopathy.

Diagnosis: Obtain a peripheral smear first and then a CBC count to rule out lymphoma. Other routine laboratory results that suggest lymphoma or leukemia are elevated lactate dehydrogenase (LDH) and hypercalcemia with suppressed parathyroid hormone.

The definitive diagnosis is to excise lesions for examination. A CT scan of the thorax, abdomen, and pelvis can be used to determine the extent of disease.

Most children with Hodgkin lymphoma have a mediastinal mass.

92. How do patients with prostate cancer present?

A patient usually presents with an elevated prostate-specific antigen (PSA) level (asymptomatically). The normal PSA level is 0.4-4 µg/dl. Prostate cancer is the second most common cause of cancer death in men. It is the number one type of cancer in men.

A definitive diagnosis is made with a transrectal biopsy of the prostate.

93. What are the risk factors for prostate cancer?

The risk factors are age >40 years, African American race, family history, and a high-fat diet.

94. Diagnosis of prostate cancer is usually via prostate screening showing an elevated PSA. True or false?

True. A **definitive diagnosis** is made with a transrectal biopsy of the prostate.

95. What are the management options for prostate cancer?

Surgery is done using an anterior abdominal approach with a nerve-sparing prostate removal technique, or, alternatively, with radiation.

Androgen deprivation therapy is the mainstay for metastatic disease. Active surveillance may be considered for patients with early-stage disease, a low PSA level, and a low Gleason score.

96. List some complications of treatment of prostate cancer.

The most common complications are erectile dysfunction and urinary incontinence; others are proctitis and diarrhea.

Prognosis depends on the stage of the cancer; an early-stage (tumor localized) Gleason score of 1-6 has a 15-year survival rate of >90%.

97. When is a reflex nuclear bone scan done in patients with prostate cancer?

A reflex bone scan is done in patients with a higher risk of metastasis such as when a Gleason score is ≥7 and a PSA level is ≥10 ng/ml. Why? The probability of metastasis is high.

98. What are the risk factors for cervical cancer?

Know the risk and protective factors for cervical cancer.

The risk factors include human papillomavirus (HPV)-11 and HPV-16, smoking, multiple sexual partners, and initial sexual intercourse at a young age.

The patient may present asymptomatically or with post-coital bleed.

Treatment: This varies depending on the stage. The options are conization, hysterectomy, radiation, and chemotherapy.

Prevention is the best cure via a Pap smear screen.

99. If a patient's Pap smear report is atypical squamous cells of undetermined significance (ASCUS) and a low-grade squamous intraepithelial lesion, what is the next step in screening?

Order an HPV test or do a follow-up in 4-6 months. If

HPV is absent or the follow-up Pap smear is normal, then do a yearly follow-up (Figure 10-9).

However, if HPV is present, or follow-up remains abnormal then perform a colposcopy.

Treat atypical areas with a loop electrocautery/electrosurgical excision procedure or cone biopsy.

Understand the workup for ASCUS and other cervical lesions.

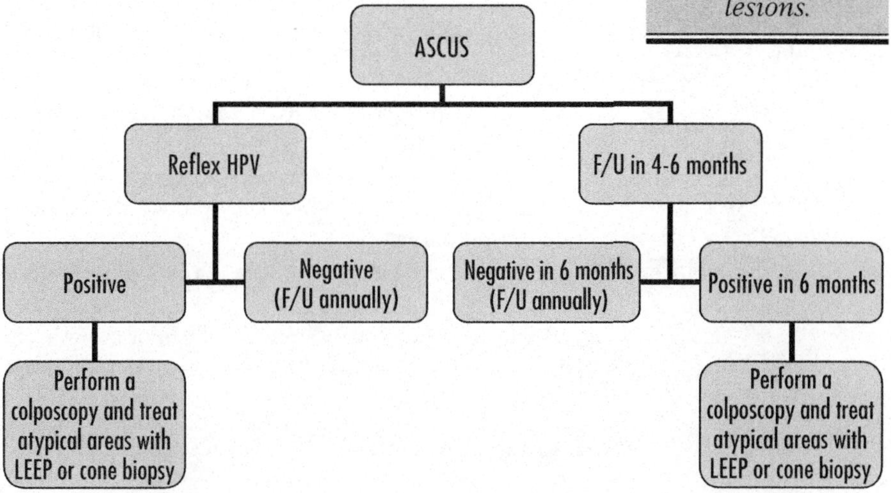

Figure 10-9. *Screening for cervical cancer with a Pap smear. ASCUS, atypical squamous cells of undetermined significance; F/U, follow up; HPV, human papillomavirus; LEEP, loop electrocautery/electrosurgical excision procedure.*

100. If a patient's report is atypical squamous cell-high grade, high-grade squamous intraepithelial lesion, what is the next step?

Go straight to colposcopy. Why? The cells are more likely to progress to cancer.

101. What are the risk factors for endometrial cancer?

The risk factors are related to estrogen exposure: obesity, ovarian cancer (granulose-theca), tamoxifen use, nulligravida, and atypical endometrial hyperplasia.

Factors that reduce the risk of endometrial cancer are related to decreased estrogen exposure: oral contraceptives and multiple pregnancies.

The patient may present with postmenopausal bleed. The first step would be to perform an endometrial biopsy or dilation and curettage.

Treatment is total abdominal hysterectomy with salpingo-oophorectomy.

102. What is the association between diethylstilbestrol (DES) and female offspring?

DES is a synthetic estrogen that was prescribed during 1938-1971 in pregnant women to prevent miscarriages and abnormal births. It was discontinued in 1971 because research indicated that it does not prevent miscarriages or abnormal births, but causes rare vaginal cancer in young girls and women who are exposed in the womb.

103. What are the risk factors for ovarian cancer?

Why are oral contraceptives protective against ovarian cancer and endometrial cancer?

The risk factors are the **BRCA** gene, a family history, and a high-fat diet.

Factors that reduce risks: oral contraceptives and multiple pregnancies. Why? They reduce the stimulation of the ovaries.

Epithelial cell ovarian cancer is the most common type.

Because of the slow progression of tumor growth, the patient usually presents at a late stage with abdominal pain and swelling.

104. List the key findings in ovarian/testicular cancer.

What is Meigs syndrome?

- Germ cell cancer: The types are choriocarcinoma, dysgerminoma (ovarian), embryonal carcinoma (testicular and ovarian), seminoma (testicular), teratoma (testicular and ovarian), and yolk sac (testicular and ovarian).
- Choriocarcinoma: An elevated serum beta human chorionic gonadotropin **(HCG) level** can provide evidence for diagnosis.
- Dysgerminoma: An elevated serum lactate dehydrogenase (LDH) test result can provide evidence for diagnosis.
- Seminoma: Elevated serum **beta HCG** and LDH levels can provide evidence for diagnosis.
- Yolk sac: An elevated serum **alpha fetoprotein** level can provide evidence for diagnosis.
- Embryonal: An elevated serum beta HCG level and, less often, alpha fetoprotein test result can provide evidence for diagnosis.
- Sex cord stroma cancer: Examples are granulosa-theca and Sertoli-Leydig cell tumors.
- Ovarian fibroma: This causes fibrosis of the ovaries. It can lead to ascites and hydrothorax (Meigs syndrome).

105. What are the management options for ovarian cancer?

Diagnosis is confirmed by laparotomy and debulking surgery that includes the ovaries, fallopian tube, omentum, part of the bowel, and appendix. Patients with a higher staged malignancy should also receive chemotherapy (platinum based).

106. What screening interval is recommended for those at high risk for ovarian cancer (BRCA gene)?

Obtain a CA-125 level and transvaginal ultrasound every 6-12 months at the age of 35, or 5-10 years younger than a family member with the earliest age of diagnosis.

107. What are possible treatment options for those with the BRCA gene and a family history of ovarian cancer?

A bilateral salpingo-oophorectomy before the age of 40 is recommended for those with a family history of ovarian cancer, especially BRCA gene carriers. This also reduces the risk of breast cancer in this patient population.

108. What is the initial evaluation of patients with breast pain (mastalgia)?

Find out whether pain is associated with menses and is bilateral or unilateral. If the patient is older than 30 years and the pain is unilateral, a mammogram should be obtained. If the patient is younger, pain is bilateral, and it is associated with menses, a sports bra or NSAIDs with reassurance should be offered.

109. How do patients with breast cancer present?

Patients usually present with an asymptomatic breast mass. Breast cancer is the most common type of cancer in women. It is the second most common type of cancer causing death in women.

The risk factors include age ≥40 years, a family history, the BRCA gene, and hormonal factors.

110. What is the most common factor that reduces the risk of breast cancer?

Use of tamoxifen is the most common factor.

111. What types of imaging are used to diagnose breast lesions?

At age ≥30 years, patients need to have a mammogram; those <30 years who are pregnant and have focal breast lesions need to have an ultrasound. Why? Young patients

Patients with BRCA gene should discuss either screening with serological tests and ultrasound or chose therapeutic intervention such as tamoxifen or invasive surgical procedures to prevent breast or ovarian cancer.

Eczematous, scaly rash with chronic ulcerations that begins in the nipple area and spreads to the areola is the hallmark of Paget disease of the breast.

Paget disease of the breast in most cases is associated with with underlying breast cancer (in situ and /or invasive).

have highly dense breast tissue. A definitive diagnosis is excision.

112. What do erythema, edema, and thickening of the skin of the breast in relatively younger patients with breast cancer suggest?

These suggest inflammatory breast cancer. If this occurs in older women, Paget disease of the breast should be considered.

113. What are the treatment options for breast cancer?

Treatment options depend on the stage of cancer. If it is an early stage (tumor <2 cm and/or no lymph node metastasis), treat with lumpectomy and postoperative radiation. Make sure you add adjuvant therapy for pre- and postmenopausal patients with a node-positive tumor and a HER oncogene-positive tumor. Why? These patients have a poor prognosis. HER-positive tumors can be treated with the **anti-HER antibody, trastuzumab**.

Give a selective estrogen receptor modulator (tamoxifen) or aromatase inhibitor (anastrozole) to patients with an estrogen-receptor-positive mass. Tamoxifen can cause thromboembolism and endometrial cancer, whereas aromatase inhibitors do not. However, like tamoxifen, anastrozole can cause osteoporosis and postmenopausal symptoms. Why? This is because tamoxifen is a partial estrogen agonist and anastrozole completely inhibits the conversion of androgen to estrogen.

114. What are known breast surgery complications?

Complications include injury to the C5-C7 nerves (anterior serratus muscle) and the long-thoracic nerve. The patient will present with a winged scapula. Lymphedema and lymphangiosarcoma are also known complications.

115. What is the recommendation for prophylactic treatment in those with the BRCA gene to prevent breast cancer?

Prophylactic treatment is a bilateral mastectomy and salpingo- oophorectomy.

116. How do patients present with fibrocystic changes?

The patient presents with breast pain that is worse during menses. On the physical examination, multiple nodular breast lesions are present. If the patient is ≥30 years old, a mammogram is needed to rule out cancer; if the patient is <30 years old, an ultrasound is adequate.

Treatment: Use of a sports bra and analgesics.

117. How do patients present with fibroadenoma?

The patient presents with a breast mass that is rubbery and mobile on examination.

Diagnosis: Ultrasound for patients who are <30 years old and a mammogram for those who are ≥30 years old.

Treatment: Follow up for enlargement of the mass; if it is 3-5 cm in size, excise it. Why? It can mimic phyllodes cystosarcoma, which can be malignant.

118. How do patients present with intraductal papilloma?

The patient presents with bloody discharge from the nipple; it is usually unilateral but it can be bilateral. Send the discharge for cytological examination to rule out papillary carcinoma.

119. What is the evaluation of a breast cyst?

A breast cyst is identified on an ultrasound.

Treatment: Fine-needle aspiration. If bloody contents are aspirated, send them for cytological examination. If clear fluid is aspirated, follow up in 3 months. If a solid cyst is present in 3 months, an excisional biopsy is required (Figure 10-10).

What is phyllodes cystosarcoma?

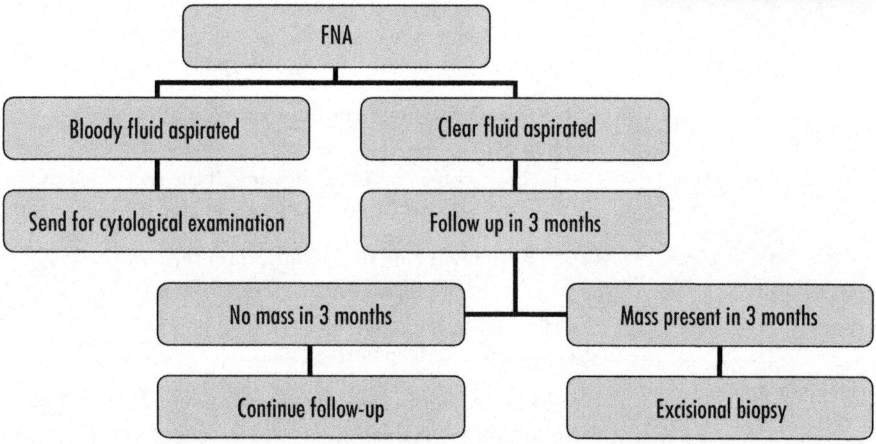

Figure 10-10. *Breast cyst evaluation. FNA, fine-needle aspiration.*

Why does left-sided colon cancer present with constipation?

120. What are the risk factors for esophageal cancer?

The risk factors are smoking, Barrett esophagus, and tylosis (an autosomal dominant condition that causes thickening of palms and soles). The patient may present with dysphagia to solids and then liquids and weight loss.

Diagnosis: Endoscopy (esophageal gastroduodenoscopy) can be used to diagnose esophageal cancer.

121. What are the risk factors for colon cancer?

The risk factors are adenomatous polyps, family history (Gardner syndrome, familial adenomatous polyposis syndrome, hereditary nonpolyposis cancer, a first-degree relative with colon cancer or an adenomatous polyp), ulcerative colitis, age ≥50, smoking, obesity, and other types of cancers such as ovarian, endometrial, and breast cancers. It is the third most common cancer in the United States.

122. What are the types of polyps?

Adenomatous polyps are preneoplastic lesions. Different types exist with varying preneoplastic predispositions. Villous adenoma polyps are much more preneoplastic than tubulous adenomas, which are more preneoplastic than tubulovillous adenomas.

123. What is the difference between left- and right-sided colon cancer?

Left-sided colon cancer will usually present as constipation (solid contents are absorbed there, and it is smaller than the left colon) or diarrhea, whereas right-sided colon cancer usually presents as an occult rectal bleed or iron-deficiency anemia in a man. HNPCC-associated cancer is more common on the **right side**.

124. What is the most common site of colon cancer metastasis?

The most common site is the **lung**, if the rectum is the site of cancer. Why? The inferior vena cava drains this site.

125. There is no role for radiation therapy in the management of colon cancer. True or false?

True. After surgical resection, adjuvant chemotherapy is used for node-positive disease.

126. What screening interval is recommended for those with hereditary syndromes of colon cancer (HNPC or FAPS)?

Start screening at age 25, or 5-10 years younger than

the earliest age of diagnosis in a family member, with colonoscopy every 1-2 years.

127. Which malignancy presents with jaundice, weight loss, and abdominal pain?

Biliary tract cancers such as cholangiocarcinoma, and head of pancreas tumors present this way. They may also present with other cholestasis signs such as dark urine, pruritus, and white stools.

128. What are the risk factors for hepatic adenoma?

The risk factors are being female and taking estrogen contraceptive pills. Hepatic adenoma can rupture and cause shock. The mass can increase during pregnancy.

Diagnosis: A CT scan confirms the diagnosis.

Treatment: Resection to prevent rupture

129. What are the risk factors for hepatocellular cancer?

The risk factors are cirrhosis or chronic liver disease from hepatitis B or C, hemochromatosis, or chronic alcohol abuse. A markedly elevated **serum alpha fetoprotein** level in a cirrhotic liver is diagnostic.

The treatment is a liver transplant.

130. What are some treatment options for hepatocellular cancer?

A **liver transplant** is the mainstay of therapy, or, if the patient is not a surgical candidate, embolization with alcohol injection/radiofrequency **ablation**.

131. What are the most common tumors to metastasize to the CNS?

The most common are lung, breast, and melanoma.

132. What is the definition of multiple endocrine neoplasia (MEN)?

What are the three Ps?

Type 1 is defined by the three Ps: Pancreatic islet tumor (gastrinoma), pituitary tumor, and hyperparathyroidism. The patient may present with a gastric ulcer in abnormal locations (e.g., jejunum) and hypercalcemia.

133. What are the clinical features of gastrinomas?

Clinical features include **multiple ulcers** in unusual locations (esophagus, jejunum). The serum gastrin level is usually >150-200 pg/ml.

134. What is the definition of type 2a MEN?

Type 2a is medullary carcinoma, hyperparathyroidism,

and pheochromocytoma. The serum calcitonin level may be elevated in medullary carcinoma. MEN 2a is associated with the RET proto-oncogene. Always remove pheochromocytoma before thyroidectomy in MEN syndrome.

Which MEN syndrome presents with marfanoid habitus?

135. Depression, dermatitis, diabetes, and DVT suggest what endocrine malignancy?

They suggest the 4Ds of glucagonoma.

136. A syndrome causing watery diarrhea, hypokalemia, and achlorhydria suggests what endocrine tumor?

This suggests VIPoma.

137. What is the definition of type 2b MEN?

Type 2b is ganglioneuroma, medullary carcinoma, and pheochromocytoma. The patient presents with marfanoid habitus. MEN 2b is associated with the RET proto-oncogene.

138. What are the complications of chemotherapy?

- Nausea and vomiting. Treatment: Administer a serotonin antagonist (ondansetron) and encourage ingestion of small, frequent meals.
- Bone marrow deficiency: The patient may present with fever only. Laboratory tests reveal neutropenia. Treatment: Granulocyte colony-stimulating factors (GCSFs) and antibiotics (e.g., cefepime) against gram-negative rods (Pseudomonas) can be considered if the patient is neutropenic and febrile.

139. List the common chemotherapy or radiation agents and attendant toxicities.

- Chemotherapy agent toxicity: Bleomycin (**pulmonary toxicity**); cisplatin (**ototoxicity, nephrotoxicity**); anthracycline such as doxorubicin (**cardiac toxicity**, dyspigmentation); cyclophosphamide (**hemorrhagic cystitis**, bladder cancer, pulmonary toxicities)
- Chest/head and neck radiation therapy: Susceptible to **solid cancers** such as breast and thyroid cancer, respectively
- Infertility due to radiation or chemotherapy regimen.
- Coronary artery disease due to radiation.

140. What is the definition of a paraneoplastic syndrome?

A paraneoplastic syndrome is a cancer syndrome that presents at different sites in the body mediated by secretions of the tumor or immune response against the tumor. A paraneoplastic syndrome can be classified into neurological, hematologic, or endocrine categories.

141. How do patients with a neurological paraneoplastic syndrome present?

Excess adrenocorticotropic hormone (ACTH) can cause Cushing syndrome, anticholinergic antibodies can cause myasthenia gravis, and anti-calcium voltage-gated antibodies can cause Lambert-Eaton myasthenic syndrome. **Lambert-Eaton myasthenic syndrome** presents as **proximal muscle weakness** with **autonomic symptoms** (dry eyes, dry mouth, and erectile dysfunction) and **absent deep tendon reflexes**. Electromyography (EMG) will show **improvement of weakness with muscle activity**.

142. How do patients with hematologic paraneoplastic syndrome present?

Hematologic paraneoplastic syndrome can manifest as coagulopathy leading to migratory thrombophlebitis (Trousseau syndrome), which is a superficial vein inflammation. On the physical examination, a cord of vessels may be felt.

What is migratory thrombophlebitis?

143. How do patients with endocrinologic paraneoplastic syndrome present?

Endocrinologic paraneoplastic syndrome can occur when parathyroid-related immunoglobulin leads to hypercalcemia.

144. What are the most common cancers that cause these syndromes on the Step 2?

- Small cell cancer: Excess ACTH and antidiuretic hormone (ADH) lead to Cushing syndrome and syndrome of inappropriate ADH, respectively. **Sensory neuropathy** can occur with small cell cancer.
- Thymoma: Anticholinergic antibodies lead to myasthenia gravis.
- Pancreatic cancer: Migratory thromboemboli lead to Trousseau syndrome.

DIC can be a prominent feature in patients with acute promyelocytic leukemia.

- Squamous cell cancer of the lung: Parathyroid-related immunoglobulin leads to hypercalcemia.
- Leukemia: Disseminated intravascular coagulopathy (DIC) can occur here.

Chapter 11
Musculoskeletal System

1. Pain over the SI joint is strongly suggestive of what?
It suggests spondyloarthropathies (Reiter syndrome, psoriatic arthritis, ankylosing spondylitis)

2. Pain over the greater trochanter by hip adduction should alert you to think of what pathological hip condition?
Consider greater trochanter bursitis.

3. Pain in the groin area, buttocks, or anterior thigh or knee should alert you to think of what pathological hip condition?
Consider hip osteoarthritis. A radiograph may show joint-space narrowing, osteophytes, and sclerotic changes.

4. What is a cause of anterior lateral thigh pain?
Meralgia paresthetica can cause anterior **lateral thigh (outer thigh) pain** that is characteristically burning in quality with paresthesia (numbness and tingling) and dysesthesia (diminished sensation). Compression of the **lateral femoral cutaneous nerve** as it courses under the inguinal ligament is the cause. It is common in patients with diabetes, who have obesity, and who are >50 years old. Tight belts or garments around the waist can also cause it. It is a self-limited condition.

The most frequently associated factors in meralgia paresthetica are diabetes, obesity and older age.

5. Nontraumatic hip pain in a patient with steroid use or a history of sickle cell disease, alcohol abuse, or gout should alert you to think of what pathological hip condition?
Consider hip osteonecrosis (avascular necrosis). Legg-Calve-Perthes disease and Gaucher disease are other

Anterior knee pain upon extension of the knee in a seated position suggests patellofemoral syndrome.

Patellofemoral pain syndrome is the most common cause of anterior knee pain, and it worsens with squatting, running, and when ascending and descending steps.

A valgus stress causes an MCL injury, while a varus stress causes a lateral collateral ligament injury.

Knee hyper-extension causes an ACL injury.

causes of hip avascular necrosis, but typically occur in the pediatric population.

6. **What is the differential diagnosis of anterior knee pain?**
   Consider patellar or bursa (which surrounds the patella) problems. If pain is deep and nonlocalized, suspect **osteoarthritis**. Other causes of anterior knee pain that is localized are gout, ACL/PCL injuries, and meniscal tears.

7. **What is the significance of Baker's cyst?**
   A Baker's cyst is caused by synovial fluid collection in the posterior knee due to osteoarthritis that has caused chronic meniscal tears.

8. **What kind of knee injury would cause a medial collateral ligament (MCL) tear?**
   An MCL tear occurs when the foot is planted with force against the lateral aspect of the knee.

9. **What kind of knee injury causes an anterior cruciate ligament (ACL) tear?**
   An ACL tear develops occurs when there is a **twisting injury** that causes medial rotation of the knee with the foot planted.

10. **What kind of knee injury causes a meniscal tear?**
    A meniscal tear occurs when a **twisting injury** of the knee elicits a **popping or tearing sound** while the foot is planted.

11. **What causes an "unhappy triad" injury?**
    This is caused by a **twisting knee injury** with force against the lateral aspect of the foot while it is planted while an individual is trying to change position. It consists of an **ACL**, an **MCL**, and a **medial meniscus injury**.

12. **What is the most sensitive test for ACL rupture?**
    The most sensitive is the **Lachman test**, in which laxity is felt while bringing the tibia anteriorly over the femur. The anterior drawer test and pivot test are other tests used to diagnose ACL injuries.

13. **What kind of knee injury causes a posterior cruciate ligament tear?**
    This is caused by a direct blow to the tibia when the knee is flexed (e.g., baseball player sliding into a catcher).

14. **What is the most common ankle injury?**
    The most common is a **lateral ankle ligament injury** (ankle sprain) due to **inversion** of the ankle joint. Patients

may present with pain and swelling of the ankle joint. Treatment is external support with an ankle brace and early mobilization. The mnemonic for treatment is PRICE: protect, rest, ice, compress, and elevate.

15. What is the differential diagnosis of heel pain?

The most common diagnosis is **plantar fasciitis**: pain with initiation of movement, especially in the morning. Others are compression syndromes (tarsal tunnel syndrome), calcaneal stress fractures (associated with repetitive exercise, e.g., running), and peripheral neuropathy.

16. What is the differential diagnosis of Achilles pain?

Consider Achilles **bursitis or tendonitis**: pain associated with poorly fitting shoes and repetitive exercise (e.g., running/jumping), respectively.

17. Great toe extension weakness is suggestive of what nerve root abnormality?

It is suggestive of an **L5 nerve root** abnormality.

18. Hyporeflexia of the patellar is associated with what nerve root abnormality?

It is suggestive of an **L4** abnormality. The mnemonic is "on all 4s."

19. Hyporeflexia of the upper extremity suggests what nerve root abnormality?

It suggests **C6 or C7** nerve root involvement. In addition, paresthesias in **the thumb** suggests C6 involvement, whereas **lateral arm** and pinky paresthesias suggests **C8** involvement.

20. A history of multiple sites of pain in the neck, chest, back, elbow, thigh, and knee with concomitant depression suggests what musculoskeletal syndrome?

This suggests **fibromyalgia**, which is a clinical diagnosis of exclusion. Be sure to rule out other causes such as depression, as well as conditions involving generalized pain such as thyroid disease, myopathies, and polymyalgia rheumatic.

21. Lateral shoulder pain worsened by reaching or raising the arm above the head suggests what pathological shoulder condition?

It suggests a **rotator cuff tear or tendonitis**; a rotator cuff tear is more suggestive if there is shoulder weakness and a positive drop-arm test with abduction.

Acute swelling (hemarthrosis) is usually present in ACL and unhappy triad injuries.

Delayed knee swelling after an injury to the knee suggests meniscal tears.

Knee locking suggests chronic meniscal tears from OA, while the feeling of giving away suggests ligamentous injury.

Positive drop arm test suggests rotator cuff injury.

A decrease in shoulder ROM due to stiffness suggests adhesive capsulitis (frozen shoulder).

22. Anterior shoulder pain worsened by lifting or raising the arm above the head suggests what pathological shoulder condition?

It suggests **bicipital tendonitis**. On palpation, there is bicipital groove tenderness; if a lump is felt in the antecubital fossa, bicipital rupture should be suspected.

23. A progressive decrease in range of motion in the shoulder joint suggests what pathological shoulder condition?

It suggests **adhesive capsulitis**. A decrease in range of motion is usually due to stiffness rather than pain on the physical examination.

24. List the differential diagnosis of anterior shoulder pain.

- Acromioclavicular syndromes: due to overuse, trauma
- Glenohumeral arthritis: usually chronic, associated with crepitations

25. What are the rotator cuff muscles?

SITS: supraspinatus, infraspinatus, teres minor, subscapular

26. How may patients present with tennis elbow?

Patients present with **lateral epicondyle pain** due to repetitive use of the elbow by pronation.

Treatment is NSAIDs and immobilization in a sling.

27. How may patients present with "trigger finger (stenosing flexor tenosynovitis)"?

Patients present with an **extensor tendon sheath** nodule or granuloma after repeated trauma to the tendon sheath, usually involving the finger, especially the thumb. Patients may report **pain** and **snapping** of the finger when it is flexed, and they may awaken with the **finger locked in the palm**. Treatment is splinting and steroid injection.

28. Wrist pain radiating to the thumb and index finger suggests what pathological wrist condition?

It suggests carpel tunnel syndrome (**median nerve entrapment**) due to repetitive wrist motion. Treat with a splint and pain control; steroid injection and surgery are last resorts. Make sure to differentiate from de Quervain's tenosynovitis, tendonitis of hand and wrist causing pain in radial side of wrist that radiates to the thumb. It is associated with repetitive use of the thumb, and it is seen commonly in women between 30-50 years of age.

de Quervain's tenosynovitis is associated with repetitive use of the thumb.

Chapter 12
Dermatology

1. What is the definition of actinic keratosis?

Actinic keratosis is a premalignant skin lesion. The patient usually presents with rough, dry lesions, which can become raised, on areas of the body such as the arms, legs, face, and head that are exposed to ultraviolet (UV) rays.

2. What do multiple red papules found on the penile shaft of young men suggest?

They suggest bowenoid papulosis, which is a benign lesion thought to be caused by HPV but which histologically resembles carcinoma in situ. It can also progress to invasive squamous cell cancer.

3. What are the risk factors for cutaneous squamous cell cancer (SCC)?

Risk factors are UV radiation, actinic keratosis, chronic osteomyelitis, burn scars, xeroderma pigmentosum, chemical agents (arsenic), organ transplant, and albinism. The patient will also present with rough, scaly material on sun-exposed skin areas.

4. How do patients present with keratoacanthoma?

The patient presents with a red, nodular lesion with a central crater that is keratin filled on sun-exposed areas. This is not a premalignant lesion, but needs to be differentiated from SCC. Rapid growth within weeks favors a diagnosis of keratoacanthoma over SCC.

SCC can be prevented with protective clothing or by using sunscreen ½ hour prior to going out in the sun.

5. What is the treatment for SCC?

The most frequently used treatment of low- and high-risk

SCC is surgical excision within a 1-cm margin of normal tissue. **Shave biopsy** can be used for diagnosis of SCC.

Prevention of all skin cancers: Wear protective clothing (e.g., long sleeves) or wear sunscreen lotion 30 minutes prior to going out in the sun.

6. How do patients with basal cell carcinoma present?

Patients are blue-eyed, blond-haired individuals with chronic burn scars or sunburns. The patient presents with a pearly, raised lesion **and telangiectasia** with an ulcerated center commonly found on the nose or inner canthi. It has low metastatic potential.

Treatment: A **shave biopsy** is preferred for diagnosis. Surgical excision, within 4-mm surgical margins, is frequently used for both high- and low-risk BCC.

7. What is the significance of the sign of Leser-Trélat (sudden appearance of multiple seborrheic keratoses)?

It is associated with a variety of malignancies, including gastrointestinal and lung cancers. Seborrheic keratoses are benign lesions with a "stuck on" warty appearance that are hyperpigmented. They can occur with skin tags and acanthosis nigricans.

Why is melanoma treated aggressively?

8. How do patients with melanoma present?

The risk factors are UV radiation exposure, a significant number of nevi, and dysplastic nevi. The patient presents with lesions with asymmetric borders in a variety of colors, with an enlarging diameter. Melanoma easily metastasizes. A **punch biopsy** is preferred for diagnosis because the depth is prognostic.

Treatment: Excision is based on the size of the lesion. If the lesion is >1 mm, excise within a 2-cm margin of skin.

What is the difference between Kaposi sarcoma in immunocompromised and immunocompetent individuals?

9. What is the pathogenesis of Kaposi sarcoma?

Kaposi sarcoma develops by fibroblastic angiogenesis. It is caused by human herpesvirus 8. A major risk factor is HIV. Those with AIDS have lesions on the GI mucosa, the skin, or the lungs, whereas those without AIDS (Jewish men) have lesions on the extremities.

10. Pruritus can be a manifestation of systemic disease. How should pruritus be evaluated?

The most common causes of pruritus are **xerosis** (dry skin) and **atopic eczema**. An evaluation for cholestasis, HIV, uremia, thyroid disease, diabetes, iron-deficiency anemia, polycythemia vera, lymphoma, and malignancy should be done if the history is suggestive.

11. What is the most common specific dermatosis of pregnancy?

The most common is pruritic urticarial papules and plaques of pregnancy (PUPP). It is characterized by erythematous papules within striae, and the most common location is the **periumbilical area** where striae have developed. It may spread to the extremities, but usually spares the face, palms, and soles. Patients present with **extreme itching during the third trimester of pregnancy**. Treatment is topical steroids.

12. What is a mnemonic for causes of eosinophilia?

The mnemonic is NAACP: neoplasm, allergy/asthma; Addison disease; collagen vascular disease, parasites.

13. Atopic dermatitis is associated with what other types of diseases?

Atopic dermatitis can be associated with asthma and hay fever.

14. Allergic contact dermatitis is a type I hypersensitivity. True or false?

False. It is a type IV hypersensitivity reaction that occurs on re-exposure to an antigen that causes a skin reaction 12-48 hours later. An example is re-exposure to the plant resin found in poison ivy, causing vesicles to develop on the skin 12-48 hours later. High-potency topical steroids can be used as treatment, or oral steroids for severe cases. This should be differentiated from irritant contact dermatitis, due to physical, mechanical or chemical irritation of the skin, such as xerosis or diaper rash in children.

What is the difference between type I and type IV hypersensitivity reactions?

15. If a young male adult who is physically active and muscular presents with acne, what cause should be considered?

Anabolic steroid use should be suspected. In women, PCOS, ovarian/adrenal tumors, and Cushing disease should be part of the differential diagnosis.

16. List some papulosquamous skin lesions.

These skin disorders are usually described as "**red and scaly**":

- Pityriasis versicolor (also called tinea versicolor)
- Pityriasis rosea

Oral lichen planus may be associated with an increased risk of oral cancer.

- Seborrheic dermatitis
- Rosacea
- Lichen planus
- Psoriasis

17. What are the defining characteristics of acne rosacea?
This may present as red, flushing, dilated blood vessels (**telangiectasia**) occurring on the face, which is worsened by heat, sunlight, and alcohol ingestion. Treat with topical metronidazole and azelaic acid cream, or oral antibiotics for severe cases.

18. What are the defining characteristics of lichen planus?
Lichen planus presents as **violaceous polygonal, flat-topped papules** and **plaques**, causing pruritus, which commonly occurs on the wrist (4P's: polygonal, pruritic, papules, and plaques). Oral lesions can be associated with oral cancer. Treatment is retinoids or topical steroids.

19. Reactivation of herpes virus from dorsal rot ganglion causes what skin lesions?
This is known as **herpes zoster**, presenting earlier in life as chicken pox. It causes **erythematous rash** leading to vesicles that occurs in a dermatomal pattern, along with pain. It is usually **unilateral** and does not cross the midline. Treatment is acyclovir within 72 hours.

20. What is the significance of herpes zoster lesions on the eyelid, eye, or forehead?
This suggests infection that involves the **ophthalmic branch** of cranial nerve V ((herpes ophthalmicus).

21. What is Hutchison's sign in reaction to herpes zoster in the setting of herpes ophthalmicus?
Vesicles occurring on the side or **tip of the nose** in the setting of herpes ophthalmicus suggest **nasociliary branch** nerve involvement of the fifth nerve.

22. What is Ramsay Hunt syndrome?
This is a herpes infection of the **ear** that involves several cranial nerves, leading to the development of **vesicles in the ear**, pain, and facial paralysis.

23. What is the approach to postherpetic neuralgia?
This is pain acquired after herpes zoster infection; treat with tricyclic antidepressants such as amitriptyline, or anticonvulsants such as gabapentin.

24. How may patients present with tinea (superficial fungal infections)?

- Skin: **Well-demarcated** border of inflammation; KOH scraping confirms the diagnosis with the presence of hyphae. **Tinea cruris** occurs on the groin; **tinea corporis** on the face, trunk, and extremities.
- Hair: **Tinea barbae**, usually associated with folliculitis and pseudofolliculitis (ingrown hair)
- Nails: **Onychomycosis**, which presents as distal nail thickening and subungal (underneath nails) debris
- Feet: Maceration between the web spaces of the digits and scaling on the sole (**tinea pedis**)

Treatment is topical azole antifungal agents for all tinea infections; oral griseofulvin is recommended for onychomycosis.

25. List some vascular dermatologic disorders.

These lesions are usually described as "**red**"; if they do not blanch, they are called purpura.

- Drug reactions
- Viral reactions
- Staphylococcal scalded skin syndrome
- Toxic shock syndrome
- Purpura
- Urticaria
- Kawasaki disease
- Erythema multiforme

26. List some vesicobullous dermatologic disorders.

These lesions are usually described as "**blisters**":

- Pemphigus vulgaris (very frequently **involves the mouth**)
- Bullous pemphigoid (oral involvement is less common)
- Dermatitis herpetiformis (associated with **celiac disease**)
- Staphylococcal scalded skin syndrome
- Erythema multiforme

27. What are the characteristics of staphylococcal scalded skin syndrome?

In staphylococcal scalded skin syndrome, the toxin causes fever and the development of red papules that become bullae and rupture, especially in the perioral and facial areas. It usually occurs in children after otitis media,

What is the ***Nikolsky sign?***

What is the difference between Stevens-Johnson syndrome and toxic epidermal necrolysis? Nikolsky sign and percentage of body surface area affected

conjunctivitis, or nasopharyngeal infection. Upon rubbing the lesion, it easily peels (Nikolsky sign). Treatment is IV nafcillin against Staphylococcus.

28. How do patients with erythema multiforme present?

The patient will present with target lesions (erythematous lesions with central papules or bullae) secondary to drugs, a virus, or Mycoplasma pneumoniae. The lesions appear on the palms, soles, and dorsum of the hands. Treatment: Discontinue drugs, if this is the cause, and administer antihistamines and steroids.

29. How do patients with Stevens-Johnson syndrome present?

Stevens-Johnson syndrome is usually caused by medications (antibiotics, allopurinol, antipsychotics, analgesics, and NSAIDs) causing necrosis and sloughing of skin. The patient presents 1-3 weeks after use of medications with fever and influenza-like symptoms and multiple bullae on the oral mucous membrane, lips, and face. Lesions involve <10% of the body surface area.

30. How do patients with toxic epidermal necrolysis present?

Toxic epidermal necrolysis presents similarly to Stevens-Johnson syndrome, with fever and rash after use of medications, but involves a greater body surface area (>30%).

Treatment of Stevens-Johnson syndrome and toxic epidermal necrolysis: Stop all suspected medications, and treat similarly to burns and staphylococcal scalded skin syndrome, with IV fluids and antibiotics.

31. Describe a skin lesion from a black widow spider bite.

Most lesions are self-limited local skin reactions; however, local skin necrosis can be rarely observed. The bite can also lead to autonomic system stimulation, causing nausea, vomiting, dizziness, tachycardia, hypertension, and diaphoresis.

32. How may patients present with brown recluse spider bite?

Most lesions are self-limited local skin reactions; however, patients can rarely present with autonomic symptoms similar to those after a black widow spider bite.

33. How may patients present with hidradenitis suppurativa?

Patients are usually less than 20 years old, **smokers**, and **obese**, with a family history of hidradenitis suppurativa. Lesions consist of **chronic draining** and nondraining sinus tracts and abscesses in the **intertriginous areas** (axillary, inguinal, and anogenital). Treatment is topical clindamycin or intralesional steroids for mild disease. Systemic antibiotics with doxycycline should be used for severe disease.

34. What is the pathophysiology of alopecia areata?

This is a T-cell mediated **autoimmune disease** causing **non-scarring hair loss**. Most patients will present with many round patches of hair loss. Alopecia areata can affect hairs in areas other than the scalp, as opposed to **androgenetic alopecia**, which will present as scalp and **frontal hair loss**. Alopecia areata can also be itchy and sometimes painful. Hair **tapering near the proximal** end is pathognomonic. Treatment is steroids in intralesional or topical form.

35. What is the pathogenesis of acne vulgaris?

Acne vulgaris is the growth of the sebaceous gland with propagation by **propionibacterium and androgens**. The most commonly affected areas are on the face, back, and chest.

Treatment: Treat mild acne (**few comedones**) with **topical retinoids**; moderate acne (**numerous comedones with pustules**) by adding topical **retinoids to topical antibiotics**; and severe acne (**pustules, abscess, and potential for scarring**) with oral retinoic acid (isotretinoin). In female patients, pregnancy tests should be performed twice before beginning isotretinoin and two methods of contraception should be used during usage. **Systemic antibiotics** (tetracycline, macrolides, or trimethoprim/sulfamethoxazole [TMP/SMX]) can be used in moderate to severe acne, and **oral contraceptives** are an option for some women with moderate acne.

Know the different treatments for various types of acne.

36. What is the definition of psoriasis?

Psoriasis is an autoimmune, systemic disease that results in the formation of **well-demarcated silvery plaques,** usually **symmetrically (both sides of the body)** on the **knees, elbows, and extensor surfaces.** It is associated with nail pitting and arthritis.

Treatment: Moistening agents, topical high-potency steroids, and vitamin D can be used for skin lesions. In more severe cases, immunosuppressive agents such as methotrexate, tumor necrosis factor inhibitors (etanercept, adalimumab, infliximab), CD2 T-cell inhibitors (alefacept), and ultraviolet B light or psoralen with ultraviolet A light (PUVA) can be used.

37. What are the defining characteristics of seborrheic dermatitis?

Seborrheic dermatitis is a **papulosquamous skin lesion** located in the sebum-rich areas of the body, including the skin, scalp, and face. It occurs as a red, flaky, dry rash **on the face, behind the ears,** and on the **scalp (cradle cap or dandruff)**. It is also associated with ***Malassezia*** in the setting of an abnormal immune response (e.g., low helper T cells). It occurs more often in **AIDS patients**.

Treatment: Treat cradle cap with baby oil and selenium shampoo and skin lesions with topical steroids.

38. What other cutaneous manifestation is caused by *Malassezia*?

What is the difference between tinea versicolor and pityriasis rosea?

It causes **tinea versicolor: hypopigmented/hyperpigmented, erythematous scaly macules** that occur in patients in warm, humid, summertime environments. When the macules are scraped and observed under the microscope with KOH, they will show short hyphae and spores ("**spaghetti and meatballs**" appearance). Also, under Wood's light, these lesions will fluoresce. Treat with selenium sulfide shampoo and azole antifungals.

39. Oval erythematous papules and plaques with a "herald" patch are suggestive of what diagnosis?

They suggest **pityriasis rosea**, which is usually asymptomatic or presents with itching, initially with a single eruption known as a "**herald**" patch that is **raised erythematous** and becomes scaly with **central clearing**. Two weeks later, oval lesions that are similar to the herald patch but smaller present on the trunk and extremities in a diagonal pattern ("**Christmas tree**" appearance). This is thought to be due to human herpes 7 (HH-7) reactivation. Treatment is reassurance or topical steroids for itching.

40. In a KOH preparation under the microscope, how may yeast (*Candida*) be differentiated from tinea?

Candida has **pseudohyphae**, branching filaments without septae, whereas tinea has hyphae (filaments with septae).

41. What is the significance of infantile hemangioma?

A benign vascular lesion, infantile hemangioma usually proliferates from birth to 1 year, remains stable for months, and then involutes. On examination, **a red, raised lesion** can be observed. Treatment is reassurance.

Infantile hemangioma usually involutes.

42. How may patients present with molluscum contagiosum?

This lesion is caused by poxvirus, leading to a **dome-shaped papule** with **central umbilication**. It is common in children and occurs on the trunk, face, and extremities.

43. What is the significance of molluscum contagiosum in adults?

It is usually associated with sexually transmitted infection via skin contact and is very common in **AIDS patients,** with a predisposition for the face. Cryotherapy can be used for treatment in AIDS patients, but the lesions self-resolve in children.

Molluscum contagiosum is a self limited infection in immunocompetent patients.

44. How do patients present with *Pthirus pubis* (crab louse) or *Pediculus humanus capitis* (head louse) lesions?

The patient presents with itching of the involved area (**usually pubic hair and axilla**) and the hair is infested with nits and lice, which are usually transmitted by **sexual contact**. Diagnosis is by identifying the lice and nits (lice eggs) in the involved area. Household contacts may be infected and need to be treated since transmission is by person-to-person contact. Screen patients for other sexually transmitted infections.

Treatment: Permethrin cream (first line) or Lindane (second line)

45. How do patients present with *Sarcoptes scabiei* **(scabies) lesions?**

The patient presents with itching and excoriations **with superficial furrows** in the **hands and wrist**. Household members may also be affected and need to be treated.

Treatment is Permethrin cream (first line) or Lindane (second line).

46. How may patients present with bed bug rash?

Patients present with a red, raised, and pruritic rash, usually in a "**linear cluster**" in exposed areas of the skin.

47. Skin is the most common nonpulmonary site involvement in *Blastomyces dermatitidis, Coccidioides immitis,* and *Cryptococcus neoformans*. True or false?

True. Lesions can range from **verrucous plaques** to **umbilicated papules**.

48. Nodules on the face and earlobes with sensory loss in the extremity lesions and a history of travel to a developing country should prompt a search for what diagnosis?

Consider leprosy, caused by ***Mycobacterium leprae***, which grows on **cooler areas** of the body, including the **skin**, **nerves**, and upper respiratory tract. Lesions can present in a variety of ways and certain clues such as absence of pain with cuts and burns, as well as travel to a developing country, should help point to the diagnosis. Transmission is via a respiratory route. Skin biopsy is diagnostic.

49. Yellow-red macules or slightly raised papules in a patient with hypertriglyceridemia are suggestive of what lesion?

They suggest **xanthomas**, which have a predilection for the **Achilles heel**, hand, patella, and neck.

50. Chronic blistering skin lesions associated with hepatitis C and alcohol abuse is suggestive of what diagnosis?

Consider **porphyria cutanea tarda**, a common cause of porphyria due to accumulation of porphyrins in the skin. It results in photosensitivity, which causes **blistering** on sun-exposed areas, usually the back of the hands. The **urine will turn pink** under Wood's lamp, indicating the presence of urine porphyrin. Serum results will also be positive for porphyrin. Treatment is hydroxychloroquine or phlebotomy.

Blistering skin lesions on the back of hands and sun exposed areas should suggest the diagnosis of porphyria cutanea tarda.

Chapter 13
Immunology

1. What is the pathophysiology of allergies?
Allergy is a type I hypersensitivity reaction. Immunoglobulin E is presensitized by antigen that binds to mast cells, which release histamines, bradykinin, and leukotriene. This leads to dilated vessels, vessel permeability, and pruritus.

2. What is the first step in the treatment of allergy?
Treatment is oral antihistamines. Why? They antagonize the release of histamine.

3. What is anaphylaxis?
Anaphylaxis is a type I hypersensitivity reaction that affects multiple systems such as the skin, the gastrointestinal (GI) tract, the pulmonary system, and the cardiac system. Anaphylaxis can eventually lead to shock.

4. What is the first step in the treatment of anaphylaxis?
The first step is administration of intramuscular epinephrine. Why? It antagonizes vessel dilation in the periphery and stimulates the heart to pump harder. Other treatment options are H1 blockers (antihistamines), H2 blockers (famotidine), and glucocorticoids.

5. How do patients present with urticaria?
The patient may present with red or pigmented well-circumscribed skin lesions secondary to type I sensitivity. **Typically transient**, the lesions last 2-24 hours.

The most common causes of urticaria are medications and food.

Subcutaneous epinephrine is the first step in anaphylaxis reaction.

What is the difference between type I and type III hypersensitivity reactions?

Treatment: Oral antihistamines for mild cases; subcutaneous epinephrine for severe forms that include anaphylaxis.

6. **How do patients with angioedema present?**
   Angioedema is urticaria that involves deeper tissues such as the tongue, lips, or pharynx. The patient presents with swelling of the lips or shortness of breath from airway swelling occlusion. The pathogenesis is a type I hypersensitivity reaction. C1 esterase inhibitor deficiency can also cause it.

   Treatment: Oral antihistamines or subcutaneous epinephrine if angioedema is severe. Steroids can increase the C1 esterase inhibitor. **Steroids** can also decrease the inflammation that occurs.

7. **Define autoimmunity syndromes.**
   An autoimmunity syndrome is an antibody directed against self, which leads to the deposition of antigen-antibody complexes in various tissues and organs It can be a **type III hypersensitivity** (Arthus reaction), or a **type II hypersensitivity** (complement or macrophage/natural killer cell-activated lysis).

8. **Describe the pathogenesis of autoimmunity syndromes.**
   The autoimmune destruction of tissues results in extracellular matrix (ECM) accumulation, leading to fibrosis (e.g., CREST syndrome or systemic sclerosis, Sjögren syndrome) and antigen-antibody complex deposition in several tissues (e.g., systemic lupus erythematosus [SLE]).

The joints and kidneys are most commonly affected in patients with SLE.

9. **How do patients with SLE present?**
   Although SLE causes antigen-antibody complex deposition in joints, skin, face, heart, kidneys, and vessels, which leads to arthralgia, myalgia, arthritis, malar rash, oral ulcers, discoid rash, heart failure, kidney insufficiency, and anemia, it commonly affects the **skin**. Joint pain (**arthralgia**) is frequently a presenting symptom of SLE.

10. **List the cutaneous manifestations in SLE.**
    - Malar rash: **butterfly rash** on face
    - Discoid lesions: scaling, atrophic, and scarring rash
    - Livedo reticularis: **net-like rash** that occurs on the extremities

- Raynaud's phenomenon: **blue-red discoloration of the digits** on exposure to cold temperatures

11. What are treatment options for SLE?

Treatment options are **NSAIDs and hydroxychloroquine** for mild disease, **cyclophosphamide** for those with end-organ damage such as renal failure; and **mycophenolate mofetil** or **azathioprine** for those who have achieved remission with cyclophosphamide.

Antimalarias (hydroxy-chloroquine) are used for skin and musculoskeletal manifestations in SLE.

12. What is the most common visceral organ affected in SLE?

The kidney is most affected. A biopsy sample is needed before treatment, however. Why? A biopsy sample will help determine the stage of kidney disease that is present because severity affects treatment type. The most common causes of death in SLE are **infections** and atherosclerosis disease. Cardiovascular disease can occur in the form of pleural disease (effusions) or **Libman–Sacks endocarditis. Neurological involvement** can also occur in the form of cognitive decline. **Hematologic involvement** can occur in the form of ITP, cytopenia, and antiphospholipid syndrome. **Pulmonary disease** can occur in the form of restrictive lung disease.

13. List the types of renal disease in SLE.

- Mesangial - class II
- Focal proliferative - Class III
- Diffuse proliferative - Class IV
- Membranous - Class V

14. What is the next step in the evaluation of a patient with SLE?

The next step after clinical diagnosis is to acquire antinuclear antibody, anti-double-stranded DNA, and anti-smith DNA test results. Low **serum C3 and C4** levels usually indicate flares of the disease.

15. Which test is the most specific for SLE?

Anti-smith DNA is most specific.

16. What yearly examination should patients on hydroxychloroquine obtain?

These patients should obtain an **ophthalmologic examination**. Hydroxychloroquine can cause irreversible retinopathy.

Patients with antiphospholipid syndrome have elevated aPTT despite the tendency for hypercoagulation.

Infants of SLE mothers can develop heart block.

Patients with Sjögren syndrome need to be followed up for B-cell lymphoma.

When a patient presents with GERD-like symptoms, make sure you rule out CREST syndrome.

17. How do patients with antiphospholipid syndrome present in pregnancy?

The patient may present with a story of **multiple spontaneous abortions** (recurrent fetal loss in the second and third trimesters) and a history of hypercoagulation (**thrombosis**).

18. Screening for anti-Ro/SSA and anti-La/SSB antibodies is indicated in all pregnant women with SLE. True or false?

True. These maternal antibodies are associated with **congenital complete heart block.**

19. What is the definition of Sjögren syndrome?

Sjögren syndrome involves the autoimmune destruction of tissues, resulting in accumulation of ECM material in the salivary glands. This leads to dry mouth and dry eyes.

The next step is look for antibodies to **Ro/SSA and La/SSB**. Definitive diagnosis is made by **labial (lip) biopsy**.

Treatment: Artificial tears, as well as saliva and mouth lubricants to manage symptoms and dental care to prevent gingival disease

Complications such as neuropathy and renal tubular acidosis can occur; monitor the patient for development of **B-cell lymphoma**.

20. What is the pathogenesis of scleroderma, or CREST syndrome?

CREST syndrome involves the autoimmune destruction of tissues, leading to ECM accumulation and fibrosis in the skin, esophagus, vessels, lungs, heart, and kidneys. The patient presents with scleroderma or thickened skin, heartburn and difficulty swallowing, Reynaud's phenomenon, interstitial lung disease (ILD), pulmonary fibrosis, and pulmonary hypertension.

The first step is to check for Anti-scl70 (topoisomerase-1) for systemic scleroderma or anticentromere for CREST syndrome. CREST stands for calcinosis, Reynaud's phenomenon, esophageal dysmotility, sclerodactyly, and telangiectasia.

Treatment: Various medications including prostacyclin, vasodilators or certain calcium channel blockers can be used to treat pulmonary hypertension; antacids and promotility drugs for heartburn and dysphagia; angiotensin-converting enzyme inhibitors for kidney disease; and cyclophosphamide for interstitial lung disease.

21. What is the major vascular manifestation associated with systemic sclerosis?

Raynaud's phenomenon, which is digital discoloration (usually the fingers) in association with cold weather, occurs in almost all patients diagnosed with systemic sclerosis. It can be treated with aspirin or calcium channel blockers.

22. What is the significance of Dupuytren's contracture?

This is characterized by **fibroblastic proliferation**, leading to palmar fascia fibrosis. It can be seen in those with diabetes mellitus, those who smoke cigarettes and use alcohol, workers who are exposed to repetitive handling tasks or vibration, and those with Peyronie's disease. Patients will present with **painless finger stiffness** on physical examination.

What is the difference between trigger finger and Dupuytren's contracture?

23. Young male smokers <40 years old who present with digital ischemia with pain and subsequent discoloration should be evaluated for what diagnosis?

Consider **thromboangitis obliterans** (also known as **Buerger's disease**), an inflammatory disease that affects small to medium-sized arteries and veins of the extremities. Patients will present with **digit ulcers or gangrene. Smoking cessation** is the only definitive treatment.

24. Patients with anti-Scl 70 antibodies are at increased risk of what manifestations?

These patients are at risk for ILD and diffuse cutaneous disease.

25. What is the definition of Behçet syndrome?

Behçet syndrome is a systemic anti-inflammatory adulthood syndrome that involves multiple ulcers in the mouth (**aphthous ulcers**), genitals, eyes (uveitis), and skin. It is due to inflammation of tissues and blood vessels. It is associated with erythema nodosum and CNS vasculitis.

Treatment: Steroids, thalidomide for oral or genital ulcers, and azathioprine for ocular involvement

In a patient with ulcers everywhere, consider Behçet syndrome.

26. What is the definition of vasculitis?

Vasculitis is an autoimmune inflammation of the vessels. Vasculitis is classified based on the size of the vessel that is involved.

Polymyalgia rheumatica is associated with temporal arteritis.

27. What is the pathogenesis of polyarteritis nodosa (PAN)?

Polyarteritis nodosa is a systemic vasculitis that affects **small** or **medium-sized arteries** in many organs, including the nervous system, kidney, and GI tract. Patients usually present with systemic symptoms such as fever, chills, weight loss, kidney failure (microaneurysms and irregular constrictions on renal arteriography is diagnostic of PAN), and blood in the stool with abdominal pain. A biopsy of subcutaneous nodule showing "onion skin" appearance is pathognomonic of PAN. Polyarteritis nodosa may be associated with hepatitis B **or C or HIV.**

Treatment: **Cyclophosphamides** if associated with hepatitis B or HIV; treat the underlying viral infection.

28. What is the pathogenesis of temporal arteritis?

Temporal arteritis affects the large arterial vessels and **carotid artery branches** and is called giant cell arteritis. A T-cell mediated reaction (**type IV hypersensitivity reaction**) causes the formation of granulomas. The patient will usually be in their sixth decade and present with headache and **jaw claudication**, **scalp tenderness**, and **fever**. Temporal arteritis can be associated with pelvic and shoulder stiffness and pain (polymyalgia rheumatica). The erythrocyte sedimentation rate (ESR) is elevated.

Complications: Temporal arteritis can cause transient blindness (carotid artery involvement) and headache (temporal artery) or optic nerve ischemia causing diplopia.

Treatment: The first step in evaluation is to treat with a high-dose steroid. Obtain a biopsy sample of the temporal artery 2 weeks later. **Low-dose aspirin** can reduce visual and cerebrovascular complications.

29. List some small vessel systemic pauci-immune vasculitides.

These vasculitides are associated with glomerulonephritis:

- Wegener granulomatosis
- Churg–Strauss syndrome (eosinophilia, asthma and vasculitis, P-ANCA and C-ANCA)
- Microscopic polyangiitis (P-ANCA)

30. What is the pathogenesis of Wegener granulomatosis?

Wegener granulomatosis is associated with necrotizing

inflammation of the **small** arterial vessels in the lung, upper and lower respiratory tract, kidneys, and GI tract.

The patient may present with hypertension, proteinuria, bronchitis, sinusitis, and blood in the urine and renal failure.

Diagnosis: The antineutrophil cytoplasmic antibodies (**C-ANCA**) test can help confirm the diagnosis.

Treatment: Immunosuppressants such as steroids and **cyclophosphamides**

What is the difference between Wegener granulomatosis and Goodpasture syndrome?

31. How do patients present with Kawasaki disease?

Kawasaki disease is mucocutaneous vasculitis in children. The patient presents with lymphadenopathy, mucocutaneous lesions (dry and fissured lips), strawberry tongue, fever, extremity edema, and hyperpigmentation.

Differentiate Kawasaki disease from scarlet fever (also has strawberry tongue) (see chapter 16).

Complications: Coronary artery aneurysm

Treatment: Aspirin or IV immunoglobulin

What is the difference between Kawasaki disease and scarlet fever?

32. How may patients present with Takayasu's arteritis?

Patients present with vasculitis of the **aortic branches**, causing **ischemia** in young **women of Asian origin**. It can also cause asymmetric hypertension and valve regurgitation. Arteriography confirms the diagnosis. Treat with prednisone.

33. How do patients with Henoch-Schonlein purpura present?

Patients are usually younger than 8 years old and present with **palpable purpura,** arthritis, glomerulonephritis, and **gastrointestinal** involvement with intussusception. The disease is self-limited.

34. What is the pathogenesis of cryoglobulinemic vasculitis?

Mixed cryoglobulinemia is associated with hepatitis C. Cryoglobulins are monoclonal or polyclonal immunoglobulins that can precipitate in a **cold environment**. They are present in various conditions, including hepatitis C, hepatitis B, plasma cell dyscrasias, or chronic inflammatory conditions.

35. How may patients present with common variable immunodeficiency?

Common variable immunodeficiency presents as impaired B-cell immunoglobulin, which leads to **frequent**

What is the difference between type II and type III hypersensitivity reactions?

Age-appropriate screening for cancer is recommended for outpatient follow-up of patients with polymyositis or dermatomyositis.

bacterial, **viral sinus**, and **pulmonary infections**. Patients will also have an absent response to immunization and a history of a family member with the disease. Obtain quantitative immunoglobulin for diagnosis. Immunoglobulin treatment is the mainstay of therapy.

36. What is the definition of connective tissue disorders?

A connective tissue disorder is an immune-mediated inflammation of striated muscle and ECM.

37. What is the pathogenesis of polymyositis?

Polymyositis is a T-helper-2-mediated immune response that activates cytotoxic cells to damage the muscle. This is a type II hypersensitivity reaction. Patients will thus present with proximal muscle weakness, weakness standing from sitting, and weakness climbing stairs.

Laboratory tests reveal elevated ESR (normal is 12-20 mm/hour in those <50 years old) and an elevated creatine kinase level. Why? These results are indicative of the inflammatory response. Look for **anti-Jo-1** antibodies. Those with anti-Jo-1 antibodies are more likely to develop ILD, arthritis, and Raynaud's phenomenon.

38. What is the pathogenesis of dermatomyositis?

Dermatomyositis is thought to be a complement-mediated/myocyte vascular inflammation. In addition to proximal muscle weakness, the patient will also develop a heliotrope rash on the face, and a papular rash on the dorsal interphalangeales (Gottron's papules). Mucosal and periungual telangiectasia can also be found in juvenile dermatomyositis.

Laboratory tests reveal elevated ESR and creatine kinase level. Why? They are indicative of the inflammatory response. Look for **anti-Jo-1** antibodies. EMG can confirm the diagnosis. Genetic risk factors are HLAQA1 and HLA-DRB1 genotypes.

39. What are treatment options for polymyositis/dermatomyositis?

Initial therapy is steroids. Refractory cases can be treated with immunosuppressants such as methotrexate and azathioprine. Complications of polymyositis/dermatomyositis may include respiratory and pharyngeal muscle weakness causing respiratory failure, pneumonia, or dysphagia.

Long-term complications of polymyositis/dermatomyositis may also include increased risk of visceral cancer; therefore, regular screening for cancer is warranted.

40. How may patients present with Adult Still's disease?
This is an inflammatory disease occurring in adolescents. They present with a **high-grade fever** of **1 week's** duration, arthralgias, myalgias, and **rash**. It is a diagnosis of exclusion. Laboratory results may reveal **leukocytosis** and **elevated serum ferritin**. Treat with NSAIDs or aspirin.

41. What is the pathogenesis of AL amyloidosis?
Amyloidosis is the deposition of insoluble proteins (e.g., monoclonal light chains) in the ECM of several organs, including heart, skin, kidney, lung, and joints. AL amyloidosis is the deposition of **monoclonal** L chain in tissues. Patients most commonly will present with **weakness** and **purpura**. Other symptoms vary widely, including heart failure (nephrotic range proteinuria), Kussmaul sign (a sign of restrictive cardiomyopathy), waxy skin, kidney failure, and arthritis (swelling of joints). Serological or tissue detection of monoclonal immunoglobulin further supports diagnosis.

Confirm the diagnosis with Congo red staining and apple-green birefringence of the biopsy sample (**abdominal fat pad aspiration**) when visualized under polarized light.

Treatment: Treat heart failure and kidney failure and the underlying causes (e.g., multiple myeloma).

42. What is the pathogenesis of sarcoidosis?
Sarcoidosis is a systemic inflammatory disease that results in cell-mediated noncaseating granuloma. It is common in African American women. Patients have involvement of the eyes, joints, lungs, skin, liver/spleen, heart, and brain. Sarcoidosis often presents with abnormal chest X-ray (CXR) findings on routine screening with bilateral hilar lymphadenopathy, which is pathognomonic. Systemic symptoms such as fever, night sweats, and weight loss are common. In Lofgren's syndrome, patients can present with arthritis, erythema nodosum (tender red lesions on the shins and legs), and bilateral hilar lymphadenopathy.

Other findings in sarcoidosis are uveitis, restrictive lung disease, cardiac granulomas, seizures, cognitive dysfunction, and liver disease. Laboratory tests may show elevated serum angiotensin-converting enzyme and

Kussmaul's sign can also be found in right sided infarction, PE, partial obstruction of the vena cavae, right sided tumors and rarely, cardiac tamponade.

A History of infiltrative disease that involves the heart muscle favors (amyloidosis, sarcoidosis) favors the diagnosis of restrictive cardiomyopathy over constrictive pericarditis

In a patient with recurrent uveitis, consider sarcoidosis.

Why is the calcium level elevated in sarcoidosis?

calcium levels. Why elevated calcium levels? Vitamin D production is increased. A biopsy of the involved tissue will reveal noncaseating granulomas.

Treatment: Steroids are used as initial therapy. Immunosuppressants such as **methotrexate** or azathioprine and anti-tumor necrosis factor (anti-TNF) agents can be used for refractory cases.

Proximal digital arthritis suggests RA, while distal digital arthritis suggests OA.

43. List significant differences between rheumatoid arthritis (RA) and osteoarthritis (OA).

Most patients with polyarticular joint pain who are older and have no evidence of inflammation will have osteoarthritis. On physical examination, obesity, **distal interphalangeal arthritis**, and **joint crepitus** are suggestive of osteoarthritis.

Joint stiffness of less than 1 hour's duration after waking up and after sitting for long periods is common in osteoarthritis. OA is a slowly progressive disease that can cause progressive joint damage and functional limitation if not aggressively treated. Quadriceps exercise can be effective for OA. Tylenol, NSAIDs, intraarticular steroids, and surgery are other treatment options for OA.

44. Evidence of weakly positive birefringent crystals is present in what inflammatory arthritis?

It is present in pseudogout, indicating accumulation of **calcium pyrophosphate crystals**. On joint X-ray, the presence of **chondrocalcinosis** (linear calcification) in the joint space is pathognomonic. It can be treated with NSAIDs and low-dose colchicine.

45. How is a patient with gout evaluated?

Gout is suggestive if patients present with **podagra** (big toe swelling); long-term gouty arthritis may cause tophaceous deposits in the skin. Those with gout usually have metabolic syndrome and hypertension and are taking diuretic (thiazide) therapy. Arthrocentesis reveals monosodium urate with **needle-shaped crystals** that are **negatively birefringent**. Treat acute episodes with NSAIDs, colchicine, or steroids. Treat chronic gout with hyperuricemia with allopurinol, probenecid, or febuxostat.

46. What is the pathogenesis of rheumatoid arthritis (RA)?

RA is an inflammation against self due to T-cell proliferation and activation of interleukin-1 and tumor necrosis factor, which affects several organs including the heart, joints, lungs, and spleen. The patient presents with arthritis (1-hour morning stiffness). The arthritis in RA is commonly red, swollen, and symmetrical, affecting mainly the small joints such as the proximal interphalangeal and metacarpophalangeal joints. Systemic symptoms include fever, weight loss, pericarditis, interstitial lung disease, and splenomegaly. Splenomegaly and neutropenia in RA is referred to as Felty syndrome.

What is the definition of Felty syndrome?

47. How may RA be diagnosed?

Diagnosis is mainly clinical. The human leukocyte antigen (HLA)-DR4 is present in some patients. Look for anti-rheumatic factor and **IgM** citrulline-containing protein in the serum. Patients with anti-citrulline antibodies and RF have a **worse prognosis.**

48. What are treatment options for RA?

Treatment: NSAIDs and early aggressive treatment with immunosuppressants (disease-modifying drugs) such as methotrexate (preferred initial therapy), sulfasalazine, and hydroxychloroquine. Cyclophosphamide can be used for those with evidence of end-organ damage such as vasculitis and mononeuritis multiplex. Antitumor necrosis factor drugs (e.g., infliximab, etanercept) are a last resort, and steroids can be used for acute flares.

49. List the complications of RA and its attendant treatment.

Complications are due **to mouth ulcers from methotrexate** and **cervical atlantoaxial dislocation** from arthritis of the cervical vertebra joint. Patients with RA are more likely to have infections, MI, stroke, and non-Hodgkin lymphoma.

Cervical atlanto-axial dislocation is a common complication of long-term RA.

50. What is the pathogenesis of ankylosing spondylitis or arthritis?

Ankylosing spondylitis is an inflammation of the sacroiliac joints due to a reaction to self. The patient will be young (usually male) and present with back pain and stiffness that is alleviated by exercise. Some patients will present with enthesitis (heel pain). Patients can also present with hip and shoulder involvement, fatigue, and weight loss. Laboratory tests may reveal anemia. Some patients will have the HLA-B27 genotype, and so

Most patients presenting with ankylosing arthritis will have the HLA-B27 genotype.

obtain genotyping test results in all patients. Make sure to obtain serological results for inflammatory markers such as CRP or ESR, which should be elevated.

51. How may ankylosing arthritis be diagnosed with imaging?

The first step is to obtain an X-ray of the sacroiliac joint to look for sacroiliitis (inflamed sacroiliac joint) and fusion of the spine ligaments (bamboo spine) (Figure 13-1).

Treatment: NSAIDs, exercise, and DMARDS such as methotrexate and sulfasalazine; anti-TNF agents for severe cases (those with spinal fusion)

52. What is a feared complication of ankylosing arthritis?

A serious complication is a vertebral fracture years later because of the destruction of the sacroiliac joints from inflammation. Uveitis, cauda equine syndrome, lung fibrosis, and aortic insufficiency due to aortitis are some known complications.

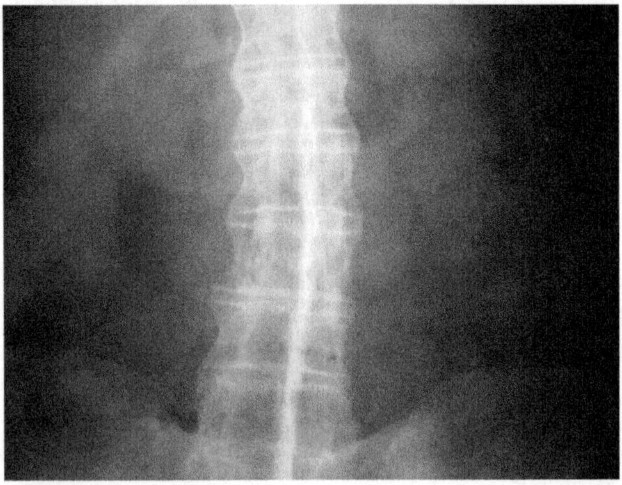

Figure 13-1. *Fusion of spine ligaments (bamboo spine).*

53. What is the definition of Reiter syndrome (now called reactive arthritis)?

Reiter syndrome is arthritis, urethritis, and conjunctivitis (mnemonic: can't see, can't pee, can't walk) secondary to reactive arthritis (due to various sexually transmitted and gastrointestinal infections, most commonly due to chlamydia arthritis). This arthritis usually occurs 1-3 weeks

Can't pee, can't see, can't walk is a mnemonic for Reiter syndrome.

after gastrointestinal/genitourinary infection due to molecular mimicry. Other extraarticular manifestations are oral ulcers, rashes such as **keratoderma blennorrhagica** (hyperkeratotic skin rash on palms and soles), and genital lesions such as **circinate balanitis** (shallow ulcers on glans and shaft of the penis). The first step is to acquire cervical, urethra, pharyngeal, and stool cultures in an attempt to identify the causative organism. **HLA B27** is present in most patients with this condition.

Treatment: NSAIDs for arthritis, sulfasalazine or methotrexate for chronic arthritis, and anti-TNF agents for refractory cases

54. What is the pathogenesis of psoriatic arthritis?

Psoriatic arthritis is a type of chronic spondyloarthropathy with inflammation to self. Patients present with pitting nails and sausage-like digits. Cutaneous manifestations (usually symmetric plaques) usually appear before joint inflammation. Treatment is similar to that of RA.

Pitting nails is associated with psoriatic arthritis.

55. In IBD, when does the flare of joint inflammation occur?

An acute flare of peripheral arthritis in IBD occurs at the same time as the flare of acute intestinal disease.

56. Anti-TNF agents can cause what type of infections?

Anti-TNF agents can cause **tuberculosis**, atypical mycobacterial disease, histoplasmosis, and listeriosis. Why? TNF blockage causes a lack of macrophages, which are needed for elimination of these intracellular organisms. These drugs can also cause **drug-induced SLE**.

57. How do steroids cause bone density loss?

Steroids prolong osteoclast lifespan and induce osteoblast apoptosis. Those taking long-term steroids should be offered prophylactic treatment for bone density loss.

58. What is a prerequisite for a bone marrow transplant (BMT)?

A sibling with **six** human lymphocyte antigen (HLA) matched markers (two HLA-A, two HLA-B, and two DRB1 loci) is preferred for BMT because this has been shown to prevent graft-versus-host disease (GVHD) and to improve graft survival; however, a sibling with a mismatched marker at one HLA locus is considered in some centers. All unrelated donors must meet a minimum

Know the prerequisite for BMT

What is the prophylaxis of acute transplant reaction?

of six matched HLA markers before donor blood can be used for transplant.

59. What is the pathogenesis of GVHD?

In GVHD, graft T cells attack host cells. **The first sign may** be a skin reaction (**purpura or skin rash**). The most common symptom is a **GI bleed**.

Treatment: Steroids to deplete the T cells or anti-thymocytes

Prevention of GVHD is done by depleting T cells from the donor with an immunosuppressant; however, a complication is BMT failure. Transfusion-related GVHD can be prevented by gamma irradiation of cellular blood components (RBC and platelets).

60. How many matched HLA markers are recommended for kidney transplant?

Six possible HLA markers need to match, and the likelihood of matching with a sibling is higher than with any other relative. Siblings have a 25% chance of having fully matched HLA, a 50% chance of having half-matched HLA, and a 25% chance of having zero matched HLA because half of the HLA antigens are inherited from each parent. It is important to match all six antigens to improve graft survival and prevent GVHD.

61. What is the pathogenesis of hyperacute organ rejection?

Hyperacute reaction occurs **minutes to hours** after the transplant of the organ, secondary to **preformed antibodies** to ABO or HLA.

Treatment: Steroids or an immunosuppressive agent

62. What is the pathogenesis of acute organ rejection?

Acute rejection occurs **days to weeks** after transplant of an organ secondary to perivascular inflammation (lymphocytes and **antibodies** are responsible). There is no known treatment, other than prevention with a cross and match.

63. What is the pathogenesis of chronic rejection?

Chronic rejection occurs **months to years** after a transplant secondary to endothelial destruction (**T lymphocytes** are responsible).

Treatment: Steroids or an immunosuppressive agent

64. What is the mechanism of action of steroids in immunosuppression?

Steroids decrease lymphocytes and interleukin-1.

65. What is the difference between hyperacute rejection reaction and cytomegalovirus infection after kidney transplant?

With a hyperacute rejection reaction, laboratory tests will show elevated creatinine and proteinuria and patients may develop oliguria.

Treatment: Steroids

With cytomegalovirus infection, the biopsy sample will show **intranuclear inclusion cells.**

Treatment: Ganciclovir

66. How do patients with a single kidney present?

Compensatory function of a single kidney may result in **massive enlargement** of the kidney. Encourage the patient to avoid contact sports. The risk of hypertension and proteinuria, especially in those with elective removal 25 years after a unilateral nephrectomy, is possible. Therefore, yearly urinalysis and follow-up is recommended. However, donors do not seem to have a risk of developing kidney disease and the **life expectancy of patients is normal.**

67. Listeria is the most common cause of meningitis in postrenal transplant patients. True or false?

True. Treat patients with suspicion of meningitis with empiric antibiotics against this organism.

68. Cytomegalovirus (CMV) is the most common opportunistic infection in renal transplant. True or false?

True. CMV usually **presents months** after transplant. Fever, headache, leukopenia, respiratory distress, and thrombocytopenia are clinical features of CMV infection.

Always think of CMV infection in a patient with renal transplant.

Chapter 14

Infectious Diseases

> *Types of pneumonia and their treatment are high yield for the exam.*

1. How do patients with pneumonia present?

The patient may present with fever, chills, rigors, and sputum production.

On examination, the patient will present with consolidation signs (decreased breath sounds, increased fremitus).

2. What is the most common cause of pneumonia?

Community acquired pneumonia is the most common cause of pneumonia in healthy patients. It is usually caused by Streptococcus pneumoniae.

Treatment includes quinolones, doxycycline, and tigecycline for monotherapy. Ceftriaxone plus azithromycin or doxycycline or a respiratory quinolone are combination options. These antibiotics cover typical organisms such as S. pneumoniae as well as atypical organisms. Patients with significant comorbid conditions, advanced age, increased respiratory rate, hypotension, anemia, or hypoxia should be admitted to the hospital because of a higher risk of mortality.

3. List specific risk factors for and treatment of types of pneumonia.

- **Alcohol: Consider anaerobic organisms, such as *Peptostreptococcus* species. Treat with metronidazole or clindamycin.**
- Smoking and alcohol use: Consider Klebsiella pneumoniae. Treat with amoxicillin.
- Immunocompromised individual: Consider CMV. Patient may present with pneumonitis. Treat with ganciclovir.

- Chronic obstructive pulmonary disease (**COPD**): Consider *Moraxella* and *Haemophilus* species. Treat with a macrolide such as azithromycin.
- Immunocompromised individual (with HIV): Patients may present with Pneumocystis jiroveci (carinii) pneumonia. If there is a positive silver stain, treat with trimethoprim/sulfamethoxazole (TMP/SMX) (Bactrim). Treat cryptococcal pneumonia with amphotericin B.
- Animal, rabbits, or farm exposure: Consider tularemia pneumonia, caused by Francisella tularensis (gram-negative bacteria). Treat with streptomycin.
- Southwestern United States: Consider coccidioidomycosis pneumonia. Treat with fluconazole.
- Previous viral infection or intravenous (IV) drug use: Consider Staphylococcus aureus pneumonia. A chest X-ray (CXR) may reveal lung cavity nodules. Treat with nafcillin.
- Elderly, air conditioning, and respiratory ventilator (water) system: Consider Legionella pneumonia (gram-negative bacteria). Treat with azithromycin.
- Soil contaminated with **bat or bird** droppings in Mississippi and Ohio river valleys or central United States: Consider histoplasmosis and blastomycosis pneumonia. Peripheral blood stain (Wright's stain) can show evidence of monocytes with numerous yeasts in histoplasmosis. Treat with itraconazole, or amphotericin B for severe or neurological symptoms.
- Young adult: Consider Mycoplasma pneumonia. Treat with azithromycin.
- Immunocompromised patients with **neutropenia and organ transplant** Aspergillosis (fungi) pneumonia: The patient will present with hemoptysis and a fungus ball (cavitation) on CXR or a "halo" sign/cavitary lesions on a CT scan. Serological antibody tests (**galactomannan**) are sensitive but less specific. Treat with voriconazole.
- Nocardia pneumonia (gram-positive rod): Examination may reveal partial acid-fast branching organisms. Treat with TMP/SMX.

Histoplasmosis and blastomycosis are common in the midwestern states in the United States along the Ohio and Mississippi river valley.

The most common radiographic findings in histoplasmosis are diffuse interstitial infiltrates

4. What is the first step in the evaluation of patients with pneumonia?

Decide if the patient needs hospitalization versus

outpatient treatment. If patients have other co-morbidities or severe pneumonia, most likely they need to be hospitalized.

5. **How is a pneumonia diagnosis confirmed?**
   Obtain sputum cultures, stain with Gram stain, and do a CXR. Once pneumonia is confirmed with a CXR, treat empirically.
   Inpatient treatment: Ceftriaxone plus a macrolide (azithromycin) is preferred, but **respiratory quinolone (levofloxacin) is an alternative.**
   Outpatient treatment: Doxycycline or respiratory quinolone.
   Always treat inpatients and outpatients empirically. After confirming the causative organism, treat with specific antibiotics as in question 3.

The presence of an infiltrate on CXR, with clinical and microbiological correlation, is the gold standard for diagnosing pneumonia.

6. **What are the complications of pneumonia?**
   Pneumonia is the most common cause of death stemming from infection.
   Pleural effusion and empyema are other known complications.

7. **What is the most common cause of pleural effusion in patients with pneumonia?**
   Consider Staphylococcus aureus as the cause of pneumonia.
   Treatment: Needle thoracotomy to identify the causative organism. Why? Pleural effusion can progress to empyema.

8. **What are the characteristics of empyema?**
   Empyema is characterized by pleural effusion fluid pH <7.0, gross pus, and positive Gram stain and culture.
   Treatment is a tube thoracostomy (chest tube).

9. **What is the pathogenesis of tuberculosis (TB)?**
   TB is an infection caused by *Mycobacterium tuberculosis* that is most prominent in the lungs and characterized by a granulomatous reaction. Usually this reaction contains mycobacteria and remains dormant for life. The patient may present with fever, chills, night sweats, and weight loss. Hemoptysis indicates severe TB.

10. **List the four ways that a patient can present with TB.**
    - Primary disease: **Acute pneumonia** or military TB due to lack of containment of the infection

- Superinfection: Reinfection with TB causing **cavity on CXR**
- Reactivation: TB years later when T-cell immunity has decreased due to old age or immunosuppression
- Advanced HIV patients may present atypically with diffuse small lung nodules on CXR (**military nodules**)

11. What are the risk factors for TB?
- Low economic social status
- Immunocompromised individual
- Smoking and alcohol use

12. What is the first step in the evaluation of patients with TB?

Obtain a sputum swab, an acid-fast microscopic smear stain to detect acid-fast bacilli (AFB), or nucleic acid hybridization of the tubercle bacillus for rapid confirmation, and a CXR. Cultures can be done, but it takes weeks to obtain results and are more sensitive than rapid tests. CXR may show upper lobe apical cavity and a Ghon complex (consolidated apical lymphadenopathy) or apical thickening and cavities in lower lobe apices. Treatment: Active TB is treated with isoniazid (INH), rifampin, pyrazinamide, and ethambutol.

13. List some extrapulmonary involvement in patients with TB.

Extrapulmonary involvement includes **lymphadenopathy**, pleural effusion, **Pott's disease** (T11, T12 vertebrae involvement), CNS, peritoneum, kidney, intestine, and genitals.

14. What magnetic resonance imaging (MRI) finding in TB meningitis is diagnostic?

Meningeal enhancement at the **base of the brain** is diagnostic.

15. What is the significance of HIV and active TB co-infection?

TB causes the HIV virus to replicate faster. Early treatment of HIV with antiretroviral drugs in those with active TB reduces mortality except in patients with TB meningitis.

IRIS usually begins within 1 week to a few months of initiating HAART.

16. What is the significance of immune reconstitution inflammatory syndrome (IRIS) in patients who are co-infected with HIV and active TB?

IRIS is an inflammatory disorder that causes worsening of the infectious process after initiation of antiretroviral therapy. Early treatment of HIV in those being treated for TB can lead to IRIS, which usually manifests as respiratory symptoms and lymphadenopathy.

17. How is asymptomatic latent TB usually diagnosed?

Latent TB is diagnosed by a routine TB skin test, a purified protein derivative given subcutaneously. Watch for a delayed reaction (type IV delayed hypersensitivity reaction).

If the skin test result is positive, a CXR is obtained, and the patient is treated regardless of CXR findings (Table 14-1).

Table 14-1. *BCG Test and Asymptomatic TB Treatment*[a]

Induration	Risk Factors	Next Step	Treatment
≥15 mm	Healthy	CXR	INH, even if normal CXR
≥10 mm	Moderate[b]	CXR	INH, even if normal CXR
≥5 mm	High[c]	CXR	INH, even if normal CXR

BCG, bacillus Calmette-Guérin; CXR, chest X-ray, INH, isoniazid, TB, tuberculosis.

a Memorize Table 14-1.

b Moderate-risk factors: Patient living in a high-risk home (nursing home or other long-term care facility), patient with chronic medical condition, health care worker, immigrants from endemic areas, intravenous drug users.

c High-risk factors: Immunocompromised individual (HIV, transplant recipient, leukemia), living with a patient with active TB, those who have received BCG (bacille Calmette-Guérin) vaccine.

18. List other non-tuberculosis mycobacterial infections.

- *Mycobacterium avium* complex: **Disseminated** infection in **AIDS patients**. Treat with ethambutol and clarithromycin.
- *M. kansasii*: Superinfection of lungs
- *M. marinum*: Infection of distal extremity (erythematous **raised skin lesions**) after **fish exposure**
- *M. fortuitum*, *M. abscessus*: Bone and skin infection after trauma

Know the various treatment options for different types of cellulitis.

19. What is the definition of cellulitis?

Cellulitis is a **non-necrotizing inflammation** of the skin and subcutaneous tissues that does not involve the fascia or muscles and usually presents as red, hot, swollen, and tender skin. Cellulitis is usually caused by a **streptococcal** or **staphylococcal** infection. Community-acquired methicillin-resistant *Staphylococcus aureus* (**MRSA**) should be considered in cellulitis with abscesses or purulent drainage.

Treatment: **Beta-lactams** are the antibiotics of choice for cellulitis. Mild cellulitis, characterized by slight warmth and minimal pain, is treated with dicloxacillin, amoxicillin, or cephalexin (Keflex); **severe cellulitis**, characterized by severe erythema, ulcers, irregular border, and severe pain, is treated with IV ceftriaxone, cefuroxime, nafcillin, or oxacillin. Cellulitis associated with **diabetic ulcers** is often polymicrobial, and so consider broad-spectrum antibiotics that target gram-positive, gram-negative, and anaerobic bacteria.

20. What are the specific antibiotics used to treat cellulitis with MRSA?

In mild cellulitis with abscess or purulent drainage, consider treating with TMP/SMX, clindamycin or doxycycline to target MRSA. In more severe MRSA cases needing IV antibiotics, some options are vancomycin, daptomycin, linezolid, and tigecycline.

21. Lymphedema is a differential diagnosis of extremity swelling and pain that should be considered when a diagnosis of cellulitis is made. True or false?

True. It can be caused by **lymphatic filariasis** (a parasitic infection common in developing countries). Cellulitis is a more common cause of lymphedema in developed countries.

22. What is the characteristic appearance of advanced lymphedema?

Lymphedema appears as nonpitting "**peau d'orange**" (orange peel) edema, caused by fibrosis of cutaneous and subcutaneous tissues. Other causes of such a skin finding are tumor, lymph node dissection, radiation, and skin trauma.

23. What are some complications of cellulitis?

Contiguous spread via lymphatic or venous systems can

cause lymphangitis, abscess, gangrene or **necrotizing fasciitis**, and septic shock.

24. What is the definition of necrotizing fasciitis?

Necrotizing fasciitis is an inflammatory infection, frequently caused by **group A hemolytic streptococci** and ***S. aureus***, which involves the deep fascia with secondary necrosis of the subcutaneous tissues. It spreads rather rapidly. A history of trauma or recent surgery is usually present. On physical examination early on, pain may be out of proportion to the lesion. Later, the area of involvement may be characterized by **bullae**, subcutaneous air, and **severe pain**. Anesthesia in the involved area may indicate subcutaneous thrombosis of blood vessels, leading to nerve fiber necrosis. CT scan or MRI finding of **gas in tissue planes** is diagnostic. Evidence of **multiorgan failure** is usually present.

Treatment: This is a surgical emergency. Aggressive debridement by surgery is required early on, in addition to broad-spectrum antibiotics.

25. How may patients present with tetanus infection?

This is caused by inoculation by *Clostridium tetani*, an anaerobic bacterium, through an **open wound**, leading to **trismus**, **opisthotonus**, **dysphagia**, and **abdominal rigidity**. It can be prevented by making sure all those with complete immunization and open wounds have been vaccinated with tetanus within the previous 5 years. Those with unknown status of immunity or with less than three doss of tetanus toxoid are given both tetanus toxoid and tetanus immune globulin.

All patients with open wounds should be screened for current tetanus immunization.

26. How are mammalian bite wounds treated?

Treat such wounds with antibiotics that target common cellulitis organisms and anaerobes. Mild bite wounds are treated with oral **amoxicillin/clavulanate**. In more severe cases, treat with IV ampicillin/sulbactam or piperacillin/tazobactam.

27. What is the definition of folliculitis?

Folliculitis is an **inflammation of hair follicles** that is caused by various infections. Acne is a type of noninfectious folliculitis whereby a keratin plug obstructs superficial follicles, causing *Propionibacterium acnes* to secrete excess fatty acids, which causes inflammation.

***Staphylococcus* infection** is the most common cause of folliculitis. Hot tube exposure can predispose to "**hot tub**" folliculitis from ***Pseudomonas* infection**.

Treatment: Superficial folliculitis is treated with antibacterial soaps; refractory deep folliculitis is treated with topical antibiotics that target gram-positive organisms. If systemic symptoms are present, treat with IV antibiotics that include coverage of methicillin-resistant organisms.

28. Furuncle is a deep folliculitis infection mostly caused by *S. aureus*. True or false?

True.

29. What is the causative agent in bullous impetigo?

Bullous impetigo is a **vesiculopustular** infection caused mostly by a group A *Streptococcus* infection (Streptococcus pyogenes and Staphylococcus aureus). It occurs in very warm, humid areas with poor hygiene. The patient, usually a child, presents with raised lesions that are golden brown upon rupture.

Treatment: Topical mupirocin is the first-line treatment; if numerous lesions are present, treat them with first generation cephalosporins such as Keflex (oral cephalexin).

QuantiFERON test is preferred in patients with a history of positive PPD skin test.

30. How do you manage a patient with a positive PPD skin test and a history of BCG vaccination or BCG as therapy for bladder cancer?

Disregard the history of BCG vaccination and treat as latent TB. In future testing, the serum **QuantiFERON** test is preferred in this patient population.

31. What is the pathogenesis of sexually transmitted diseases (STDs)?

STDs cause infection of the mucosa of the genital tract that can extend to the inner genital organs.

32. What are the risk factors for STDs?

- Multiple sexual partners
- Prostitution
- Unprotected sexual intercourse

33. How do patients with gonococcal urethritis present?

The patient may present with genital discharge and dysuria and women may have purulent vaginal discharge on the pelvic examination.

The next step is to obtain urine samples or a swab of the urethra or vaginal wall to look for gonorrhea or chlamydia. Send serological samples to test for herpes and syphilis.

Treat empirically with IM ceftriaxone and azithromycin or doxycycline as an alternative. Why? Neisseria gonorrhoeae is a gram-negative diplococcus and chlamydia is covered by azithromycin or doxycycline. Acquire consent for HIV testing. Gonococcal urethritis can be complicated by monoarticular or migratory arthritis tenosynovitis and maculopapular rash, which are suggestive of disseminated gonococcal infection (DIG). Obtain cultures of rectum, pharynx, blood, and joints for diagnosis of DIG.

Why is gonococcal urethritis treated with ceftriaxone?

Gonococcal urethritis can be complicated by monoarticular arthritis and maculopapular rash.

34. How do patients with chlamydial urethritis present?

Approximately half of the patients present asymptomatically. Chlamydial urethritis is usually seen on a routine screening test.

Treatment: Azithromycin or doxycycline. Why? Chlamydia trachomatis is an obligate intracellular organism.

Which STD is usually asymptomatic?

Why is chlamydial urethritis treated with azithromycin?

35. How do patients present with pelvic inflammatory disease?

The patient presents with fever and abdominal pain. The patient will have cervical motion tenderness on physical examination.

Treatment: A single intramuscular dose of ceftriaxone and oral doxycycline for 14 days. If it is a severe case, with sepsis and vomiting, admit the patient to the hospital and treat with intravenous (IV) cefotetan or cefoxitin and IV doxycycline for 14 days.

36. List common ulcerated genital infections and associated findings.

- Herpes simplex virus (most common): **Vesicles**
- Primary syphilis: Three weeks after sexual intercourse, **painless**, **heaped borders** and indurated
- Lymphogranuloma venereum: Nonpainful transient ulcer, followed by bilateral **inguinal lymphadenopathy**, HIV patients
- Chancroid (*Haemophilus ducreyi*): Nonindurated **painful ulcer** with exudative base and inguinal lymphadenopathy
- Granuloma inguinale (donovanosis): **Painless beefy red** ulcers that form from **pseudo-buboes** common in tropics.

Which ulcerative lesions are painful and which are painless?

What is the difference between chancroid lesions and lymphogranuloma venereum?

Why is the VDRL or FTA-ABS test not performed for primary syphilis?

Rule out HIV in patients with lymphogranuloma venarum.

Why is penicillin used for neurosyphilis in patients who are allergic to penicillin? ***Penicillin is most effective.***

New-onset or changing murmur and fever are the most common findings in endocarditis.

37. What is the pathogenesis of syphilis?

Syphilis is an infection of the genital tract by the spirochete Treponema pallidum. Primary syphilis presents as a painless chancre on the genitals.

The first step in primary syphilis is to scrape and perform dark-field microscopy to identify the spirochetes. Do not perform the Venereal Disease Research Laboratory (VDRL) test or the fluorescent treponemal antibody-absorption (FTA-ABS) test in primary syphilis. Why? The results will be negative because antibodies take weeks to appear in serum.

38. How do patients with secondary syphilis present?

It occurs 2 to 8 weeks after the primary lesion. There is a widespread hematogenous spread of infection to many organs, including the skin, lymph nodes, and liver. The patient may present with a maculopapular rash on the palms and soles, with condyloma latum (warty wet lesion.) The first step is to obtain a VDRL test followed by an FTA-ABS test to confirm.

39. How do patients present with tertiary syphilis?

Patients present with neurological disease of the posterior or dorsal spinal columns (tabes dorsalis). Other organs affected include the heart (aortic root dilation) and bone (defects).

The first step is to obtain a VDRL test and to confirm with an FTA-ABS test. VDRL in cerebral spinal fluid (CSF) confirms neurosyphilis.

40. What are the treatment options for syphilis?

For primary and secondary syphilis, penicillin G can be used or doxycycline for patients who are allergic to penicillin, but for neurosyphilis, penicillin must be used regardless of allergies.

41. What is the definition of endocarditis?

Endocarditis is an infection of the endocardium of the heart valves. The patient may present nonspecifically with fever and weight loss.

42. What are the risk factors for endocarditis?

- Prosthetic heart valves
- Congenital heart defects
- IV drug use

Diagnosis: On the physical examination, the findings that are diagnostic include a new-onset murmur, immunological reactions (Janeway lesions and Osler node), and a hemorrhagic reaction (Roth spots). Complications in the form of systemic emboli from the vegetation fragments can damage blood vessels within various organs, including brain (stroke, paralysis), eye (blindness), spleen (splenic infarct), kidneys (renal infarct), pulmonary (hypoxia), and heart (myocardial infarction). Janeway lesions are nontender erythematous lesions on the palms and soles, and an Osler node is a tender nodule on the tip of the finger.

43. What are the organisms found in infectious endocarditis?

The most common cause of nonprosthetic valve endocarditis is Streptococcus species (including S. mutans and S. viridans). Staphylococcus, Enterococcus, and HACEK organisms (Haemophilus species, Actinobacillus actinomycetemcomitans, Cardiobacterium hominis, Eikenella corrodens, and Kingella species) may cause endocarditis. ***Staphylococcus aureus*** is the most common organism in those with **IV drug use**. IV drug endocarditis frequently involves the **tricuspid valve**.

The first step in diagnosing endocarditis is to obtain blood cultures and an echocardiogram (a transesophageal echocardiogram is more sensitive for diagnosis of endocarditis). Treat empirically with vancomycin (against Staphylococcus, Streptococcus, and Enterococcus) and cefepime (against gram-negative bacteria).

Staphylococcus aureus is the most common organism that can cause IV drug use endocarditis.

44. Libman-Sacks endocarditis is frequently an asymptomatic noninfectious endocarditis seen in systemic lupus erythematosus (SLE) patients. True or false?

True. Usually they are large verrucous lesions on the valve and asymptomatic, but they can fragment and cause systemic emboli and infective endocarditis.

45. How do patients with meningitis present?

Patients present with infection of the meninges. The patient may present with fever, headache, stiff neck, and sometimes photophobia and maculopapular rash.

46. List the causes of meningitis and common associations.

- Streptococcus pneumonia: Most common cause of **bacterial meningitis**

Why is ceftriaxone effective in treating meningitis?

- Meningococcemia: Look for petechiae and purpura rash in patients. In recurrent *Neisseria meningitidis* infection, screen for **complement deficiencies**.
- Group B strep meningitis: Common in **neonates**
- Aerobic gram-negative bacilli (including *Pseudomonas aeruginosa*) meningitis: Common in **hyperinfection syndrome** of **disseminated strongyloidiasis**
- Haemophilus influenzae: Consider this in patients with incomplete immunization.
- Listeria monocytogenes: This is common in elderly patients, infants, and renal transplant patients after consuming milk, cheese, raw vegetables, and coleslaw.
- Viral (herpes simplex virus [HSV]): HSV-1 is common in young adults. It is associated with **seizures** and **temporal enhancement** on imaging. CSF polymerase chain reaction (PCR) assay is diagnostic. Treat with acyclovir empirically. Resistance to acyclovir can be treated with foscarnet.
- Lyme disease: This is caused by Borrelia burgdorferi, a spirochete, and is common in individuals exposed to ticks. Treat meningitis with ceftriaxone.
- Syphilis: Secondary syphilis can cause meningitis.
- Cryptococcus: This is common in immunocompromised patients (e.g., AIDS patients). CSF with evidence of cryptococcal antigen is diagnostic. **India ink gram-positive stain** with evidence of encapsulated yeast organisms can also be used for identification. Treat with amphotericin B and flucytosine.

47. How is meningitis diagnosed on physical examination of the patient?

On the physical examination, look for neck stiffness, Brudzinski sign, and Kernig sign. Brudzinski sign is involuntary lifting of the legs on lifting the patient's head. Kernig sign is flexion of the hip and knee and subsequent extension that leads to painful resistance.

If the history and the findings from the physical examination are typical of meningitis, the first step is to obtain blood cultures, then to administer antibiotics, and then to obtain cerebral spinal fluid (Table 14-2). Why antibiotics first? Meningitis can be life-threatening; thus, waste no time.

48. What is hypoglycorrhachia?

Hypoglycorrhachia is a low glucose level in cerebrospinal

fluid (CSF), which occurs in bacterial, mycobacterial, mycoplasmal, and fungal meningitis. A CSF-to-serum glucose ratio of <0.4 is diagnostic. Normal CSF-to-serum ratio is 0.6.

Table 14-2. *CSF Laboratory Results for Meningitis*[a]

Organism	WBC Count (cells/μL)	Glucose (mg/dl)	Cells	Protein (mg/dl)
Virus	Increased (<250)	Normal	Lymphocytes	Increased (<200)
Bacteria	Increased (>1000)	Low (<40)	PMNs	Increased (>200)
Mycobacterium tuberculosis, *Cryptococcus*[b] (granulomatous diseases)	Increased	Low	Mononucleo-cytes	Increased

CSF, cerebral spinal fluid; PMN, polymorphonuclear neutrophil; WBC, white blood cell.

a Memorize Table 14-2. Normal CSF values: WBC 0-5, glucose 50-75, protein 15-40.

b WBC, glucose, and protein are only slightly abnormal with mononuclear predominance.

49. What is the empirical treatment for meningitis?

Treat meningitis with broad-spectrum cephalosporin (ceftriaxone, cefotaxime, ceftazidime, cefepime). Add ampicillin if the patient is elderly (>50 years old), or an infant (0-3 months old), **or immunocompromised** to work against Listeria monocytogenes and Haemophilus influenza (infants only). Add vancomycin in all patients if you suspect staphylococci and penicillin-resistant S. pneumoniae.

Steroid treatment can be added if suspicion for bacterial meningitis is high because it reduces meningeal inflammation after antimicrobial-induced lysis of meningeal organisms.

50. When is prophylaxis of meningitis initiated?

Exposure to a patient who has meningitis can be treated with rifampin or ciprofloxacin.

51. In all types of meningitis, always consider using broad spectrum cephalosporin (e.g., ceftriaxone). True or false?

True. Why? Ceftriaxone and other broad spectrum cephalosporin penetrate the blood-brain barrier and are active against the most common cause of meningitis (*S. pneumoniae*).

What is the benefit of steroid treatment for meningitis in children?

52. What complication of meningitis is feared?
Residual neurological defects can occur.

53. How do patients with viral encephalitis present?
Patients present with infection of the brain parenchyma. The patient may present with personality changes, fever, headache, nausea and vomiting, memory loss, and photosensitivity.

Some common causes are arboviruses such as the **West Nile virus** (associated tremors, myoclonus, **paralysis**, and parkinsonism), the varicella zoster virus (grouped vesicles in dermatomal pattern), and the herpes simplex virus (associated seizures and focal deficits). If encephalopathy is caused by the herpes simplex virus, temporal lobe dysfunction (edema or enhanced contrast activity in this region **on brain imaging**) will be present. Treat according to underlying causes (e.g., treat HSV with acyclovir).

54. MRI is more sensitive than CT scan for diagnosis of brain abscess. True or false?
True. MRI may show early signs such as cerebritis and a spread to ventricles and the subarachnoid space.

55. List some predisposing conditions for brain abscess.
Predisposing conditions include sinusitis, dental work, penetrating head trauma, otitis media, lung abscess, and endocarditis.

What is the difference between HIV and other immunodeficiency syndromes?

56. How do patients present with acute HIV infection?
Acute presentation: The patient may present with fever, chills, lymphadenopathy, and a viral-like infection. Test results for HIV are usually negative for HIV antibodies or indeterminate for Western blot, but **HIV RNA** results are positive.

57. What is the current definition of AIDS?
AIDS is defined as a CD4 count of <200 cells/mm3 or the development of an opportunistic infection.

58. What are risk factors for HIV?
- Anal receptive sex is still the most common risk factor.
- Unprotected sex
- IV drug use

59. What is the first step in the diagnosis of HIV?
Perform an enzyme-linked immunosorbent assay (ELISA) test and then a Western blot test to confirm.

60. When is treatment initiated in patients with HIV?

In 2012, antiretroviral therapy was recommended for all HIV-infected patients, including asymptomatic patients, regardless of immune status. Two nonnucleoside reverse transcriptase inhibitors plus a protease inhibitor or a nonnucleoside reverse transcriptase inhibitor are used in combination.

All HIV infected patients should be treated.

61. HIV lipodystrophy is associated with HIV-protease inhibitor. True or false?

True. It is a combination of fat loss in the limbs and fat accumulation in the abdomen. This can lead to hyperlipidemia and insulin resistance.

62. What are the various opportunistic infections in AIDS?

- Toxoplasmosis: The patient will present with a ring-enhanced lesion in the brain. Treat with sulfadiazine and pyrimidine.
- PCP pneumonia: The patient may present with a CXR finding of interstitial infiltrates. Treat with Bactrim. Add adjunctive steroids if PO2 <70 mm Hg or A-a gradient >35.
- Cytomegalovirus (CMV): The patient may present with end-organ damage or **retinitis**. Laboratory tests will show intracellular inclusion cells **and multinucleated giant cells**. Treat with ganciclovir.
- Esophagitis: The patient may present with pain on swallowing. The most common cause is Candida; therefore, the first step is to treat with an antifungal drug (azole). If this fails, then do a biopsy to rule out HSV-1 or CMV. Both viruses have inclusion bodies, but CMV has a larger inclusion body.
- ***Cryptococcus*** **meningitis**

63. What are preventive therapies against opportunistic infections in patients with AIDS?

- CD4 count <200 cells/mm^3: For Pneumocystis pneumonia, administer TMP/SMX (Bactrim (trimethoprim/sulfamethoxazole, TMP/SMX), dapsone, or atovaquone.
- CD4 count <100 cells/mm^3: Administer TMP/SMX or pyrimethamine for ***Toxoplasma*** (against toxoplasmosis).
- CD4 count <50 cells/mm^3: For Mycobacterium avium complex (MAC), administer macrolide

E. coli o157:H7 is an entero-hemorrhagic E.coli that causes HUS.

(azithromycin); perform a dilated retinal examination every 6 months for **CMV** retinitis.

64. What are the prophylactic vaccines required for patients with HIV?

- Hepatitis A
- Hepatitis B
- Influenza
- Pneumococcal vaccine
- Measles-mumps-rubella (MMR), if CD4 count >200

65. What are some important conditions that need to be screened for in patients with HIV?

Screen for hepatitis C, hepatitis B, and cervical cancer; do a PPD skin test for TB.

66. What are the risk factors for gastroenteritis and the causative organisms?

- Unpasteurized milk: **Listeriosis**
- Norovirus: Prominent vomiting plus diarrhea and **outbreaks**
- Child daycare centers: Shigella (gram-negative rod)
- Poultry: Campylobacter jejuni (gram-negative rod) and **nontyphoid salmonellae**
- Trip to Mexico/Caribbean and ground beef: Escherichia coli (gram-negative rod)
- Salad and mayonnaise: Staphylococcus aureus (gram-positive cocci in clusters)
- Unclean drinking water (hikers who drink water in the wilderness), fecal–oral route (child daycare centers): Giardiasis diarrhea is usually >10 days with weight loss from malabsorption caused by Giardia lamblia, an enteric protozoan.
- E. coli o157:H7: An enterohemorrhagic E.coli that causes hemolytic uremic syndrome
- Yersinia enterocolitica (gram-negative rod): Causes pain in right lower quadrant and mesenteric adenitis, mimicking appendicitis
- Antibiotic use: ***Clostridium difficile*** diarrhea
- Vibrio parahaemolyticus: Associated with bloody diarrhea and **ingestion of seafood**
- Vibrio cholera: Associated with explosive diarrhea and **outbreaks**
- Consumption of undercooked or uncooked **fish**: *Diphyllobothrium latum* (fish tapeworm) can present

with nonspecific diarrhea and megaloblastic anemia with **vitamin B12 deficiency**. Prevalent in northern Europe and Japan. Stool microscopy identifies egg in stool. Treatment is praziquantel.

67. Severe chronic diarrhea associated with cryptosporidiosis is found in what patient population?

It is found in HIV patients.

68. What are the most common causes of infectious chronic diarrhea?

The most common causes are intestinal **amebiasis and protozoal species** such as *Giardia*, *Cryptosporidium*, and *Isospora*.

69. What is the pathogenesis of a hydatid cyst?

A hydatid cyst forms when eggs of Echinococcus are ingested by humans via a sheep host. The eggs form a cyst (or cysts) in the liver that becomes calcified.

Serological analysis can confirm the diagnosis. A computed tomography (CT) scan of the liver can aid in diagnosis by showing a cystic mass.

Treatment: Albendazole

What is the difference between hydatid cyst and amebic abscess?

70. How may an ascariasis infection present?

It is caused by Ascariasis lumbricoides, an intestinal roundworm prevalent in tropical regions, usually acquired via ingestion of eggs in contaminated soil and water and usually asymptomatic. It can present with symptoms when worm larvae migrate through the lungs (cough) or adult worms develop in the intestine (intestinal obstruction, nutritional deficiency). Stool microscopy can identify eggs. Treatment is albendazole.

71. Perianal itching that occurs predominantly at night is characteristic of which infection?

It is characteristic of infection with Enterobius vermicularis (pinworm), which is ingested by scratching the perianal region and transferring eggs to the mouth or from person to person. Infection can also cause abdominal pain. Diagnosis is via cellophane tape against the perianal area and looking for eggs. Treatment is albendazole.

72. What is the significance of loiasis?

Also known as African eye worm, loiasis is endemic to central and West Africa, caused by a nematode known as Loa loa. Most patients will present with subcutaneous swellings (Calabar swellings) and migration of the worm in the conjunctiva. Treatment with diethylcarbamazine can precipitate encephalitis or shock.

73. Where is an amebic abscess acquired?

An amebic abscess from Entamoeba histolytica can be acquired from central or south America. It causes inflammatory diarrhea and a liver abscess.

Serological analysis can confirm the diagnosis. A CT scan of the liver can aid in diagnosis by showing a mass.

Treat with metronidazole.

An MRI is the preferred study for the diagnosis of osteomyelitis.

74. What is the pathogenesis of osteomyelitis?

Osteomyelitis is an infection that originates most commonly in the metaphyseal region of bone. Why? This is an area of blood stasis. The patient will present with a limp, or pain around the involved area, and fever.

An X-ray will be diagnostic after a week. An MRI/CT scan or a bone scan/**indium labeled leukocyte scan** is diagnostic in the first 24-48 hours. **MRI is preferred.** If hardware (metal, pacemaker, stent) is present, a **bone scan** can be used. Treatment: Surgery for debridement and biopsy for identification of causative pathogens prior to empiric treatment with vancomycin and piperacillin-tazobactam or ampicillin/sulbactam

Staphylococcus aureus is the most common cause in all ages. If a patient has sickle cell anemia, suspect Salmonella, as it is the most common cause in this group. Treat these patients with ceftriaxone.

75. What is the differential diagnosis of liver abscess (pyogenic abscess) seen on imaging?

Most pyogenic liver abscesses are due to **biliary tract infection** or **infections** via the portal or hepatic vein. Common organisms are *E. coli*, *Klebsiella*, and streptococcal species. Suspect **amoebic abscess** in those from developing countries or with fever, respiratory symptoms (cough), and gastrointestinal symptoms (abdominal pain). IV antibiotics and eventual percutaneous drainage is needed.

76. Pseudomonas aeruginosa (gram-negative rod) is the most common cause of osteomyelitis or soft tissue infection in patients that have been punctured by a nail. True or false?

True. Ciprofloxacin, with or without ceftazidime or cefepime, is active against Pseudomonas. Other types of puncture wounds should cover S. aureus or beta-hemolytic streptococci.

What is the difference between the ROM in osteomyelitis and that of septic arthritis?

77. What is the pathogenesis of septic arthritis?

Septic arthritis is an infection in the joint space. **Intravenous drug users** and patients with prior **joint surgery**, prior damaged joints, and **diabetes** are at risk. The patient presents with severe **monoarticular** pain and significant reduction in ROM.

The first step is to perform an arthrocentesis to analyze synovial fluid. Synovial fluid is diagnostic if **>100,000 leukocytes/ml**. ***Staphylococcus aureus*** is the most common cause of native joint septic arthritis.

Treat these patients with empiric IV ceftriaxone plus IV oxacillin or vancomycin for a minimum of 4 weeks.

If you suspect N. gonorrhoeae, perform blood, cervical, nasopharyngeal, and stool cultures.

78. List the risk factors for septic arthritis and the organisms responsible.

- Intravenous drug users: **Suspect *Pseudomonas*.**
- Cat bite: Suspect *Pasturella multocida*.
- Immunosuppressed: Suspect mycobacterial, fungal, and viral organisms.
- Prosthesis: Suspect ***Staphylococcus epidermidis***.

79. What are the treatment options for osteomyelitis?

Treatment options include empiric vancomycin plus or minus ceftriaxone IV. Once blood culture results confirm the organism, treat with IV antibiotics for a total of 4 weeks.

80. PCP pneumonia prophylaxis with TMP/SMX should be offered to those taking steroids for the long term. True or false?

True.

81. Neuraminidase inhibitors can be given to immunosuppressed patients exposed to influenza within 48 hours for prophylaxis. True or false?

True.

82. PPD skin testing is indicated before beginning treatment with an anti-TNF agent. True or false?

True. If skin induration is >5 mm, then treat.

Avoid steroids in patients with strongyloidiasis to avoid hyperinfection syndrome.

83. Varicella immunoglobulin is given only in what situations?

Varicella vaccine is given within 3 days in those exposed to contagious varicella without a prior history of the vaccine. If contraindicated (i.e., pregnancy, immunosuppressed), then give varicella immunoglobulin.

84. List some viruses that can cause hemorrhagic fever.

- Dengue fever: A small RNA virus transmitted by **mosquitoes**, it may present as **high fever** and nausea/vomiting associated with **petechial** hemorrhages. Laboratory results reveal **leukopenia** and **thrombocytopenia**.
- Lassa fever, Ebola fever, and Bolivian fever may present the same way.

85. What virus may be reactivated in those with a renal transplant?

Polyomavirus BK, which is acquired asymptomatically in childhood, may be reactivated. It can present as nephropathy and mental status change.

86. What virus may be reactivated in those with HIV or in patients with stem cell transplants?

Polyomavirus JC may be reactivated. It can cause leukoencephalopathy. Patients can present with severe dementia and white matter abnormality on imaging.

87. How may patients present with strongyloidiasis (caused by *Strongyloides*)?

Patients may present with pulmonary, intestinal, or CNS symptoms, as the organism is a nematode that remains dormant for years in the gastrointestinal tract, but in immunosuppressed patients, it migrates to the **lungs** and **brain**. Treat it with ivermectin. A **hyperinfection syndrome** in which patients present with exaggerated symptoms can occur in those **taking steroids**.

88. What is the significance of herpes labialis infection (cold sores)?

An immunocompetent patient may present with cold sores, fever, and blisters, which usually resolve in 7-10 days. Acyclovir can improve healing by 1 day. In immunosuppressed patients, acyclovir can help heal within 10-14 days.

89. How may patients present with Lyme disease?

Lyme disease is common in areas with a deer population.

- Early presentation (3-30 days): **Erythema migrans rash** (erythematous rash with central clearing) and nonspecific viral-like syndrome
- Disseminated (weeks to months): **CNS** (meningitis), facial palsy, heart block
- Late (years): **Monoarticular arthritis**

Erythema migrans is diagnostic of early lyme disease.

90. What are diagnostic tests for Lyme disease?
Serology ELISA and Western blot are diagnostic.

91. What are treatment options for Lyme disease?
Treat it with ampicillin, amoxicillin, ceftriaxone, or doxycycline, but **doxycycline** is preferred. Individuals exposed to patients with Lyme disease are treated prophylactically with doxycycline.

92. List some vector-borne diseases and areas of predominance.

- Babesiosis: Transmitted by the *Ixodes* tick, it is a protozoan-borne illness. It is endemic to the **northeastern United States**, especially Rhode Island and New England. Intracellular organisms in RBCs are usually present as basophilic inclusion bodies. The presence of inclusion bodies characterized by **Maltese cross Maltese cross formations** inside RBCs is pathognomonic. Treatment is atovaquone and azithromycin or clindamycin and quinine. Always consider **Lyme disease and anaplasmosis** in patients with babesiosis, since they share the same tick vector (*Ixodes scapularis*).
- Ehrlichiosis: Bacteria that resemble *Rickettsia* are transmitted by the lone star tick. Ehrlichiosis is endemic to the **southeastern**, **south central**, and **eastern** United States. Treatment is doxycycline.
- Rocky mountain spotted fever: This is transmitted by the dog tick *Dermacentor variabilis* in the **southeastern and south central United States**.
- Lyme disease: This occurs between May and November, peaking in June or July. It is present in **most states**, but is more common in the **Midwest** and **eastern** United States.
- Malaria: This is mostly caused by the protozoan *Plasmodium falciparum*, transmitted by mosquitos in **Africa**, leading to fevers, rigors, headache, and hemolytic anemia. Severe illness can lead to hypoglycemia,

Rose spots are salmon-colored spots on the abdomen and trunk.

lactic acidosis, and cerebral malaria (confusion, seizures, coma, death). When it causes anemia, a peripheral smear can detect **intracellular (RBC) parasites, which presents as inclusion bodies inside RBCs.** Treat with quinine plus doxycycline, pyrimethamine-sulfadoxine, or clindamycin.

- *Borrelia hermsii*: This is caused by a spirochete that causes **relapsing fever** (e.g., fever for 5 days, and then symptom free for another 5 days). It is a tick-borne illness common in **mountainous areas** of the **west** and desert areas of the **southwest** United States. Treatment is doxycycline or tetracycline.

93. List some endemic regions and parasitic or bacterial diseases.

- Leishmaniasis: Endemic to Latin America and the **Middle East** (soldiers from Iraq), it is transmitted by the **sandfly**, infecting hematopoietic cell lines and causing mucocutaneous lesions, leukopenia, fever, and splenomegaly. Treat with amphotericin B.
- Typhoid fever: *Salmonella typhi* is transmitted by fecal or oral routes or in contaminated water. It is endemic to **Asia** (China, Pakistan, India, Bangladesh), **Africa**, and the **Caribbean**. Patients present with **high fever**, abdominal pain, rash (**rose spots**), relative **bradycardia**, and splenomegaly over 1-3 weeks. Treat with broad-spectrum antibiotics.
- Schistosomiasis: *S. mansoni* causes intestinal and liver disease; it is transmitted by a fluke trematode. Endemic to **tropical** or subtropical areas, the **Caribbean**, and the **Middle East**, it is transmitted in **fresh water**, with symptoms occurring 4-8 weeks after contact.
- *S. haematobium*: This causes **hematuria**, bladder ulcers, and risk of **bladder cancer**. Treatment is praziquantel.
- Cysticercosis: It is caused by the larval stage of the tapeworm of *Taenia solium* (**pork tapeworm**), transmitted fecal-orally by those that have ingested **undercooked pork**. It is endemic to **Central and South America**, sub-Saharan Africa, India, and Asia. Symptoms are due to cysts formed by *T. solium* in several tissues, causing **neurocysticercosis** (intracranial cystic masses with calcifications that can cause **seizures**) and ocular, muscular, or cardiac cysticercosis. Treat

neurocysticercosis with anticonvulsants and antiparasitic agents (albendazole or praziquantel).

- Leptospirosis: Caused by a spirochete, *Leptospira interrogans*, it is transmitted by contaminated soil or by rodents to people while they **perform outdoor activities**. The symptoms are nonspecific myalgia, fever, and rigors. It is common in **southern** and **pacific coastal states** (most common in **Hawaii**) in the United States or the tropics.

94. What is a Jarisch-Herxheimer reaction?

This reaction consists of symptoms such as fever, rigors, myalgias and hypotension, which occur a few hours to 24 hours after treatment of spirochete or bacterial infections with antibiotics. It is thought to be related to inflammatory cytokines. Antipyretics can be used for treatment.

95. List the key findings for viral exanthems.

- Mumps: This is associated with **parotid swelling** and **orchitis.**
- Measles (rubeola): A maculopapular rash that starts on the forehead, and then moves to the face, torso, and extremities in 24-48 hours. It is associated with **Koplik spots (oral white papules on buccal mucosa lesions that are pathognomonic),** coryza, and conjunctivitis. **Vitamin A** can help in the treatment of measles.
- Rubella: The patient presents with a **maculopapular rash** and posterior cervical lymphadenopathy.
- Roseola (human herpesvirus 6): A high fever that appears and completely resolves followed by the appearance of rash is diagnostic.
- Chickenpox (varicella virus): This presents as a rash in **various stages of healing** with a **vesicular**, crusting, and **erythematous rash**.
- Small pox (variola virus): Caused by a double-stranded DNA orthopox virus, symptoms include high fever, vomiting, headache, abdominal pain, and maculopapular rash or pustules on the face and extremities. Give a vaccination to persons exposed and immunoglobulin to pregnant or immunosuppressed patients.

96. What is the differential diagnosis of maculopapular rash and fever?

Consider enterovirus, meningococcemia, human monocytic ehrlichiosis, and Rocky Mountain spotted fever (RMSF).

What are Koplik spots?

Resolved fever followed by rash is characteristic of what viral exanthem?

Smallpox was eradicated in 1979 but it can be used as a potential bioterrorism agent as it has a high mortality rate.

In smallpox, the rash (exanthem) often comes later, after the onset of lesions in the mucous membranes (enanthem), and constitutional symptoms.

The rash in rocky mountain spotted fever usually appears between the 3rd and 5th day and begins with a red, blanching rash.

97. A tick-borne disease associated with rhabdomyolysis, thrombocytopenia, leukopenia, and transaminitis suggests what type of maculopapular rash and fever?

It suggests ehrlichiosis or anaplasmosis (usually no rash). Always consider ehrlichiosis and anaplasmosis in patients with RMSF.

98. What are the clinical features of Rocky Mountain spotted fever?

This is a tick-borne disease with a **triad** of fever, rash, and a history of tick bite. It is caused by *Rickettsia rickettsii* (a gram-negative, obligate intracellular coccobacillus).The patient presents with **fever** and a **maculopapular** rash (purpura and petechia) that extends from the extremities (wrist and ankle) to the head and trunk **rapidly over hours**. Treatment is doxycycline.

99. List some potential bioterrorism agents.

- Anthrax: Caused by aerosolization of the bacteria *Bacillus anthracis*, it can cause **skin necrosis** and **intestinal** and **pulmonary** hemorrhage. Treatment is fluoroquinolone or doxycycline.
- Bubonic plague: Transmitted by rat fleas or aerosolization of the bacteria *Yersinia pestis* (gram-negative coccobacilli), it can result in **cutaneous lesions** in the form of extremely **tender masses** (buboes) and **hemoptysis**. The inhaled form can cause severe sepsis and pneumonia. Treatment is streptomycin.

100. List the common causes of skin lesions that occur during travel abroad.

Common causes of skin lesions are as follows:

- Cutaneous larva migrans: It is the most common **migratory skin infection** caused by hookworms. Hookworms create a serpiginous (**snake-like) eruption** on the skin of the feet, thighs, or buttocks by penetrating the skin. Humans are infected by contact with **contaminated soil**. Self-limited or treatment with albendazole.
- Dengue fever: This causes **petechia or a hemorrhagic rash** with severe itching toward the end of the febrile period.
- Skin abscess, insect bites
- Leishmaniasis: Symptoms can range from localized lesions, papules that turn into **painless ulcers**

with heaped up edges, mucosal lesions, and diffuse cutaneous lesions, which are nodules that do not ulcerate. Biopsy will reveal Leishman-Donovan bodies (amastigotes).

101. Recurrent infections with bacterial and fungal infections that are severe should prompt testing for what congenital disorder?

Consider chronic granulomatous disease, a genetic disorder with a defect in phagocyte NADPH oxidase, which results in defective phagocytes that commonly affect the lung, skin, lymph nodes, and liver. Neutrophil function testing by a nitroblue tetrazolium reduction test is diagnostic. Lifetime prophylaxis with antibiotics and antifungals is indicated.

Nitroblue tetrazolium reduction test checks for NADPH oxidase activity, which is absent in chronic granulomatous disease.

102. Recurrent sinopulmonary infections that are severe should prompt testing for what primary immunodeficiency?

Consider primary humoral immune deficiency with impaired B cells and antibody production causing susceptibility to encapsulated bacteria (Streptococus pneumonia, Haemophilus influenzae) and viruses.

Examples of primary humoral syndromes are X-linked agammaglobulinemia (male patients with recurrent otitis media and enteroviruses); common variable immunodeficiency (low IgG, IgA, and/or IgM); and hyper IgM syndromes (normal or elevated serum IgM and deficiency in IgA, IgG, and IgE).

Chapter 15
Neurology

Ten percent of patients with myasthenia gravis have associated thymoma.

1. What is the definition of Guillain-Barré (GB) syndrome?

Guillain-Barré syndrome is an ascending paralysis due to demyelization of the peripheral nerves. The patient will present with extremity weakness after a viral illness, **immunization**, or surgical procedure. On the physical examination, the deep tendon reflexes are diminished. A deadly complication is respiratory depression.

Treatment: Intravenous immunoglobulin for acute GB; steroids for chronic GB

2. What is the definition of myasthenia gravis?

Myasthenia gravis is an autoimmune disease that affects the neuromuscular junction in which antibodies against acetylcholine bind to postsynaptic receptors, causing generalized muscle weakness. Diagnosis is made by **Tensilon (edrophonium) test** and serological test for **acetylcholine receptor antibody** and confirmed with an EMG. **EMG** will show further worsening in muscle weakness with repetitive nerve stimulation while the **tension test** will show improvement in muscle weakness with drug infusion.

Most patients present initially with ptosis. After diagnosis, the next step is to obtain a chest X-ray (CXR). Why? Ten percent of patients with myasthenia gravis have associated thymoma.

Treatment: Steroids, pyridostigmine (acetylcholinesterase inhibitor). Intravenous immunoglobulin can be used for those with severe respiratory muscle weakness and dysphagia, and thymectomy can be used for thymoma.

3. How may patients present with muscle dysfunction (myopathy)?

Patients may present with muscle weakness in the lower extremities (difficulty climbing stairs or difficulty going from sitting to standing) or upper extremities (difficulty raising objects above head). These are examples of proximal muscle weakness.

4. What is the most common cause of myopathies?

The most common cause is **proximal muscle weakness.**

5. What is the most common presentation of rhabdomyolysis?

Rhabdomyolysis indicates muscle destruction, with patients commonly presenting after **rigorous exercise** with **cola-colored urine**, which indicates myoglobin release. Other causes of rhabdomyolysis are drugs, electrolyte abnormalities, alcohol, inflammatory myopathy, and infections.

The major causes of myopathy are inflammatory disorders, metabolic disorders (glycogen storage diseases), endocrinopathies (thyroid dysfunction or Cushing's syndrome), drug and toxins, infections and rhabdomyolysis.

6. What type of myopathies may present with constant muscle weakness?

Congenital myopathies such **as muscular dystrophies** manifest as nonprogressive weakness that is constant over many years. Look for dysmorphic features. Inflammatory myopathies such as polymyositis/dermatomyositis can also present as constant weakness.

7. When a patient presents with periodic muscle weakness, what is this suggestive of?

Periodic muscle weakness or paralysis is suggestive of **mitochondria myopathies**, which cause muscle channel abnormalities, and metabolic myopathies such as **lipid storage diseases** and acid maltase deficiency.

8. Systemic myopathies can cause cardiac diseases and respiratory failure. True or false?

True. **Myotonic dystrophy** and some muscular dystrophies can cause arrhythmias and congestive heart failure, and some **metabolic myopathies** and **myotonic dystrophy** can cause respiratory failure by causing diaphragmatic weakness.

9. What common drug agents can cause myopathies?

- Steroids: Cause proximal muscle weakness

- HMG-CoA inhibitors (statins): Cause proximal muscle weakness, myalgias, and cramps

10. List the three different manifestations of neuropathy (nerve dysfunction).

- Motor nerve involvement: Presents as muscle weakness
- Sensory nerve involvement: Presents as numbness, tingling, pain
- Autonomic nerve involvement: Presents as orthostatic hypotension, impotence, arrhythmias, bladder dysfunction

11. In a patient with muscle weakness, how does the physical examination differentiate between neuropathy and myopathy?

- Proximal muscle weakness: Usually myopathy
- Segmental weakness: Usually neuropathy (anterior horn cell), multiple myotomes in many distributions
- Task-specific fatigable weakness: Usually neuropathy, neuromuscular transmission abnormality
- Sensory abnormality: Neuropathy
- Diminished reflexes: Neuropathy

Polyneuropathy is neuropathy affecting the peripheral nerves.

12. What is the most common cause of hereditary neuropathy?

Charcot-Marie-Tooth disease is most common, in which patients present in the **first decade** with clumsiness and neuromuscular findings such as distal muscle atrophy, weakness, sensory loss with pes cavus (high arches), and hammertoes.

13. What are the two types of neuropathies?

- Axonal neuropathy: Most weakness in distal extremity
- Demyelinating neuropathy: Most weakness in proximal, distal, and facial muscles

14. The major risk factor for botulinum toxin is an infant who ingests honey. True or false?

True. The patient presents with rapidly progressing paralysis **and cranial nerve abnormalities** within hours of ingesting honey containing a neurotoxin produced by *Clostridium botulinum*, a gram-positive spore-forming bacterium. The toxin can also be transmitted in food, or

The hallmarks of NF1 are cafe au lait spots and neurofibromas.

by growth of the organism in wounds or in the intestine. A major complication is respiratory depression.

15. List the key findings in some cutaneous-neurological syndromes.

- Neurofibromatosis 1: Mutation in *NF1* gene, a tumor suppressor gene causing multiple **café au lait spots (6-7 spots) and two or more neurofibromas,** which are diagnostic. It is also associated with iris hamartoma **(Lisch nodules), optic glioma,** inguinal or axillary freckles, bone abnormalities, and presence in a first-degree relative.
- Neurofibromatosis 2: A chromosome 22 gene is affected, causing multiple CNS tumors. The most commonly associated tumors are bilateral acoustic neuromas **(eighth nerve masses)**. Cutaneous findings can occur in the form of subcutaneous nodules or plaque-like lesions (swelling of peripheral nerve).
- Tuberous sclerosis: Autosomal dominant defect in tumor suppressor gene causes **cerebral** and **cerebellar tubers**. Dermatologic findings, such as ash green patches (hypopigmented spots), shagreen patches (**connective tissue nevus** thickening of the skin), and angiofibromas (flesh-colored papules on the malar region of the face), help point to the diagnosis. The patient has associated infantile spasms (jerky movements in the neck or extremities). Treat infantile spasms with adrenocorticotropic hormone. Obtain renal ultrasound to look for renal angiomyolipomas.
- Von Hippel-Lindau (VHL) syndrome: Autosomal dominant inheritance of tumor suppressor gene causing various benign and malignant tumors, including retinal **hemangioblastoma** (orange yellow tumor on funduscopy), cerebellar hemangioblastoma, renal cell cancer, pheochromocytoma, endolymphatic tumors of the middle ear, pancreatic tumors, and epididymal and broad ligament cysts. There are no cutaneous findings in VHL syndrome.
- Sturge-Weber syndrome: Embryonal abnormality in neural crest cells causing a **port-wine stain** (facial angioma) on the face in the first division of the trigeminal nerve and **hemangioma** in the brain. Most patients have **glaucoma.** The patient will present with seizures, visual changes, **and intracranial calcifications.**

- Osler-Weber-Rendu syndrome: Autosomal dominant condition that causes **mucocutaneous hemorrhagic telangiectasias, epistaxis,** and **arteriovenous malformations** in lungs, CNS, liver, and intestinal tract.

16. What is the differential diagnosis of acute onset cerebellar ataxia?

Alcohol abuse, vitamin B12 deficiency; medication toxicity; toxic agents; cerebellar stroke; basilar meningitis (e.g., TB or listeria); cerebellitis (e.g., varicella zoster virus, rubeola, JC virus, or pertussis), cerebellar abscess

17. What is the differential diagnosis of chronic cerebellar ataxia?

Consider neurodegenerative ataxia and hereditary ataxia.

18. In patients younger than 30 years old, what form of chronic cerebellar ataxia should be considered?

Friedreich ataxia should be considered. This is an autosomal recessive condition caused by excessive **trinucleotide repeats** that leads to demyelination of nerve fibers with **slowly progressive** ataxia and **peripheral neuropathy**, muscle weakness, areflexia, and extensor reflexes of the extremities, which lead to the patient being wheelchair bound before age 45. It has the same spinal cord pathology and symptoms as subacute combined degeneration.

19. What are the types of seizure disorders?

Partial

- Simple partial: The patient may present with motor, sensory, and psychotic acts with no loss of consciousness. It is the only seizure disorder with **no loss of consciousness.**
- Complex partial: **Automatisms** without direction occur (e.g., repetitive acts with no purpose) with loss of consciousness. The patient may have olfactory **hallucinations** or strange feelings prior to episodes (e.g., smelling burnt rubber).

Generalized

- Absent seizures: Patients have a **blank stare** associated with loss of consciousness. An electrocardiogram shows **three wave-spike-wave patterns** in 1 second. Treatment: Ethosuximide or valproic acid
- Tonic clonic: Sustained **contractions** alternating with **stiffness**. Tonic clonic is associated with **bowel** and

What is the only seizure disorder without loss of awareness?

What is the difference between prophylactic and abortive therapy for migraine?

urine incontinence, irregular breathing, and a postictal phase of fatigue. Treatment: Anticonvulsant

Complication of seizure disorders: Status **epilepticus**. This is a continuous seizure activity lasting **more than 30 minutes**.

Juvenile myoclonic seizures (rapid jerks) are a subset of generalized seizures in adolescence that occur soon **after awakening** and are precipitated by alcohol, **sleep deprivation**, and flickering lights. It can occur with other seizure disorders. Treatment is lamotrigine or valproic acid.

20. What are causes of headache?

- Migraine: **Unilateral headache** associated with nausea, vomiting, and photosensitivity. It is alleviated by rest or lying down in a quiet, dark room. Treat it with NSAIDs (abortive), selective serotonin (5HT1) agonists (abortive) or opioid agonists (abortive), beta-blockers (prophylactic), calcium blockers (prophylactic), or topiramate (prophylactic).
- Tension headache: **Diffuse headache** associated with stress, neck pain, and constant headache. Treat it with NSAIDs.
- Pseudotumor cerebri: Intracranial benign hypertension seen in **overweight women** associated with corticosteroid and tetracycline usage. Patients may present with new-onset **non-throbbing headache** worsened with cough or position. It may also cause transient vision loss, diplopia, or sixth nerve palsy. On the physical examination, **papilledema** is noted. The lumbar puncture shows **elevated cerebrospinal fluid pressure**. Treat with serial lumbar punctures or acetazolamide.

21. What are the most common primary headaches?

Migraine and menstrual migraine, medication overuse, tension, and cluster headaches are most common.

22. Percutaneous estradiol to suppress menses and used through the menses is effective for menstrual migraines. True or false?

True. A low estrogen level prior to menses is thought to contribute to menstrual migraines. Naproxen and certain triptans other than sumatriptan can also be used. Oral contraceptives are contraindicated in migraines.

23. Patients who use medications for headaches more than 2 days week are at increased risk for medication overuse headache. True or false?

True. Patients may present with headache **soon after waking up** and medication may reduce headache, but not completely relieve it.

24. Cluster headache, like migraine headache, can cause autonomic symptoms. True or false?

True. Both types of headache can cause **rhinorrhea, nasal congestion**, and **ptosis**, but cluster headaches usually lasts 15 minutes to 3 hours, whereas migraines last 4 to 72 hours. Patients with cluster headaches usually do not have pain between episodes. In addition, cluster headaches **worsen with rest** and patients cannot sit still.

25. Differentiate cluster headaches from trigeminal autonomic cephalalgias.

Trigeminal autonomic cephalalgias such as paroxysmal hemicranias present **similarly to cluster headaches** and are differentiated on the basis of duration (last 15 minutes) and frequency (occur about 10 times a day). Treat paroxysmal hemicranias with indomethacin, and cluster headaches with 100% oxygen (acute therapy) or verapamil and prednisone (prophylactic therapy).

What is the difference between cluster headache and migraines?

26. Vascular loops of blood vessels compressing the trigeminal nerve can cause trigeminal neuralgia. True or false?

True. Patients with **trigeminal neuralgia** may present at age >40 years with sharp stabbing facial pain that lasts seconds to minutes brought on by chewing, brushing, or face washing. Most cases are idiopathic. If it presents at a younger age, look for secondary causes such as vascular loop compression or multiple sclerosis.

Treat with an anticonvulsant such as carbamazepine.

27. Which condition may present with unilateral headache or orbital pain associated with Horner's syndrome?

Internal **carotid artery dissection** may present this way. It usually occurs after head and neck trauma, but can be spontaneous. Dissection can also lead to carotid thrombus occlusion or distal arterial branch embolus occlusion to cause a stroke.

Anisocoria that is more in the dark (small pupil with dilation lag and ptosis) may suggest sympathetic dysfunction.

Anisocoria tha is greater in the light (large pupil is abnormal, ptosis/ ophthalmoplegia) suggests 3rd nerve palsy.

28. How may neck trauma lead to Horner syndrome?

Neck trauma may cause carotid dissection as a result of sympathetic chain transection. Examination of the patient reveals the presence of anisocoria as a dilation lag in the affected smaller pupil in darkness. Greater anisocoria in darkness is characteristic of sympathetic dysfunction.

29. Unilateral severe headache in a young patient with risk factors for thrombosis should be worked up for what condition?

Consider cerebral venous sinus thrombosis.

30. What are the various mechanisms of action of anticonvulsant medications?

Most anticonvulsants work by blocking sodium-dependent voltage channels (carbamazepine, phenytoin) or calcium-dependent channels (ethosuximide); activating GABA activity (benzodiazepine, phenobarbital); or by a mixture of these mechanisms (valproic acid, topiramate). The mechanism of action of levetiracetam is unknown; gabapentin and pregabalin inhibit voltage-gated calcium channels.

31. What are some anticonvulsant drugs that are not metabolized in the liver?

An anticonvulsant drug not metabolized in the liver is levetiracetam (Keppra). It is excreted unchanged in the urine. Pregabalin and gabapentin also do not have significant metabolism in the liver and can be used in those who have liver disease.

32. Which antiepileptic medication may worsen generalized absence and myoclonic seizures?

Carbamazepine may worsen these seizures.

33. What is the strategy for treating status epilepticus?

Initial therapy: Benzodiazepine plus phenytoin

If this fails, consider initiating phenobarbital. If seizures persist, initiate a phenobarbital coma by administering a phenobarbital drip.

34. Which antiseizure drug is most likely to cause thrombocytopenia and hepatotoxicity?

Valproic acid can cause these conditions.

35. Which antiseizure drugs can cause hyponatremia?
Carbamazepine and oxcarbazepine are more likely to cause hyponatremia. This is due to increased responsiveness to ADH, and it is considered a form of SIADH.

36. What adverse effect of topiramate should the patient be aware of?
Topiramate, a carbonic anhydrase inhibitor, can cause nephrolithiasis. Advise the patient to drink plenty of fluids.

37. Alcohol degeneration usually involves the vermis of the cerebellum. True or false?
True. The patient may present with truncal ataxia.

38. What myopathic systemic disease causes diabetes (hyperglycemia), frontal balding, mental retardation, and gastrointestinal symptoms?
Myotonic dystrophy causes these signs and symptoms. It is an autosomal dominant condition that involves both skeletal and smooth muscles as a result of a trinucleotide repeat mutation (not to be confused with muscular dystrophy).

39. What are the causes of bilateral facial palsy?
Lyme disease, sarcoidosis, and metastasis cause bilateral facial palsy.

40. What is the most common cause of cauda equina syndrome in immunocompromised patients?
Cytomegalovirus is the most common cause.

What percentage of AIDS patients develops cytomegalovirus polyradiculitis?

2%

41. On a radiograph, what is the differential diagnosis of a peripherally enhancing brain lesion?
A meningioma appears homogeneous, whereas an abscess is ring enhancing. Figure 15-1. Consider toxoplasmosis (usually in HIV patients and usually with **fever, headache, altered mental status**, and focal neurological deficits), active granulomas, lymphoma (usually homogeneously enhancing), primary glial tumors (usually heterogeneously enhancing), and metastasis (**multifocal**).

42. What is the proper treatment for meningioma?
Serial brain imaging is used to follow up a meningioma. There is no need to surgically resect unless it is causing compressive symptoms, including seizures, headache, and papilledema (Figure 15-1).

Visual hallucination is very common in Lewy body dementia.

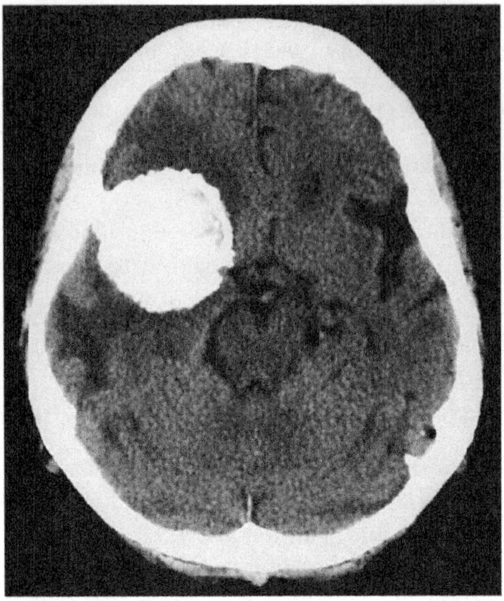

Figure 15-1. *Meningioma. Homogeneous calcified mass.*

43. What defines Wernicke-Korsakoff syndrome?

Wernicke-Korsakoff syndrome comprises short-term **memory loss**, ophthalmoplegia (**nystagmus**), ataxia, and neuropathy. Always consider in individuals with chronic alcohol abuse.

44. What is the definition of Lewy body dementia?

Lewy body dementia comprises rigidity (parkinsonian features) and dementia with extraordinary sensitivity to antineuroleptics. **Visual hallucinations** are very common. Antineuroleptics such as haloperidol may worsen rigidity and cause personality changes. Treatment is cholinesterase inhibitors (rivastigmine).

45. What criteria are used to establish the diagnosis of Alzheimer's dementia?

Criteria include **memory impairment** early on, cognitive **impairment in language**, and **executive function** impairment later on. Symptoms are usually **insidious** and interfere with social functioning. Diagnosis is clinched after ruling out systemic diseases as causes.

46. What are the most common causes of non-Alzheimer's dementia?

The most common causes are **vascular dementia**, **Lewy body** dementia, and **frontotemporal** dementia.

47. The triad of gait abnormality, urinary incontinence, and dementia suggests what cause of dementia?

This suggests normal pressure hydrocephalus (NPH). A CT or MRI scan will show evidence of ventriculomegaly. Treatment is high-volume lumbar puncture.

48. If a patient presents with an early-onset slowly developing impairment in personality, what type of dementia should be considered?

Consider **frontotemporal dementia**. Patients can present with early impairment in executive function such as making decisions and planning.

49. Dementia occurring rapidly in weeks to months suggests what form of dementia?

This suggests prion diseases, frontotemporal dementia, Lewy body dementia, supranuclear palsy, or corticobasal degeneration.

50. Dementia associated with myoclonus is associated with what form of dementia?

This is associated with prion diseases (**Creutzfeldt-Jakob disease**). It is also associated with other visual, extrapyramidal, and oculomotor symptoms. EEG shows evidence of **periodic biphasic** or **triphasic sharp wave** complexes. Elevated CSF 14-3-3 protein may be seen.

51. What are treatment options for Alzheimer's disease?

Treatment options include **cholinesterase inhibitors** such as donepezil, rivastigmine, and galantamine for **mild** to moderate dementia, or ***N*-methyl-d-aspartate receptor antagonists** such as memantine for **moderate to severe dementia**. Treat concomitant depression and psychosis with antidepressants and antipsychotics.

52. List the examination findings present in upper motor neuron (UMN) disease.

Signs are usually due to lesions above the anterior horn cells of the spinal cord (corticospinal tracts or cortical cells of origin) and include hyperreflexia, extensor plantar response (upgoing toes), and motor weakness of the extensor or flexor extremities. Examples include acute stroke syndromes, and lesions of the spinal cord.

What is a mnemonic for UMN/LMN lesions? ***Toes up is indicative of UMN; toes down is indicative of UMN.***

Poliomyelitis is a classic example of an LMN lesion.

53. List the examination findings in lower motor neuron (LMN) disease.

Findings, which are due to lesions at the **anterior horn cells** of the spinal cord or at the motor nuclei of the cranial nerves, include segmental weakness according to innervated muscles, hyporeflexia, hypotonia, fasciculations, and muscle atrophy. Cranial nerve findings are dysphagia, ptosis, and extraocular muscle involvement. Examples of anterior horn cell lesions include **poliomyelitis**, familial spinal atrophy, lead poisoning, and West Nile virus and other viruses.

54. How may patients present with amyotrophic lateral sclerosis (ALS, or Lou Gehrig's disease)?

Patients may present with gradual onset of muscle weakness in one or more regions without sensory loss associated with symptoms, of lower and upper motor neuron signs. A glutamate antagonist such as riluzole can be used to alleviate symptoms.

55. List some causes of spinal cord lesions.

Causes include infectious processes such as epidural abscess, chronic trauma, tumors, congenital leukodystrophies, cervical spondylosis, and demyelinating disorders such as multiple sclerosis.

56. How may patients present with spinal cord compression?

Patients present with signs of both upper motor and lower motor neuron disease.

57. What areas in the spinal cord does vitamin B_{12} deficiency affect?

It affects posterior columns, which causes loss of vibration, proprioception, and position sense.

58. What is the preferred imaging in spinal cord lesions?

MRI is preferred. **CT scan** with IV contrast or **myelography** is used if MRI is contraindicated. Lumbar puncture is used in those with possible demyelinating/inflammatory lesions.

59. How may patients present with multiple sclerosis?

Patients may present with neurological dysfunction in the CNS (brain, brainstem, and spinal cord) due to **demyelinating lesions** that are **random** and **asymmetric**.

Spinal cord lesions are primarily in the cervical segments. Multiple sclerosis can frequently present as vision loss due to **optic neuritis**. MRI may reveal **white matter lesions** perpendicular to the ventricles. CSF studies may reveal elevated immunoglobulin-albumin ratio or **oligoclonal bands**. Treatment ranges from steroids to plasmapheresis for severe refractory disease.

Spinal cord Lesions in multiple sclerosis are primarily in the cervical segments.

Lesions in multiple sclerosis are a combination of UMN and LMN.

60. What demyelinating white matter brain lesions are separate in time and space?

The brain lesions of multiple sclerosis are separate in time and space.

61. How may patients present with transverse myelitis?

Patients may present with inflammatory lesions in the spinal cord, causing spinal cord dysfunction, with **myelopathy** signs such as motor weakness, sensory abnormalities referable to the spinal cord, and **bladder and bowel dysfunction**, which usually **progresses over hours to days.** A **well-defined sensory level** below which sensation of pain and temperature is lost is suggestive of myelopathy. This differentiates myelopathy form peripheral neuropathy or CNS lesions as the cause of weakness.

62. What are some causes of transverse myelitis?

This is usually due to an **autoimmune disease** occurring after an infection or vaccination (most common cause in children), or is an acquired demyelinating disease (multiple sclerosis).

63. List the key findings in neuro-ophthalmology.

- Lesions in the optic nerve: Patients may present with central scotoma, visual acuity defect, and relative afferent pupillary defect.
- Lesions in the optic tract, optic radiations (parietal and temporal lobe): Patients may present with homonymous (contralateral) hemianopsia.
- Lesions in the optic chiasm: Patients may present with bitemporal hemianopsia.
- Lesions in the occipital lobe: Patients may present with homonymous hemianopsia with macular sparing.

64. What is the definition of internuclear ophthalmoplegia?

Internuclear ophthalmoplegia is an ipsilateral medial longitudinal fasciculus (MLF) lesion, common in patients

Recognize the symptoms of internuclear ophthalmoplegia.

with multiple sclerosis. When attempting a lateral gaze, the patient is unable to adduct the affected eye and nystagmus may be present in the contralateral eye; however, adduction on convergence is normal because this does not rely on MLF.

65. Which metabolic dysfunctions are associated with ocular cherry-red spots in the macula on ophthalmic examination?

Associated with cherry-red spots are Niemann-Pick disease (autosomal recessive, lysosomal storage disorder with loss of motor skills in the first month of life, hepatosplenomegaly, and difficult feeding), Gaucher disease (lysosomal storage disease with glucosylceramide enzyme accumulation in liver, spleen, and bone marrow with consequent hepatosplenomegaly, bone pain, and thrombocytopenia), and Tay-Sachs disease (autosomal dominant glycolipid storage condition with progressive weakness, hypotonia, and hyperreflexia at 2-6 months of age).

66. Multiple sclerosis causes what type of bladder incontinence?

Multiple sclerosis causes spastic urge incontinence. Why? It is thought to be due to an upper motor neuron lesion.

67. Diabetes causes what type of bladder incontinence?

Diabetes causes atonic overflow incontinence. Multiple sclerosis can also cause atonic urinary incontinence in the late course of the disease. Why? It is thought to be due to a lower motor neuron lesion.

68. What characteristics of Huntington disease are useful for diagnosis?

In Huntington disease, there is an early onset of dementia (in the 40s) and personality changes. It is also associated with **involuntary movement** disorder with **chorea**, **dystonia**, **bradykinesia**, and abnormal postural reflexes. A chromosome 4 mutation and triple CAG repeats are specific findings.

69. What drugs can cause Parkinson disease?

Metoclopramide (antiemetic) and antidopamine agents can cause Parkinson disease.

70. Progressive supranuclear palsy is a parkinsonism disorder with vertical gaze abnormality, gait impairment,

and bulbar symptoms (dysphagia, dysarthria). True or false?

True.

71. Parkinsonism plus cerebellar ataxia and pyramidal signs (flexor or extensor motor weakness) suggests what?

This suggests **multiple system atrophy**, which has prominent autonomic dysfunction early on.

72. What is the significance of Kayser-Fleischer rings?

Kayser-Fleischer rings are found in Wilson disease, an autosomal dominant condition with abnormal copper absorption. Other manifestations are dysarthria, dystonia, resting or intention tremor, chorea, and ataxia.

73. What is the pathogenesis of idiopathic Parkinson disease?

Parkinson disease is caused by the degeneration of dopamine neurons in the substantial nigra of the pars compacta. Extrapyramidal features (rigidity and tremors) are usually asymmetric. Treat with dopaminergic agents such as levodopa/carbidopa, dopamine agonists (younger patients), and MAO-B inhibitors (selegiline). Anticholinergic agents (benztropine) can be used as second-line therapy in those with difficult to control tremors.

Extrapyramidal features in idiopathic Parkinson are usually asymmetric.

74. What are long-term complications of levodopa?

Complications are **dyskinesias** and **motor fluctuations** ("wearing off' or "on-off" effect, in which the medication wears off before the next scheduled dose), which are difficult to resolve. Therefore, consider other first-line alternatives to control symptoms prior to levodopa to delay these adverse effects.

75. What are the clinical features of limbic dysfunction?

Features included behavioral, psychiatric, cognitive, memory dysfunction, and seizures.

76. What evaluation is diagnostic of limbic dysfunction?

- MRI shows **medial temporal** abnormalities.
- **CSF is bland**, but with mild pleocytosis with lymphocytic predominance and mildly elevated proteins.

77. What is the initial treatment for acute cerebral vascular accident (stroke)?

After stabilization (airway, breathing, circulation), obtain a **CT scan** of the brain without contrast. Administer a tissue plasminogen activator if the patient presents within 3-4 hours of onset of symptoms and thrombolysis is not contraindicated (e.g., elevated blood pressure [BP], massive infarct, hemorrhagic bleed).

78. What is the first step in the evaluation of a stroke or transient ischemic attack (TIA)?

The first step is to obtain a Doppler ultrasound of the carotid arteries to evaluate the extracranial vessels for possible intervention. Also obtain an echocardiogram to look for the embolic source, as well as a brain MRI/MRA to look for small strokes and thromboembolism that may be missed with a CT scan.

79. In patients with asymptomatic carotid stenosis, when is carotid endarterectomy (CEA) recommended?

It is recommended when carotid stenosis is >70%. If carotid stenosis is >60% and the patient is **symptomatic**, CEA should be performed.

80. What treatment regimen are patients with stroke or TIA given on discharge?

Patients are given antiplatelet therapy such as clopidogrel (Plavix), dipyridamole, and aspirin, as well as anti-cholesterol drugs such as statins. Why? Most of these patients have atherosclerosis.

When is BP treated in patients with acute ischemic stroke?

81. In patients with acute ischemic infarct stroke, how is blood pressure controlled?

Most guidelines recommend that blood pressure not be treated acutely in ischemic stroke unless systolic BP is ≥220 mm Hg and diastolic BP is ≥120 mm Hg.

82. What is the definition of malignant hypertension?

This is a syndrome of hypertensive emergency (BP systolic ≥180 mm Hg and diastolic BP ≥120 mm Hg with end-organ damage) associated with retinal hemorrhages, exudates (lipid exudates), or papilledema. It may also be associated with renal failure. The treatment goal in a hypertensive emergency is lowering diastolic BP to 100 mm Hg within 2-6 hours and the initial BP fall not being more than 25% of the initial value.

83. Hypertensive encephalopathy is a syndrome of hypertensive emergency. True or false?

True. It consists of brain edema caused by hyperperfusion from severe hypertension.

84. What brain structures are most commonly affected by hypertensive hemorrhage?

The basal ganglia, thalamus, pons, and cerebellum, in that order, are most commonly affected.

85. In patients with an intracranial hemorrhagic hypertensive bleed, how is blood pressure controlled?

Maintain BP at 160/90 (mean arterial pressure of 110mm Hg). Why? You are trying to avoid hypoperfusion (BP that is too low) and at the same time prevent elevated intracranial pressure (BP that is too high).

86. How may patients present with intracranial hemorrhage?

Patients may present with **sudden onset** of symptoms and progression of focal neurological deficits in minutes to hours.

87. List the brain vascular territories and symptoms manifested after a stroke.

- Middle cerebral artery (most common stroke artery): Weakness in **contralateral face/arm>leg**, aphasia, sensory deficit, and field cut
- Deep/lacunar arteries (small vessels): Contralateral pure motor or sensory deficit or **clumsy-hand dysarthria** syndrome
- Posterior cerebral artery: Contralateral **field cut**
- Basilar artery: Visual deficits, ataxia, **crossed** sensory, and motor deficit
- Vertebral artery: Lower **cranial nerve deficits**, ataxia, and sensory deficits (**crossed**)
- Anterior cerebral artery: Contralateral leg weakness

88. What do crossed sensory deficits imply?

They imply pain and temperature deficits on one side of the face and the opposite side of the body. This is most common in **Wallenberg syndrome** (also known as **lateral medullary syndrome**), usually due to posterior inferior cerebellar artery (PICA) insufficiency. Symptoms are similar to those of vertebral artery stroke.

89. How may patients present with lower cranial nerve deficits?

Patients may present with dysphagia, dysarthria, tongue deviation, and palate deviation.

What is the difference between the clinical features of ischemic stroke and hemorrhagic stroke?

Reduction of intracranial pressure is the aim of medical therapy for intracranial hemorrhage.

90. Which medical therapy is useful in intracranial hemorrhage?

Useful therapy includes sedatives, osmotic diuretics (mannitol), and hyperventilation to PCO2 of 30 mm Hg.

91. Where is the most common site of subarachnoid hemorrhage (SAH)?

SAH most commonly results from rupture of aneurysms of the **circle of Willis**. Irritation of the meningitis will cause a **stiff neck**. The most common site is the origin of the anterior communicating artery (**ACA**), followed by the posterior communicating artery (**PCA**), and then the middle cerebral artery (**MCA**). The mnemonic is, with each acronym spoken as two syllables, **AICA, PICA, MICA**. A CT scan of the brain is the first step in the initial evaluation; if the results are negative, a lumbar puncture is performed with CSF analysis for **xanthochromia**. Treatment is surgical clipping or coiling.

92. The appearance of thousands of red blood cells (RBCs) in CSF is diagnostic of what condition?

A high RBC count in the CSF is diagnostic of subarachnoid hemorrhage. Differentiate from **traumatic lumbar puncture** by comparing tube 1 with tube 4. A traumatic tap will show a significantly diminished RBC count in tube 4 compared with tube 1.

93. What is the differential diagnosis of chronic pain syndrome?

Consider neuropathic pain, post-stroke phantom limb pain, reflex sympathetic dystrophy, or compressive neuropathy.

94. Swelling, vasomotor instability, skin changes, and bone demineralization suggests what kind of chronic pain syndrome?

These suggest reflex **sympathetic dystrophy**, which occurs after injury, surgery, or a vascular event. Treat with bisphosphonates.

Chapter 16
Pediatrics

> *Know the various age groups associated with orthopedic deformities.*

1. What abnormality is present in developmental dysplasia of the hip (DDH)?

In DDH, the hip joint is loose where the head of the femur and the acetabulum meet.

The risk factors are the position of the fetus in utero, breech position, and family history of DDH.

2. What is the Barlow test?

This test is a physical examination maneuver used to diagnose DDH.

In the Barlow test (adducting the hip with posterior pressure on the hips), a clunk should be heard as the hip subluxes out of the acetabulum.

3. What is the Ortolani test?

This is a physical examination used to diagnose DDH.

In the Ortolani test (abducting the hip while placing anterior pressure on the greater trochanter), a clunk is heard as the hip is reduced into the acetabulum.

4. What is the Galeazzi sign?

This test is a physical examination used to diagnose DDH.

The Galeazzi sign (patient is supine and hips and knees are flexed) is positive in a child if one leg appears shorter than the other. A clunk sound is similar to turning a light switch on or off.

5. What imaging is used to diagnose DDH?

DDH is usually diagnosed by age group. The patient is usually a few weeks old and asymptomatic (usually detected at newborn hip examination and examination at two weeks of age). Walking age children may present with a limp. Ultrasound may show a shallow acetabulum. An X-ray is not useful until the patient is 4-6 months old.

Treatment is a Pavlik harness.

6. **What is the definition of spondylolisthesis?**
Spondylolisthesis is a congenital disorder of the vertebrae causing forward displacement of one vertebra over another (e.g., L5 over S1). On examination, the displacement is palpable as a step-off (Figure 16-1).

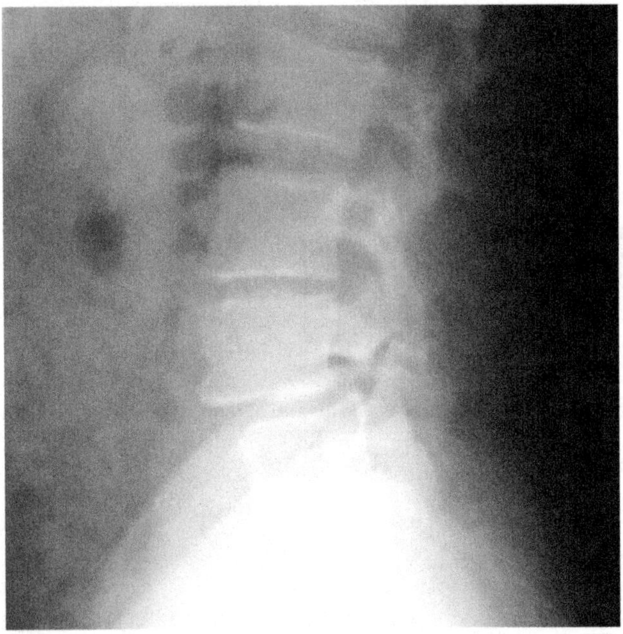

Figure 16-1. *L5/S1 spondylolisthesis. L5 is displaced forward over S1.*

In children with a limp, the location of pain does not always suggest the location of pathology.

7. **How do patients with Legg-Calvé-Perthes disease present (avascular necrosis of the femoral head)?**
The patient is usually 3-10 years old and presents with hip pain or pain referred to the knee and or a limp.

The physical examination reveals that the range of motion of the hip is reduced in all directions. An X-ray of the hip may show collapse of the femur head. A bone scan may show reduced blood flow in the femur head.

Treatment is braces to hold the femur in place.

8. What is the definition of a slipped capital femoral epiphysis?

The femoral neck separates from the femoral head. An X-ray shows a wide epiphysis plate. The patient is usually obese and at puberty.

Treatment: Surgery (osteotomy) to repair the defect

9. How do patients present with metatarsus adductus?

Patients present with a forefoot that turns inward only. The patient may present with a limp and pain.

Treatment: Stretch exercises and a brace for the most severe cases because metatarsus adductus is self-resolving

What is the difference in treatment for metatarsus adductus and clubfoot?

10. What is the definition of talipes equinovarus (clubfoot)?

Clubfoot is metatarsus adductus, medial rotation of the tibia, and fixed plantar flexion of the foot.

Unlike metatarsus adductus, clubfoot is not likely to self-resolve; therefore, treatment is immediate braces before the age of ambulation.

11. What is the definition of Osgood-Schlatter disease?

Osgood-Schlatter disease consists of tibial tubercle swelling due to infrapatellar tendon inflammation. The patient presents as a highly active adolescent who has undergone a rapid growth spurt, with knee swelling and pain.

What is the age range of patients presenting with Osgood-Schlatter disease?

The physical examination reveals that the tenderness and swelling is localized to the tibia tuberosity.

Treatment: Rest, ice application, stretching, analgesics, and compression with a protective pad

12. What is the treatment approach to patients with idiopathic scoliosis?

The patient with scoliosis that is <25 degrees should be advised to perform routine exercises.

The patient with scoliosis that is >25 degrees should be treated with a spine brace in children with an immature skeleton until the skeleton has matured.

Patients with scoliosis >45 degrees should be treated with surgery to fuse the spine if the bone remains immature or when progression or associated pain occurs when the bone has matured.

13. Localized pain and swelling for weeks to months, associated with minor trauma in children, should point to what pathological condition?

Consider Ewing's sarcoma, a bone and soft tissue tumor, or osteosarcoma. Other findings are fever, fatigue, and weight loss. An X-ray of the long bone will show an "onion peel" appearance indicative of periosteal elevation. Biopsy is used for definitive diagnosis. Surgery and radiation can be used to treat localized disease and chemotherapy for metastasized disease.

14. What is the most common primary bone malignancy of children and adolescents?

The most common is osteosarcoma. Patients will present with localized bone pain going on for months, which usually begins after an injury. However, unlike Ewing's sarcoma, there are no systemic symptoms such as fever, weight loss, or fatigue. Laboratory results may show elevated alkaline phosphatase and LDH levels and an increased erythrocyte sedimentation rate (ESR). An X-ray may show both lytic and sclerotic bone (from periosteal elevation). Biopsy is used for definitive diagnosis. Unlike treatment for Ewing's sarcoma, chemotherapy is used in all stages of osteosarcoma in combination with surgery, radiation, or both. Without chemotherapy, most patients will develop metastatic disease.

15. What are the pediatrics vaccination recommendations?

See Table 16-1.

Table 16-1. *Pediatrics Vaccination Recommendations (2011)*[a,b]

Vaccine	Vaccination Schedule
Hepatitis B[c]	At birth, 1-2 months old, and 6-18 months old
Rotavirus	At 2, 4, and 6 months old
Hib (*Haemophilus influenzae* type B)	At 2, 4, 6, and 12-15 months old
PCV (pneumococcal conjugate vaccine)[d]	At 2, 4, 6, and 12-15 months old
IPV (inactivated polio virus)	At 2, 4, 6-18 months, and 4-6 years old
DTaP (diphtheria and tetanus toxoids and acellular pertussis)[e]	At 2, 4 , 6, 15-18 months, and 4-6 years old
MMR (measles-mumps-rubella)[f]	At 12-15 months and 4-6 years old
Varicella[f]	At 12-15 months and 4-6 years old
Influenza	>6 months old
Hepatitis A[g]	>12 months old, two doses 6 months apart

a Contraindications to vaccination: fever, anaphylaxis, encephalopathy, seizure, and previous hypotension within 7 days of vaccination.
b Meningococcal conjugate vaccine (MCV): Administer two doses at least 8 weeks apart to individuals who are 2-10 years old with persistent complement deficiency or who are asplenic, and one dose every 5 years thereafter. Administer two doses to HIV-positive patients who have been previously vaccinated with MCV. Administer one dose to individuals up to age 10 years who travel to endemic areas or during outbreaks. For adolescents, administer MCV at 11-12 years, and again at 16 years, or one dose at 13-18 years old, or one dose to previously unvaccinated college freshmen living in a dormitory.
c Hepatitis B: In infants of mothers with hepatitis B, give hepatitis B immunoglobulin in addition to hepatitis B vaccine. In adults, administer three doses to those previously not vaccinated.
d PCV: The minimum age for pneumococcal polysaccharide vaccine (PPSV) is 2 years. For individuals 6-18 years old, administer one dose of PCV to those with asplenia or complement deficiencies, HIV infection, cochlear implants, or CSF leak. A single revaccination with PPSV in 5 years should be given to those aged 19-64 with asplenia, chronic renal failure, or other immunocompromising conditions.
e DTaP: The vaccine should be given at 11-13 years old. For those aged 11-18 who have not received a dose of DTaP, give one dose followed by a DT booster every 10 years.
f MMR and varicella vaccines are contraindicated in pregnancy. MMR: In adults, administer two doses 4 weeks apart to those previously not vaccinated. Varicella: Varicella zoster virus is transmitted by direct contact with vesicles or airborne inhalation of droplets. For those without evidence of immunity at >13 years old, administer two doses of varicella vaccine 4 weeks apart.
g Hepatitis A: In adults, hepatitis A vaccine is recommended for those with increased risk of infection. Administer two doses 6 months apart.

Conjugate pneumococcal vaccines should be given to patients who are <5 years old.

What are posterior urethral valves?

What is vesicourethral reflux?

16. What is the causative organism in hand-foot-and-mouth disease?

The causative organism is **coxsackievirus A and B**. The patient presents with herpangina (**vesicles** that rupture to form ulcers on the **soft palate**) and vesicles on the **palms and soles**. Treatment: Hand-foot-and-mouth disease is self-limiting.

17. What is the causative organism in scarlet fever?

Scarlet fever is caused by GAS, *Streptococcus pyogenes* (gram-positive spherical bacteria that occur in chains). The patient will present with a **sandpaper rash that extends from the neck** to the extremities in association with pharyngitis, **strawberry tongue,** and fever.

Treatment is with penicillin.

18. How do pediatric patients with a urinary tract infection (UTI) present?

The patient presents with dysuria, frequency, and urgency. Fever may be the only sign in infants and young children.

Unlike the case for certain adults, urine is cultured to confirm the diagnosis. Pyuria (≥5 WBC/hpf or ≥10 WBC/mm^3) and significant bacteriuria (≥100,000 CFU/ml of uropathogenic bacteria) are needed to make a diagnosis.

Renal and bladder ultrasound are used in children with a first febrile UTI at <2 years old. A voiding cystourethrogram is used in children of any age with two or more febrile UTIs or with renal disease, urologic disease, poor growth, or hypertension. Why? Imaging is used to look for underlying causes such as posterior urethral valves (obstructive congenital defect in the male urethra) or vesicourethral reflux (retrograde movement of urine due to an incompetent vesicoureteral valve). Risk factors for UTI in children are genetic factors, urinary tract anomalies, bowel and bladder dysfunction, vesicourethral reflux, sexual activity, and bladder catheterization.

The most common organism causing UTI is Escherichia coli.

UTI in children can be treated with amoxicillin, nitrofurantoin, Bactrim (trimethoprim/sulfamethoxazole [TMP/SMX]), fluoroquinolones or third-generation cephalosporins (recommended as first-line empiric therapy in those without genitourinary abnormalities).

Antibiotic prophylaxis is recommended in children with a higher grade vesicourethral reflux. The more severe forms of vesicourethral reflux or those refractory to treatment can be treated with surgery.

19. What is the definition of cryptorchidism?

Cryptorchidism is undescended testes. Most will descend at the age of 12 months, and so do not refer the child for treatment until then.

Treatment: Orchiopexy

Complications of cryptorchidism:

- Infertility
- Testicular cancer
- Testicular torsion

Why should one not treat undescended testes?

20. The treatment of cryptorchidism eliminates the risk factor of testicular malignancy. True or false?

False. Orchiopexy is performed for undescended testes to allow for malignancy screening, the preservation of fertility, and hormonal production.

21. What is the definition of enuresis?

Enuresis is lack of bladder control in a child >5 years old. The first step is to obtain urinalysis to rule out UTI. Treatment: This can be in the form of a nighttime alarm or an intranasal antidiuretic hormone.

Patients <5 years old do not qualify for the diagnosis of enuresis.

22. List the pediatric developmental milestones.

See Table 16-2.

23. What is the definition of pervasive disorders?

A pervasive disorder is an impairment of social and communication skills with the presence of stereotypical behaviors.

- Autism: The patient develops abnormal communication skills, engages in self-destructive behaviors, and is socially withdrawn. Treatment: Behavior-modification techniques
- Asperger syndrome: It is a less severe form of autism with intact communication skills **early on**. Treatment: Same treatment as for autism

What is the difference between autistic disorder and Asperger syndrome?

24. What are the defining characteristics of Rett syndrome?

Rett syndrome involves regression of development after reaching 1 year of age, which is associated with microcephaly and autism-like traits.

Table 16-2. *Pediatric Developmental Milestones*

Age	Social	Gross Motor	Language	Fine Motor
1-4 months	Alerts to sound	Lifts head up, rolls	Coos, smiles	Follows objects to midline
6 months	Stranger recognition	Sits unsupported	Looks around to voice	Moves object from one hand to the other
9 months	Plays pat-a-cake	Crawls	Says mama, dada	Pincer grasp
12 months	Parallel play	Walks unassisted	One-step command	Feeds self messily
24 months	Parallel play	Walks up the stairs	Two-word sentences	Undresses self
3 years	Cooperative play	Rides a tricycle	Three-word sentences	Draws circle

25. What are the characteristics of attention deficit hyperactivity disorder (ADHD)?

ADHD is characterized by hyperactivity and inattentiveness. The patient may be either predominantly hyperactive (unable to sit still in class) or inattentive (unable to pay attention to details). An associated conduct disorder is present in many patients.

Treatment: Stimulant (dextroamphetamine and amphetamine, or methylphenidate)

Complications of ADHD treatment: Anxiety and insomnia from the stimulant medications

26. How does a parent who is suspected of child abuse usually present?

Parents will present with an inconsistent history and delay in seeking treatment for the child.

The physical examination reveals multiple lesions that are at different stages of healing.

The first step is to obtain an X-ray to look for fractures and a computed tomography scan and funduscopy to rule out shaken baby syndrome (subdural hematoma, retinal hemorrhages). A circumpapillary retinal ridge on retinal examination is pathognomonic.

Treatment: Report to social services immediately.

27. How does a patient with mild mental retardation (MR) present?

The patient is educable to high school level, able to hold vocational jobs, and able to function. IQ is 50-70.

28. How does a patient with moderate MR present?

The patient is able to perform self-caring activities (bathing, brushing, dressing), but unable to live alone. The patient often lives in a long-term care facility. IQ is 35-50.

29. How does a patient with severe MR present?

The patient is placed in a long-term care facility early on, unable to perform self-caring activities. Severe MR is usually associated with physical disabilities. IQ is <20-35.

30. What is the definition of intussusception?

Intussusception is a telescoping of one part of the intestine into another, causing deprivation of blood and leading to ischemia and necrosis. This is usually the ileum into the cecum. Intussusception can be propagated by Peyer patches, polyps, or Hirschsprung disease. **Rotavirus vaccine** is associated with intussusception.

The patient will present with intermittent, crampy abdominal pain (drawing of legs toward abdomen) and vomiting. Stools may consist of mucus mixed with blood (currant jelly stools). Why? This represents necrotic sloughing of the bowel.

The first step is to obtain an air, contrast or saline enema, to untwist the bowel and usher in supportive treatment with intravenous (IV) fluids. An enema is both a diagnostic and therapeutic procedure.

31. What is the definition of pyloric stenosis?

Pyloric stenosis is an abnormal muscular growth in the gastric outlet that can lead to gastric outlet obstruction. The patient will present with multiple episodes of nonbilious vomiting that is forceful at 2-3 months of life. On the physical examination, an epigastric mass is felt.

Treatment is IV fluids initially because of multiple vomiting episodes. Pyloromyotomy is the definitive treatment after the patient is stabilized.

32. Infantile hypertrophic pyloric stenosis has been associated with orally administered erythromycin for pertussis in infants <2 weeks old. True or false?

True. In patients <1 month old, an oral macrolide antibiotic

What disorder is commonly associated with ADHD?

What are features of shaken baby syndrome?

Know the sequence and nature of pain in patients with intussusceptions.

What imaging is both diagnostic and therapeutic of intussusceptions?

(e.g., azithromycin) is an alternative to erythromycin in the treatment or prophylaxis of pediatric pertussis.

33. What is the pathogenesis of malrotation?

In malrotation, the gut does not rotate correctly during development, causing abnormal posterior fixation of the mesentery, which can cause twisting of the small bowel, leading to obstruction.

The patient will present with bilious vomiting and abdominal distention on examination. The first step in diagnosis is to obtain a plain radiograph of the abdomen such as an abdominal X-ray, which will show a "double bubble" sign: air in the stomach and intestine (first part of the duodenum). An upper GI series is the best test for diagnosis. Treatment is emergency surgery to avoid ischemic bowel (Figure 16-2).

Down syndrome is associated with duodenal atresia.

34. What is the pathogenesis of duodenal atresia?

Duodenal atresia is stenosis of the duodenum secondary to lack of recanalization during development.

The patient presents with bowel obstruction signs such as bilious emesis and an inability to pass meconium after birth; however, meconium may remain in the distal bowel beyond the obstruction. It is often associated with other malformations, including gastrointestinal (biliary atresia, agenesis of gallbladder), cardiac, renal, and vertebral abnormalities. Patients with duodenal atresia may also have Down syndrome.

On the physical examination, abdominal distention may be seen with palpable bowel loops. A plain radiograph may show a double bubble sign.

Treatment is emergency surgery to avoid ischemic bowel (Figure 16-2).

What is the most commonly involved area in Hirschsprung disease?

35. What is the pathogenesis of Hirschsprung disease?

Hirschsprung disease is the lack of innervation to a portion of the colon, usually in the rectosigmoid area, leading to fecal accumulation and obstruction.

The patient presents with an inability to pass meconium for the first 24 hours after birth.

On the physical examination, there are no feces in the rectum, the internal sphincter is unable to relax, and a rectal biopsy sample shows no ganglia.

Treatment is elective surgery.

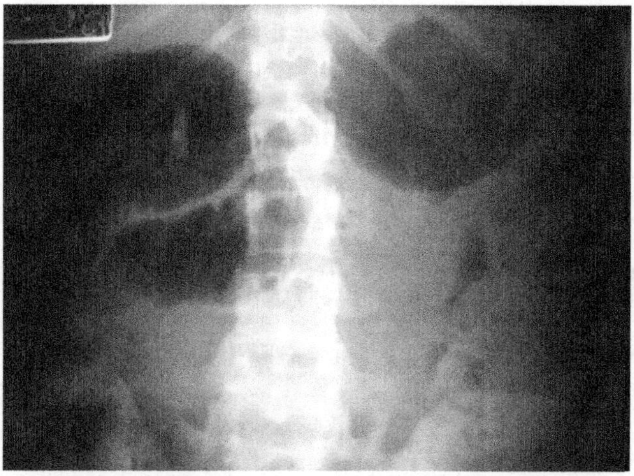

Figure 16-2. *Double bubble sign, indicating distention.*

36. What is the pathogenesis of Meckel diverticulum?

Meckel diverticulum is a remnant omphalomesenteric duct with ectopic gastric tissue. The patient will be a child who presents with a painless melena. Diagnosis is made by a 99m technetium pertechnetate radionuclide scan, which identifies gastric mucosa.

Treatment is to resect the diverticulum.

37. What is the definition of necrotizing enterocolitis?

Necrotizing enterocolitis is an ischemic or necrotic bowel in premature infants. The patient presents usually after the first feed with abdominal pain, vomiting, and bloody stools.

An abdominal X-ray shows air in the lumen or wall of the small intestine (pneumatosis intestinalis).

Treatment: Bowel rest and nothing by mouth. If air is found under the diaphragm, indicating a ruptured bowel, a surgical consult is needed for emergency surgery.

38. How may cystic fibrosis present in neonates?

Cystic fibrosis is associated with duodenal stenosis.

The patient may present with meconium ileus (inability to pass meconium in the first 24 hours). Cystic fibrosis is associated with duodenal stenosis. Clinical disease is present in multiple organs, including the pancreas, lungs, and male reproductive tract, and the patient will have an elevated sweat chloride level (>60 mmol/L).

Older children may present with complications such as failure to thrive, respiratory symptoms (productive cough, wheezing, dyspnea)fatty stools that are foul-smelling, hemoptysis, bronchiectasis, and pneumothorax.

39. What is the definition of the Apgar score?
The Apgar is a scoring system used to predict immediate survival (not long term) of a newborn. It is performed at 1 and 5 minutes after birth (Table 16-3).

Table 16-3. *APGAR Score*[a]

Apgar	0	1	2
Appearance	Cyanotic	Cyanotic extremities	Pink all over
Pulse	Absent	<100 beats/min	>100 beats/min
Grimace	Absent	Weak cry	Active cry
Activity	Absent	Slightly flexed	Active movement
Respiration	Absent	Weak	Strong

a An Apgar score of 8-9 is normal.

40. What are the risk factors for birth trauma?
The risk factors are large head size, a large-for-gestational-age infant, prolonged labor, vacuum extraction, and shoulder dystocia.

41. What is the definition of cephalohematoma?
Cephalohematoma is a subperiosteal hemorrhage that does not cross suture lines. On the physical examination, discoloration may or may not be seen on the scalp. A CT scan is helpful in making the diagnosis.

Treatment: None. The condition is self-resolving.

42. What is the definition of caput succedaneum?
Caput succedaneum is the swelling of the scalp that crosses suture lines, above the periosteum, which can cause molding of the head, leading to an abnormal head shape. On the physical examination, some discoloration may be seen.

Treatment: None. The condition is self-resolving.

43. Kernicterus is a dreaded complication of hyperbilirubinemia. True or false?
True. Hemolytic anemias, birth traumas (e.g., cephalohematoma), polycythemia, and bilirubin conjugation defects are some of the causes of hyperbilirubinemia. Severely high bilirubin results in the deposition of unconjugated bilirubin in regions of the basal ganglia, hippocampus, substantia nigra, and brainstem, causing neurotoxicity.

Treatment: Exchange transfusion is used for treatment of kernicterus, and phototherapy is used for severe hyperbilirubinemia to prevent bilirubin toxicity.

44. When is a fractured clavicle seen in neonates?

A fractured clavicle usually occurs in neonates with shoulder dystocia or who have mothers with diabetes. On the first-day neonatal examination, a fractured clavicle may be missed. It is usually caught 3-6 weeks later when a callus has formed and a crepitus is heard. No treatment is needed, as it is self-resolving.

What is the difference between cephalohematoma and caput succedaneum?

45. What is the cause of Erb palsy?

Erb palsy is secondary to excessive stretching of the neck during birth. The upper root of the brachial plexus is affected (C5-C6). The patient presents with waiter's tip position (arms extended, wrist flexed, internally rotated and supinated). On the physical examination, the Moro (startle) reflex is lacking.

Treatment: None. Erb palsy is self-resolving.

46. What is the definition of shoulder dystocia?

Shoulder dystocia is defined as the need for additional obstetric maneuvers to deliver the fetus during vaginal delivery because the shoulders are impacted at the pelvic inlet. Clinical diagnosis is made when the fetal head retracts (turtle sign) during vaginal delivery.

47. What is the initial step in managing shoulder dystocia?

Ask the mother to maintain an optimal position for delivery with her buttocks at the edge of the bed, and then perform the McRoberts maneuver (which flexes the maternal thigh against the abdomen). Ask an assistant to apply suprapubic pressure with the palm or fist. If these procedures are unsuccessful, use other invasive procedures to ensure delivery of the fetus.

48. What is the Zavanelli procedure?

After all procedures have failed to deliver the fetus, place the fetal head back into the pelvis and proceed with a cesarean delivery.

49. What is the common causative organism in neonatal sepsis?

Early sepsis occurs within the first 3 days of birth. Late sepsis occurs within 4-90 days of life and can be caused by a focal infection (meningitis, osteomyelitis). Meningitis in infants is mostly caused by a group B streptococci infection and osteomyelitis is mostly caused by

The most common cause of neonatal sepsis is group B streptococci.

Staphylococcus aureus. Early sepsis is caused by maternal vertically transmitted bacteria and is usually due to group B streptococci and E. coli infection.

The patient with sepsis may present with fetal and neonatal distress; temperature instability (fever); or respiratory, gastrointestinal, and neurological abnormalities.

Treatment: Early sepsis is empirically treated with IV gentamicin plus broad-spectrum penicillin to cover gram-negative and gram-positive bacteria after full evaluation. Late sepsis is empirically treated with broad-spectrum antibiotics on the basis of the type of infection suspected after full evaluation.

50. What is the evaluation of pediatrics patients who present with a fever of unknown cause?

- Patients <2 months old: Workup includes complete blood cell (CBC) count, urinalysis, urine and blood cultures, and lumbar puncture; administer IV antibiotics while waiting. **Why?** Search for an occult infection because patients at this age are highly susceptible to infection.
- Patients 2-12 months old: A lumbar puncture, blood culture, and CBC is warranted only if the patient is lethargic, irritable, or inconsolable. A chest X-ray (CXR) should be ordered if focal rales, nasal flaring, retraction, or hypoxia is present, and a stool culture should be obtained if there is diarrhea. Why? The most common cause of fever in this age group is viral infections. Urinary tract infection is also common in the age group <6 months old.

51. What is the pathogenesis of respiratory distress syndrome (RDS or hyaline membrane disease) in preterm infants?

RDS in preterm infants is due to the lack of surfactant, causing atelectasis with consequent respiratory distress.

Treatment: Respiratory support via noninvasive positive-pressure mechanical ventilation or invasive mechanical ventilation via low tidal volume ventilation; and surfactant therapy. Extracorporeal membrane oxygenation (ECMO) can be used in severe or refractory RDS.

Prevention: Prevent preterm delivery or administer steroids to pregnant women less than 34 weeks of gestation at high risk for preterm birth.

52. In term neonatal patients with acute respiratory failure, ECMO can be used. True or false?

Persistent pulmonary hypertension is the most common cause of acute respiratory failure in neonates, which can be idiopathic or due to meconium aspiration , hyaline membrane disease, sepsis, congenital diaphragmatic hernia. ECMO can be used after failure of conventional therapies.

53. What are the two types of neonatal jaundice?

Physiological and pathological are the two types of neonatal jaundice.

Physiologic: Causes of physiological jaundice are a combination of normal neonatal alterations, including early red blood cell destruction, reduced clearance of bilirubin from the liver, and increased enterohepatic circulation of bilirubin. This type of jaundice usually shows mildly elevated indirect or unconjugated serum bilirubin levels after the first 24 hours of birth and resolves within the first 1 to 2 weeks of age. Routine workup should be done for anemia and hemolysis. Treatment: Routine follow-up and phototherapy for severe forms

Pathological: Causes of pathological jaundice are due to pathologic conditions that cause increased bilirubin production (hemolysis), reduced clearance (Gilbert or Crigler Najjar syndrome), and increased enterohepatic circulation of bilirubin (breast milk jaundice) or neonatal cholestasis due to infections, congenital anomaly, neonatal hepatitis, alpha-1 anti-trypsin deficiency, familial cholestasis, and parenteral nutrition. This type of jaundice occurs within the first 24 hours of birth (due to hemolysis) and lasts longer than 2 weeks. If neonatal jaundice fits these criteria, a workup is warranted. If jaundice lasts longer than the first 2 weeks of age, the first step in evaluation is to obtain total and conjugated serum bilirubin levels. If unconjugated bilirubin is slightly elevated, then jaundice is likely due to breast milk jaundice. However, if conjugated bilirubin is elevated (≥20% of the total bilirubin), then search for infection and common causes of neonatal cholestasis. If the unconjugated serum bilirubin level is severely elevated, then a workup for anemia and hemolysis should be pursued.

What are the differences between physiological and pathological jaundice?

Coxsackievirus can cause dilated cardiomyopathy.

54. Biliary atresia (congenital bile duct anomaly) is a cause of elevated direct or conjugated bilirubin levels when considering a workup for pathological jaundice. True or false?

True. Primary green dentition is commonly associated with biliary atresia. Biliary atresia and neonatal hepatitis are the most common causes of neonatal cholestasis. Elevated serum GGTP raises concern for hepatobiliary disease and in this case can suggest biliary atresia. Diagnosis of biliary atresia is made by an abdominal ultrasound.

55. Why is iron-deficiency anemia the most common cause of anemia in infants?

Iron-deficiency anemia is common because of the lack of iron supplements, especially in infants taking whole milk (non-formula cow's milk) within the first year of life (breast milk contains more iron than does non-formula cow's milk).

Treatment: Oral iron replacement pills

56. What are some mandatory newborn screening tests?

In the United States, universal screening for newborns varies by state, but all states screen for hypothyroidism and phenylketonuria. Nearly all states screen for galactosemia and hemoglobinopathies. Why? Early treatment can make a significant difference.

57. List the key findings in pediatric syndromes.

- Beckwith-Wiedemann: Macrosomia (gigantism), omphalocele, macroglossia, hyperinsulinemia
- Gastroschisis: Defect in the abdominal wall causing extrusion of intestines not covered with the peritoneum
- Omphalocele: Defect in the medial abdominal wall causing extrusion of abdominal contents, not just intestines, covered with the peritoneal sac
- Dilated cardiomyopathy: The most commonly asked about viral cause of dilated cardiomyopathy in infants is coxsackievirus. Patients present with heart failure and abnormally dilated chambers of the heart. Treat heart failure and other symptoms.

58. List the key findings in neuropediatrics.

- Spina bifida occulta: Abnormal vertebral arch, failure of fusion of the vertebral bodies dorsal to the spinal cord. In occulta, the overlying skin is intact. Physical examination may reveal minor abnormalities in the overlying skin which may include dimple, hemangioma, lipoma, hyperpigmentation. It is usually benign and asymptomatic.

- Meningocele: The overlying skin is not intact, causing herniation of meninges tissue through the vertebrae and skin. Surgical closure is the treatment of choice.
- Myelomeningocele: Herniation of meninges and spinal cord through the vertebrae and skin. Surgical closure is the treatment of choice.
- Arnold Chiari II malformation: This is usually associated with a myelomeningocele. It causes hydrocephalus by downward displacement of the inferior cerebellar vermis, tonsils and medulla through the posterior fossa, which causes obstruction of cerebrospinal fluid flow through the posterior fossa. Arnold Chiari I (obstruction of the posterior fossa by cerebellar tonsils) is usually asymptomatic and Arnold chiari III (inferior displacement of the cerebellar with cervical or occipital encephalocele) is rare (Figure 16-3).
- Kawasaki disease: Oculomucocutaneous vasculitis. The risk of coronary artery aneurysm is high. Treatment: Treat coronary artery aneurysm with aspirin and IV immunoglobulin.
- Cerebral palsy: Neuromotor injury most commonly due to birth anoxia. The patient will present with hemiplegia, quadriplegia, or hyperreflexia. The most common type is spastic; therefore, on examination, most patients will be found to have hyperreflexia. Associated defects include sensory problems (vision, hearing), low IQ, and gastroesophageal reflux disease. Treatment: Treat underlying problems.

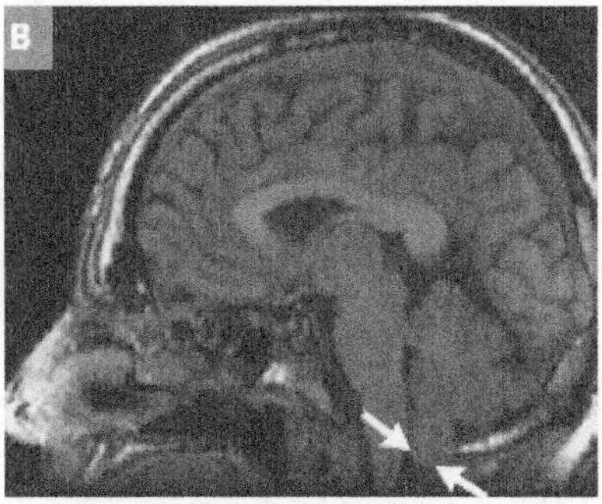

Figure 16-3. *The arrow shows tonsillar herniation (Type 1 Arnold Chiari malformation).*

The overlying skin in spina bifida occulta may be diagnostic.

What is the most common cause of failure to thrive?

59. What is the definition of Reye syndrome?

Reye syndrome is an encephalopathy in children associated with the use of aspirin following a viral illness, especially varicella or influenza A or B. Hepatic enzyme levels are elevated from hepatic dysfunction and mental status is altered.

60. How do patients with intraventricular hemorrhage present?

Intraventricular hemorrhage presents in premature infants. It can cause scarring and obstruction of the arachnoid villi, leading to hydrocephalus and widening of the ventricles.

61. What is the definition of failure to thrive?

Failure to thrive is a drop in weight below 2% on the growth chart on more than one occasion, or falling below the previous stable weight (a rate of change that causes decrease of two or more major percentile lines e.g., from 50th to 10th).

Other definitions are weight less than 80 percent of ideal weight, decreased weight for length, and weight gain less than expected for age.

An extensive workup may be needed to rule out organic causes (gastrointestinal tract, cystic fibrosis). However, the most common cause is nonorganic (e.g., neglect).

62. What are the most common causes of liver failure in children?

The most common causes are **drugs**, including acetaminophen, and then metabolic disorders, viruses (herpes and hepatitis viruses), and ischemia such as Budd-Chiari syndrome (hepatic vein thrombosis with portal hypertension, hepatic congestion, and elevated bilirubin level).

63. When is the differential diagnosis of metabolic causes of acute liver failure?

Defects in the **fatty acid oxidation pathway** can lead to accumulation of fatty acids and organ dysfunction, presenting as hypoglycemia, liver disease, hypoketosis, myopathy, or cardiomyopathy.

64. Long-chain fatty acid accumulation is more severe than short chain. True or false?

True. An example of long-chain fatty acid accumulation is **carnitine enzyme deficiency**.

65. What is the order of secondary sexual development (puberty) in males?

The earliest secondary sexual characteristic in the maturation of boys is an increase in testicular growth, followed by penile enlargement and the appearance of pubic hair. Tanner stages describe the stages of pubic hair, breast, and genitalia development, with stage one indicating prepuberty and stage five indicating adult development (Table 16-4).

Table 16-4. *Tanner stages of secondary sexual characteristics*

Boys	Girls	Boys and girls (pubic hair)
1-Prepubertal	Prepubertal	Prepubertal; no pubic hair
2-Scrotum and testes enlargement	Breast and papilla form a mound	Sparse hair at base of penis/labia
3-Penile enlargement	Enlargement of breast	Darker, coarser, and coiled hair[a]
4-Increase in size of penis	Secondary mound by areola and papilla	Hair spreads but not to thigh
5-Adult genitalia	Mature stage; projection of papilla	Hair spreads to medial thigh

a Hair spreads sparsely over the junction of pubic hair.

66. What is the order of secondary sexual development (puberty) in females?

The earliest secondary sexual characteristic in the maturation of girls is breast growth (thelarche), although some girls may present with pubic hair (pubarche) first. Menarche occurs later, on average 2 years after the onset of puberty, and peak height velocity occurs prior to menarche (Table 16-4).

67. Why is sexual development in this order?

An estrogen spurt early in puberty causes breast growth and bone fusion; later, androgen causes pubic hair development.

68. What is the definition of constitutional delay?

Constitutional delay is a delay in growth that results in delayed puberty and bone growth, with eventual growth normalization. A family history of constitutional delay is usually present. This is a diagnosis of exclusion and should be ruled out only if organic causes have been ruled out with laboratory tests, including testosterone, FSH, and LH levels, to exclude gonadal failure. Also rule out medications and systemic diseases that could cause it.

Treatment: Expectant observation or low-dose sex steroids if short stature is causing psychosocial distress.

What is the dreaded complication of constitutional delay? ***Delayed bone growth***

Height spurt occurs before pubarche, but height peak occurs after pubarche.

69. What is the definition of precocious puberty?

In precocious puberty, secondary sex characteristics appear in girls before they are 7 years old and in boys before they are 9 years old. It is caused by transient secretion of gonadotropins, causing elevated LH levels, and advanced bone growth.

The parent will present with a daughter who has an enlarged breast bud and other secondary sexual characteristics at the age of 7 years.

The first step is to order baseline levels of LH, with or without GnRH stimulation to search for causes, then check for advanced bone growth. If advanced bone growth is present, administer a gonadotropin-releasing hormone (GnRH) analogue (leuprolide); otherwise, follow up accordingly.

70. What is the definition of premature adrenarche or thelarche?

They are both considered incomplete precocious puberty. Premature adrenarche is the premature secretion of adrenal hormones due to premature adrenal gland function. The patient with premature adrenarche could present as a 7- to 8-year-old girl, usually African American, who presents with axillary hair and/or pubic hair. The cause of premature thelarche is unknown. Serum estradiol is usually normal, and the condition presents with isolated breast development in Black or Hispanic girls in the first two years of life or at six years of age. Reassurance and routine follow-up is the treatment.

Treatment: The first step in premature adrenarche is to check for other causes of virilization by obtaining hormonal studies including DHEA and 17hydroxyprogesterone and testosterone; otherwise, follow up accordingly with reassurance.

What is the difference between anorexia nervosa and bulimia nervosa?

71. What are two defining characteristics of anorexia nervosa?

Anorexia nervosa is characterized by low body weight (body mass index [BMI] <18.5 kg/m2) and amenorrhea.

The patient can present with hyperkinesia (excessive exercise), starvation, or purging.

72. What are two defining characteristics of bulimia nervosa?

Bulimia nervosa is characterized by normal body weight or slightly overweight (BMI >25 kg/m2) and binging. It is associated with obsessive compulsive disorder. The patient can present with hyperkinesia, purging, or fasting. Make sure you differentiate it from anorexia nervosa.

73. What are pathognomonic signs of bulimia nervosa?
Signs of bulimia nervosa are calluses on the back of the hand, parotid gland enlargement, and lanugo hair (as part of the body's response to insulate itself because of low body fat).

74. What are the definitions of overweight, obesity, morbid obesity, and underweight?

- Overweight: BMI >25 kg/m2
- Obesity: BMI >30 to 39.9 kg/m2
- Morbid obesity: BMI >40 kg/m2
- Underweight: BMI <18.5 kg/m2

75. What is a mnemonic for cyanotic heart diseases?
A mnemonic is all T's:

- Transposition of great vessels
- Truncus arteriosus
- Tetralogy of Fallot
- Total anomalous pulmonary venous connection
- Tricuspid valve abnormalities

76. What are some clinical features of cyanosis?
Features include blue skin color in the nail beds, tongue, and mucous membranes and digital clubbing. **Central cyanosis** is due to decreased oxygen saturation level and **peripheral cyanosis** is due to increased extraction of oxygen from the tissues as a result of decreased hemoglobin and hematocrit. Patients with **cyanotic congenital heart disease** have central cyanosis.

What is the difference between central and peripheral cyanosis?

77. Eisenmenger syndrome is a common cause of cyanosis in infants. True or false?
False. It is a common cause of cyanosis in adults.

78. What is the pathogenesis of truncus arteriosus (TA)?
In truncus arteriosus, the great vessels (pulmonary trunk and aorta) have not divided, leaving one great vessel that mixes systemic and pulmonic blood, causing cyanosis. The patient presents with cyanosis weeks after birth and has an associated ventricular septal defect (VSD) (holosystolic murmur at the left sternal border) with or without a diastolic murmur. EKG is normal for a neonate (right ventricular predominance) and CXR shows increased heart

What cyanotic heart disease is associated with mothers who are diabetic?

Why does peripheral resistance or systemic vascular resistance alleviate tetralogy of Fallot?

size and pulmonary vascular markings. An absent thymus can be found in TA associated with DiGeorge syndrome.

79. What is the pathogenesis of transposition of the great vessels?

In transposition of the great vessels, the pulmonary artery originates from the left ventricle and the aorta originates from the right ventricle, creating a parallel system. A VSD or patent ductus arteriosus (PDA) is needed to mix pulmonary and systemic systems, causing cyanosis. The patient presents with cyanosis at birth. It is associated with having a mother who is diabetic. EKG is normal for a neonate, and CXR shows cardiac enlargement and increased pulmonary vascular markings.

Treatment: Treat immediately with prostaglandin E (PGE) to maintain a patent PDA.

80. What is the pathogenesis of tetralogy of Fallot?

Tetralogy of Fallot consists of four anatomic defects, including pulmonary stenosis, VSD, right ventricular hypertrophy, and an overriding aorta that causes a right-to-left shunt, leading to cyanosis. The patient will present with "Tet spells" (acute episodes of difficulty breathing), cyanosis, and systolic murmur in the left-mid to upper sternal border radiating posteriorly from right ventricular outflow obstruction, with low peripheral resistance. The knees-chest position, or anything that increases peripheral resistance, forces blood flow through the pulmonary system, thereby relieving cyanosis. EKG is normal for a neonate or shows right ventricular hypertrophy. CXR shows a "boot-shaped" heart with an upturned apex and decreased pulmonary vascularity.

81. Patients with conotruncal abnormalities (tetralogy of Fallot, pulmonary atresia, and truncus arteriosus) should be screened for what chromosomal abnormality?

Screen for 22q11.2 microdeletion. Their offspring have a markedly increased chance of having tetralogy of Fallot.

82. What are the most common acyanotic congenital heart diseases?

The most common diseases are atrial septal defect (ASD) and VSD.

83. What is the pathogenesis of ASD?

ASD creates a left-to-right shunt due to an abnormality in the interatrial septum. On examination, the patient may have a systolic ejection murmur and an S2 split that is fixed. History of heart failure in childhood or atrial fibrillation as an adult can occur. Most patients will be asymptomatic. The most common form is **ostium secundum** defect located in the middle of the atrium. EKG and imaging may show **right-side enlargement**.

Treatment: The asymptomatic secundum type should not be treated; symptomatic patients with volume overload of the right side and paradoxical embolus should be treated surgically.

What is the difference in presentation of ASD in children vs. adults?

84. What is the significance of patent foramen ovale (PFO) in adults?

PFO is an interatrial **right-to-left shunt** remnant pathway for placenta transfer of blood to fetus. In those with unknown causes of stroke, PFO is a potential cause of paradoxical embolus, especially when associated with atrial septal aneurysm.

85. What is the pathogenesis of a VSD?

A VSD is a left-to-right shunt due to an abnormality in the interventricular septum. The patient usually presents with congestive heart failure symptoms and in worse condition than a patient with ASD. On the physical examination, a holosystolic murmur is heard in the left parasternal space, a thrill is felt, and a parasternal heave may be felt. The most common type of VSD is the muscular form, which is more likely to close spontaneously. EKG and CXR findings vary based on the severity of the defect, and a large VSD, on EKG and CXR, would typically show **left-sided enlargement** from volume overload.

86. In general, small VSD should be followed and large VSD should be closed surgically. True or false?

True. Large VSD causes **pulmonary hypertension** and pulmonary vascular disease, leading to reversal of left-to-right shunt (**Eisenmenger syndrome**). Maintain a PDA in those with irreversible pulmonary vascular disease that could eventually lead to right-to-left shunt.

87. What is the initial evaluation in a patient suspected of having pulmonary hypertension from congenital heart disease?

Patients with pulmonary hypertension may present with **peripheral cyanosis and clubbing**. Physical examination

Turner syndrome is associated with the coarctation of the aorta.

may reveal **left parasternal heave,** a **palpable second heart sound,** and a **systolic ejection murmur** in the pulmonic area from pulmonary hypertension. In Eisenmenger syndrome, there may be **differential clubbing** and **cyanosis** (lower extremities > upper extremities) due to deoxygenated blood being shunted past the level of the subclavian artery from the pulmonary trunk to the aorta by a PDA. Obtain a **CXR,** which may show **prominent central pulmonary vasculature** and "pruning" (shortening of peripheral pulmonary arteries) and a right atrial abnormality from volume overload.

88. What is the pathogenesis of coarctation of the aorta?

Coarctation of the aorta is stenosis of the descending aorta just distal to the left subclavian artery, leading to hypertension in the upper extremities and **reduced blood pressure** in the lower extremities.

On the physical examination, in addition to a **systolic murmur,** a radial-femoral delay is felt. A PDA may be present to maintain systemic flow. This condition is associated with Turner syndrome, **Shone syndrome** (aortic stenosis, mitral stenosis, bicuspid aortic valve, and aortic regurgitation), and cerebral aneurysm. CXR may reveal **rib notching** due to formation of systemic collaterals.

Treatment: Maintain the PDA with PGE1 in infancy prior to surgery for coarctation.

89. What is the pathophysiology of a PDA?

This is a **left-to-right shunt** at the pulmonary level (aorta to pulmonary artery) that presents as a **continuous murmur** that can lead to **volume overload**. PDA repair should be avoided in those with severe pulmonary vascular resistance. Otherwise, percutaneous intervention should be considered in adults; indomethacin, a prostaglandin inhibitor, is routinely used in premature infants. Those with severe pulmonary vascular resistance and/or right-to-left shunt are more likely to develop Eisenmenger syndrome and may need PDA to maintain cardiac output.

90. What are the indications for closure of a PDA in patients?

Indications for PDA closure are significant left-to-right shunt in patients who are symptomatic, volume overload, mild to moderate pulmonary arterial hypertension, and previous endocarditis.

91. PDA is associated with maternal rubella infection. True or false?

True.

92. How do patients present with trisomy 13 (Patau syndrome)?

The patient presents with a defect in the prechordal mesoderm, causing defects in the **midface**, **eye**, and **forebrain**; holoprosencephaly; microphthalmia; deafness; and cleft lip and palate. Other defects are polydactyl and congenital heart defects. Most patients die within first month of life.

93. How do patients with trisomy 18 (Edwards syndrome) present?

The patient presents with a small jaw (micrognathia), small mouth, narrow head, low-set ears, rocker bottom feet, and congenital heart disease (ASD, VSD). Most patients die within a year.

94. How do patients present with trisomy 21 (Down syndrome)?

Dysmorphic features predominantly affect the head and neck. The patient presents with a palmar crease, epicanthal folds, slanted palpebral fissures, a flat nasal bridge, excessive skin in the head and neck, a short neck, cognitive impairment, space between the first and second toes, congenital heart defects, and gastrointestinal defects (duodenal atresia). Leukemia, and dementia can present later in the fifth decade of life. Many have a reduced life expectancy.

95. What is the pathogenesis of Turner syndrome?

Because of chromosome genotype 45 XO, patients lack an ovary and have no estrogen; therefore the follicle-stimulating hormone (FSH) level is elevated. The patient presents with short stature, a webbed neck (from excess skin in neck), congenital lymphedema (hand and feet edema), and gonadal dysgenesis. Turner syndrome is associated with coarctation of the aorta and bicuspid aortic valve; endocrine (type 2 diabetes), renal (horseshoe kidneys), and gastrointestinal abnormalities (IBD); and neoplasia.

Why is FSH elevated in Turner syndrome?

96. What is the pathogenesis of Klinefelter syndrome?

An XXY genotype causes a reduced testosterone level and therefore the GnRH level is elevated. It is associated

What is the difference between Marfan's syndrome and Ehlers-Danlos syndrome?

later in life with changes that involve the long bone, breast, and lungs, resulting in a tall stature, increased **length of arms** and legs, breast cancer, bronchitis, emphysema, and germ cell tumors. Klinefelter syndrome is the most common cause of chromosomal male infertility.

97. What is the pathogenesis of Prader-Willi syndrome?

Prader-Willi is the deletion of the paternal chromosome in chromosome 15. The patient presents with infantile hypotonia, both primary and secondary hypogonadism, and excessive eating. Hypogonadism laboratory results will show low serum LH and high FSH levels. Obesity is present as the child develops because of overeating. Most deaths result from complications of obesity, including sleep apnea, diabetes mellitus, and atherosclerosis.

98. What is the pathogenesis of Angelman syndrome?

Angelman syndrome is deletion of maternal chromosome 15. The patient presents with ataxia, tiptoeing, and seizures ("happy puppet").

99. What is the pathogenesis of fragile X syndrome?

Fragile X syndrome is the microdeletion of the X chromosome. The patient presents with macroorchidism (enlarged testes), macrognathia (a large jaw), and large ears.

100. What are the clinical features of Marfan's syndrome?

Marfan's syndrome is an autosomal dominant condition due to a mutation of the **fibrillin-1 gene**, causing excess linear bone growth and **joint laxity** that manifests as tall stature, long digits, arm span length greater than height, and superior lens dislocation. **Mitral valve prolapse** is frequently present. Aortic root disease, such as **aortic root dilation, regurgitation, and dissection,** is a main cause of complications and death. Other minor defects are skin striae, a high arch palate, and joint hypermobility.

101. What is a connective tissue abnormality that leads to predominant hyperelasticity, increased fragility of the skin, and hypermobility of joints?

Ehlers-Danlos syndrome results from a collagen abnormality. Serious cardiovascular complications such as rupture of large and medium-sized arteries without dissection can be seen.

102. What is an inherited connective tissue condition with multiple fractures with minimal or no trauma?

This is **osteogenesis imperfecta** (OI), caused by a mutation in type I collagen. Clinical features vary, but include **excess or atypical fractures**, short stature, scoliosis, **blue sclerae**, hearing loss, hyperelasticity of the skin, and basilar skull fracture. Differentiate it from child abuse (trauma in various stages of healing) by looking for other clinical features in OI.

103. Macrocrania (enlarged skull with frontal bossing), severe macromelia (short limbs), and a small trunk are associated with what connective tissue condition?

These are associated with **achondroplasia**, an inherited condition that can be caused by a mutation in type II collagen. It can be associated with occasional fractures.

What is the difference between constitutional delay of growth and achondroplasia?

Chapter 17

Pregnancy, Peripartum, and Postpartum

1. **What is the first step in the initial prenatal visit?**
The first step is to order tests for complete blood cell count, Rapid Plasma Reagin (RPR) or VDRL, rubella titer, hematocrit, Rh type, chlamydial and gonorrheal smear, and Pap smear (if not done within last 6 months).

2. **What is the first step in the subsequent prenatal visit?**
Check the following at subsequent prenatal visits:
Weight: Gain of 25-30 pounds throughout pregnancy is ideal.
Vitals: Measure blood pressure to rule out preeclampsia or chronic hypertension; order ultrasound to check fetal heart rate and nuchal translucency and to confirm dates and well-being; and order urinalysis to check for infection, glucose, and proteins.

3. **What is the first step in second-trimester screening?**
The first step is to offer an aneuploidy screening test in all women before 20 weeks of gestation, with a serum alpha-fetoprotein (AFP) test or triple screening (estriol, human chorionic gonadotropin [B-HCG], and AFP), as well as genetic testing. The AFP level is elevated in neural tube disorders and decreased in Down syndrome.

AFP is down in Down syndrome.

4. **What is the first step in third-trimester screening?**
The first step is oral glucose loading to test for gestational diabetes (1 hour 50 g oral glucose test). Culture for group B streptococci; if the result is positive, treat with penicillin. Administer RhoGAM (anti-Rh antibody) to patients with Rh-negative blood.

The most common cause of abnormal AFP is inaccurate dates.

5. How is an abnormal AFP result worked up?

When serum AFP is low, the next step is to order ultrasound to confirm dates. Why? **Inaccurate dates** are the most common cause of an abnormal AFP result. If the dates are accurate, check amniotic AFP levels. Why? The amniotic AFP level is more specific.

6. What hormonal laboratory tests are diagnostic of Down syndrome in utero?

B-HCG and inhibin levels are elevated, whereas estriol and AFP levels are decreased in Down syndrome.

Why is chorionic villous sampling excellent for early diagnosis of fetal disorders?

7. What are the ways to obtain a prenatal diagnosis?

A prenatal diagnosis can be made by obtaining fetal tissue or blood samples via:

- Amniocentesis: Performed after 15 weeks of gestation
- Chorionic villous sampling: Performed after 9 weeks of gestation; excellent for early diagnosis
- Periumbilical fetal blood sampling

8. Always administer RhoGAM after amniocentesis and other fetal diagnostic procedures to Rh-negative mothers. True or false?

True. Why? Any procedure that causes transplacental hemorrhage can cause fetal-maternal blood mixing.

9. What is the definition of term premature rupture of the membranes (PROM)?

What are the nitrazine, fern, and pool tests?

Rupture of the membranes at term is premature if it occurs beyond 37 weeks of gestation or at least 1 hour before labor. The patient will present with a gush of fluids from the vagina without having contractions. Vaginal examination may show fluid from the cervical os. Assess fetal well-being with a nonstress test, BPP, and ultrasound. The results of the nitrazine test (cervical smears turn nitrazine paper from yellow to blue), fern test (cervical smears form a fern-like pattern), and pool test (pooling of fluid in the vagina) will be positive. Ultrasound may show oligohydramnios.

Treatment: Induction of labor is preferred in term PROM over expectant management because of susceptibility to infections. The risk of infections guides treatment.

10. What is preterm premature rupture of the membranes?

Preterm premature rupture of the membranes occurs at less than 37 weeks of gestation.

Treatment: Expectant management is preferred over induction of labor. The risk of prematurity is what guides management. Treat with antibiotics prophylaxis and delayed labor. Delay labor with tocolysis and administer steroids for lung maturity.

11. What are complications of rupture of the membranes?
Chorioamnionitis is the most common complication. **Vasa previa** (abnormally transversed fetal vessels covering the internal cervical os) may be compressed and may rupture, leading to **fetal distress without maternal distress.**

12. How do patients with chorioamnionitis typically present?
Patients usually present with maternal fever, fetal or maternal tachycardia, purulent or foul-smelling amniotic fluid, uterine tenderness, and maternal leukocytosis. The most important risk factors include prolonged labor and prolonged rupture of membranes. Patients are at risk for postpartum endometritis.

Treatment: IV gentamycin and ampicillin, or rapid delivery if fetal compromise occurs.

What is the difference between chorioamnionitis and post-partum endometritis?

13. When a patient presents with a prolonged stage of labor or arrest of descent, three factors need to be considered. True or false?
True. The strength of contractions, size of the pelvis, and size of the fetus need to be considered.

14. How is gestational diabetes diagnosed?
Diagnosis is made on the basis of an oral glucose tolerance test (OGTT). If plasma glucose measured 1 hour after a 50-g loading dose is ≥140 mg/dl, an OGTT is performed.

15. How is OGTT performed?
An oral glucose load of 100 g is given and the plasma glucose is measured at 1 hour, 2 hours, and 3 hours. If it is ≥180, 155, or 140 mg/dl, respectively, then the diagnosis is made.

16. Patients with gestational diabetes are at increased risk of developing diabetes years after diagnosis. True or false?
True. At approximately 10 years, 50% develop diabetes.

17. What is the sequence of events when a patient presents with prolonged labor or arrest of descent?
The first step is to evaluate for adequate contractions (normal contractions occur every 2-5 minutes and are

regular). Proportionate pelvic size and fetal size would have been investigated prior to term by previous birth (for pelvic size) and ultrasound (for fetal size).

Treatment: If contractions are inadequate, oxytocin is given. A cesarian section (C-section) may be indicated for disproportionate pelvis and fetal size or if oxytocin fails.

18. What defines the first stage of labor?

The first stage is the time of onset of contractions to complete cervical dilation, and it is divided into the **latent** and **active** phases.

- Latent phase: Onset of labor; cervical dilation and effacement is **gradual** at <1 cm/hour. Cervical dilation reaches 4-5 cm.
- Active phase: Increased contraction, frequency, intensity, and duration; cervical dilation is **more rapid** and occurs at a rate of at least 1 cm/hour. Cervical dilation reaches 5-6 cm.

What is the first step in the management of patients with prolonged latent stage of labor?

19. What is the current approach to a prolonged latent stage of labor?

The average duration of the latent phase of labor in nulliparous and multiparous women is 6.4 and 4.8 hours, respectively, but an abnormally long latent phase is >20 hours in nulliparous and >14 hours for multiparous women.

Treatment: For women who are tired and uncomfortable, the first step is therapeutic rest with morphine. Once she is rested, if labor does not progress, try oxytocin.

20. What is defined as a prolonged active phase of labor?

Contemporary studies have shown that it may take more than **3 hours** to progress from 5 to 6 cm, regardless of parity.

Administer oxytocin and wait 4 hours with adequate contractions, or 6 hours without adequate contractions, before proceeding to operative delivery.

21. Hypocontractile uterine cavity is the most common cause of a prolonged or arrested phase of labor. True or false?

True. This is why an oxytocin trial is usually given.

22. What is defined as a first-stage arrest of labor?

This is defined as cervical dilation ≥6 cm dilation and ruptured membranes with the following:

- No cervical change ≥**4 hours** with adequate contractions
- No cervical change ≥**6 hours** without adequate contractions

23. What is defined as a prolonged second stage of labor?
Contemporary studies have shown that the second stage can last up to 3 hours with anesthesia and nulliparity. The American College of Obstetricians and Gynecologists recommends that no intervention should be done as long as there is a reassuring fetal heart rate and some degree of progress. Induction does not affect the progress of the second stage of labor.

Understand indications for labor induction.

24. What defines the second stage of labor?
This is defined as the time from complete cervical dilation to delivery of the fetus.

25. What defines a second-stage arrest of labor?
This is defined as no progress (descent or rotation):

- Nulliparous women: ≥**4 hours** with epidural anesthesia or ≥3 hours without epidural anesthesia
- Multiparous women: ≥**3 hours** with epidural anesthesia and ≥2 hours without anesthesia

26. What are indications for labor induction?

- Post-term pregnancy
- Preeclampsia, eclampsia, and HELLP syndrome
- Non-reassuring fetus
- Fetal growth restriction
- Premature rupture of the membranes
- Twins
- Chorioamnionitis
- Abruptio placentae

27. The probability of induction is less likely in the latent stage of labor and more likely in the active phase of labor. True or false?
True.

28. How do patients present with preterm labor?
The patient will present with irregular contractions that result in a change in cervical dilation on the pelvic examination prior to 37 weeks of gestation.

What is the mechanism of tocolytic agents?

Treatment: Tocolysis, using beta agonists (Terbutaline), prostaglandin analogue inhibitors, magnesium sulfate, or

What is the mechanism behind early deceleration?

When is delivery mandatory in a biophysical profile?

What is the mechanism of variable deceleration?

What is the mechanism of late deceleration?

calcium blockers. These drugs all act to reduce calcium to delay labor. Administer steroids for lung maturity.

29. What is a non-stress test (NST)?

An NST is indicated for high-risk groups (diabetes, hypertension, post-term pregnancy, fetal growth restriction, multiple gestation, premature rupture of membranes, absent or decreased fetal movements) during the third trimester. NST measures the heart rate of the fetus and determines whether there is fetal distress. Two consecutive heart rates, each 15 beats/minute above baseline and lasting 15 seconds, are reassuring.

30. What is the definition of a biophysical profile?

A biophysical profile is a combination of four tests used to monitor fetal well-being in high-risk groups. The profile includes NST, fetal tone, fetal breathing, and amniotic fluid (2 points for each). A normal score is 8-10. If the score is <4, delivery is mandatory.

31. What is the definition of fetal deceleration?

Fetal deceleration occurs when the fetal heart rate decreases from baseline gradually or suddenly and may or may not coincide with maternal contractions. Bradycardia is fetal heart rate <110 beats/minute and tachycardia is >160 beats/minute. Normal fetal heart rate is between 110 to 160 beats/minute.

32. What is the definition of early deceleration?

Early decelerations occur at the same time as uterine contractions. They indicate compression of the fetal head (increased vagal stimulation). Since they are common in the second stage of labor and quickly resolve, no treatment is needed.

33. What is the definition of variable deceleration?

Variable deceleration occurs at different times with contractions and indicates umbilical cord compression. It is common in the second stage of labor and quickly resolves. No treatment is needed.

34. What is the definition of late deceleration?

Late deceleration occurs at peaks of contractions, indicating uteroplacental insufficiency. It is an ominous sign and the most common cause is hypoxia.

Treatment: Oxygen

35. What are the risk factors for oligohydramnios?
The risk factors are post-term pregnancy, renal agenesis, and premature rupture of the membranes. Oligohydramnios is diagnosed via the amniotic fluid index (AFI). An AFI of <4 cm is diagnostic.

Treatment: Depends on the cause. Enhance fetal maturity with steroids if preterm delivery is expected.

36. What are the risk factors for polyhydramnios?
The risk factors are diabetes and fetal intestinal obstruction. An AFI of >25 cm is diagnostic; the size being greater than the dates on the physical examination is also diagnostic. Treatment: Depends on the cause. Enhance fetal lung maturity with steroids if preterm delivery is expected.

37. What is the definition of post-term pregnancy?
Post-term pregnancy is defined as pregnancy ≥42 weeks. Risk factors are anencephaly and hypopituitarism.

Treatment is to monitor with a biophysical profile and NST twice a week. If ≥41 weeks of gestation, induction is recommended.

38. What are ways to reduce HIV transmission to an infant from an HIV-infected parent?
Antiretroviral therapy, excluding efavirenz (toxic in pregnancy), is recommended during pregnancy, labor, and delivery. After birth, if the mother feeds the infant with breast milk, prophylaxis is needed with antiretroviral drugs postpartum for 28 weeks in the parent or infant to reduce HIV transmission during breast feeding.

39. What is a common complication of post-term pregnancy?
A common complication is meconium aspiration. The patient presents with respiratory distress, tachypnea, retractions, and dry and peeling skin.

Treatment: Suction meconium at birth.

40. How do patients with endometritis present?
Endometritis can be divided into pregnancy related and pregnancy unrelated, the latter called pelvic inflammatory disease. In pregnancy (postpartum endometritis), patients usually present with postpartum fever, chills, lower abdominal pain (**uterine tenderness**), and foul-smelling postpartum lochia. Laboratory tests show

Why is there a delayed onset of deceleration in late-onset deceleration? ***Maternal contractions cause reduced blood flow, causing the fetus with underlying hypoxia to respond with decelerations.***

What is the most common causative organism of endometritis? polymicrobials

What intracranial lesion is seen on toxoplasmosis?

Blueberry muffin is a mnemonic for what neonatal infection?

evidence of **leukocytosis**. Risk factors for postpartum endometritis include C-section, premature rupture of the membranes, and prolonged labor.

Treatment: Combination clindamycin and penicillin for postpartum endometritis to target *Clostridium perfringens* and polymicrobials.

41. When is herpes simplex treated in pregnancy?

Treat herpes simplex only when lesions are seen on the genitals.

Treatment: Acyclovir. A C-section is preferred over vaginal delivery to prevent vertical transmission to the fetus.

42. How do infants with human immunodeficiency virus (HIV) present?

The infant may present with persistent candidiasis, lymphadenopathy, fever, sore throat, and diarrhea. C-section is the preferred mode of delivery. Why? HIV can be transmitted via vertical transmission to the fetus.

43. What are the risk factors for infant toxoplasmosis?

The risk factors are mother's exposure to cat feces and ingestion of inadequately cooked meat. Look for intracranial calcifications on magnetic resonance imaging (MRI) of the neonate.

Treatment: Spiramycin. Why? It is safe in pregnancy. Sulfadiazine and pyrimethamine can be used as alternatives.

44. Why do we treat asymptomatic urinary tract infection (UTI) during pregnancy?

During pregnancy, the progression of an untreated UTI to sepsis and pyelonephritis is more likely.

Treatment: Amoxicillin or nitrofurantoin. Why? They are both safe treatments in pregnancy.

45. What should be looked for in a neonate with cytomegalovirus (CMV) infection?

Look for petechiae and purpura, deafness, and cerebral calcifications on MRI in the neonate.

Treatment: Ganciclovir

46. What are clinical manifestations of rubella?

Look for purpuric rash (blueberry muffin), deafness, heart defects (the most common is PDA or pulmonary artery stenosis), and cataracts in the neonate.

Treatment: Postpartum vaccination

47. When is neonatal hepatitis B virus treated?

When a neonate's mother tests positive for hepatitis B surface antigen, treat the neonate with hepatitis B surface antigen vaccine and immunoglobulin on the first day of delivery.

48. When is maternal varicella virus treated?

It is treated in pregnant women who are exposed without prior vaccination. The first step is to provide prophylaxis with varicella immunoglobulin (VariZIG). If symptoms develop after giving VariZIG, then treat with acyclovir. Prophylaxis with VariZIG is also indicated in neonates whose mothers have signs and symptoms within 5 days before delivery or 2 days after delivery, premature infants who are exposed, and immunocompromised persons who are exposed and were previously not vaccinated due to contraindication.

49. How is diabetes treated in pregnancy?

Patients with diabetes are kept on insulin throughout pregnancy; no oral agents are used. Why? Oral agents are not safe in pregnancy.

50. How do neonates with Rh incompatibility present?

The second-born infant will present with hydrops with an Rh-negative mother who is not pretreated with RhoGAM.

When the titer of anti-Rh antibody is elevated in a pregnant woman, follow up to check that hemolysis has taken place by doing an amniotic fluid spectrophotometry test to check for bilirubin levels. Also take a periumbilical blood sample to check for anemia.

51. ABO incompatibility does not result in serious hemolysis in pregnancy. True or false?

True. Why? Most ABO antibodies are mainly of the IgM subtype and do not cross the placenta, exceptions being type O mothers with type A and B infants or, rarely, type A mothers with type B infants. This is because there is a higher percentage of the IgG subtype than normal in these subsets of patients. However, since fetal red blood cells (RBCs) have less expression of A or B antigens, the reaction is less severe. In addition to RBCs, several tissues in the body have surface A or B antigens, and so the maternal antibodies that are able to cross the placenta bind to only a few fetal RBC binding sites.

IgM antibodies do not cross the placenta.

Why does pregnancy predispose women to cholestasis?

Why is there normal TSH in pregnancy?

What is the difference between symmetric and asymmetric IUGR?

52. How do patients present with cholestasis of pregnancy?

The patient will present with itching that is predominantly on the palms and soles of the feet and worse at night. Jaundice is sometimes seen. Laboratory evidence shows elevated total bile acids and transaminases. Liver ultrasound is unremarkable.

Treatment: A bile binder, such as cholestyramine or ursodiol, can alleviate symptoms.

53. What is the cause of cholestasis in pregnancy?

More cholesterol is produced in pregnancy due to the increased amount of estrogen, leading to an increased production of bile acids.

54. How do healthy individuals maintain euthyroidism during pregnancy?

An increased thyroxine-binding globulin (TBG) level leaves more binding sites for free thyroid hormone, decreasing serum-free thyroid hormone. Normal individuals are able to secrete more thyroid hormones to match the increased level of TBG.

55. Which thyroid medication is preferred in pregnancy for treatment of hyperthyroidism?

Propylthiouracil is preferred.

56. Why may the dose of thyroid medication be increased during pregnancy in hypothyroid women?

Hypothyroid women are unable to increase secretion of thyroid hormones to match the increased level of TBG.

57. HCG can stimulate the TSH receptor, causing suppressed TSH in pregnancy. True or false?

True. No therapy is indicated.

58. How do patients present with uterine rupture?

Uterine rupture is secondary to trauma or vaginal birth after prior C-section. The patient will present with vaginal bleeding, abdominal pain, fetal distress, hypovolemia, and recession of the presenting part during labor.

59. How is intrauterine growth retardation (IUGR) determined?

IUGR is measured by biparietal or abdominal circumferential diameter. It can be symmetric or asymmetric. Symmetric body size occurs if it is caused before 28 weeks of gestation by chromosomal abnormalities and intrauterine infections. Asymmetric body size occurs after 28 weeks of gestation as a result of maternal diseases such as hypertension, preeclampsia, and diabetes.

60. How does breech presentation present?

On the physical examination of the patient, the vertex (cephalic) is palpated at the fundus. If a breech presentation is diagnosed before 37 weeks of gestation, do not treat it. Why? It will reverse itself before 37 weeks.

Why is breech presentation not treated before week 37 of gestation?

61. What is the birth control method of choice in the postpartum period?

A progesterone-only pill (progestin) is used if sexual intercourse is desired. Why? Estrogen inhibits lactation but progesterone does not.

62. What is the definition of lochia?

Lochia is the normal vaginal bleed after birth. It presents as sweet smelling with small blood clots. It is never foul smelling.

63. How do patients present with engorged or plugged breasts postpartum?

Patients report diffuse breast tenderness 24-72 hours after birth as a result of milk letdown. The treatment is removal of milk by good feeding technique, analgesics and an ice pack. Plugged ducts are localized area of milk stasis that cause distention of breast leading to breast pain, palpable lump and tenderness. Treatment is frequent feeding and analgesics for pain.

Differentiate engorged or plugged breasts from mastitis.

64. What is the definition of mastitis?

Mastitis is a focal infection of the breast, as opposed to engorgement and plugged ducts, which are diffuse. The associated focal inflammatory changes are erythematic, with warmth and swelling. The presence of systemic symptoms such as fever, and myalgia differentiate mastitis from engorged or plugged ducts.

Treatment: Dicloxacillin or antibiotics against S. aureus. Why? Staphylococcus aureus is the most common cause.

65. How do patients present with hyperemesis gravidarum?

Nausea and vomiting often resolve in the 16th week of gestation. When it persists beyond the 16th week, and there are electrolyte disturbances, the patient needs treatment.

What is the most common cause of PPH?

Treat with frequent, small dry meals; antiemetics; and rehydration therapy.

66. What is the definition of postpartum hemorrhage (PPH)?

In vaginal delivery and in C-section, a blood loss of >500 ml and >1000 ml, respectively, is considered PPH.

Causes: Cervical hemorrhage, uterine atony, coagulopathy, retained products of conception, and placenta accreta.

Uterine atony is the most common cause of PPH. On examination, the patient with uterine atony will have a boggy uterus.

Treatment of uterine atony: Oxytocin to stimulate the uterine muscle.

67. What is the definition of gestational trophoblastic disease (molar pregnancy)?

A molar pregnancy is an abnormal proliferation of trophoblastic tissue during gestation.

The risk factors are nulligravida and a young age at pregnancy.

The patient will present with early gestation bleeding and, on abdominal examination, the abdominal size is greater than dates. Other nonspecific symptoms are nausea, vomiting, and dizziness.

Diagnosis: Laboratory tests reveal an extremely elevated B-HCG level (>100,000 mIU/ml).

Treatment: Remove the contents regardless of the gestational age.

A major complication of molar pregnancy is persistent molar pregnancy.

68. How do patients with metastatic trophoblastic disease present?

Trophoblastic disease can occur in the form of choriocarcinoma or other forms. The patient may present the same way as in molar pregnancy.

The most common place to first metastasize is the lungs; therefore, watch out for shortness of breath.

Treatment: Combination chemotherapy

69. How is recurrent miscarriage (loss of three or more consecutive pregnancies) evaluated?

The first step is to evaluate for antiphospholipid syndrome, thyroid dysfunction, and obtain imaging (sonohysterography, hysterosalpingography) to evaluate uterine cavity and shape. Prenatal karyotyping of one partner (more often the woman) may be considered to look for chromosomal abnormalities.

Parental karyotyping is considered in recurrent miscarriage workup, if serological tests are normal.

Chapter 18

Preventive Medicine

1. Never give live vaccines to immunocompromised patients. True or false?
True.

2. List all live vaccines.
- Measles-mumps-rubella (MMR)
- Varicella
- Yellow fever
- Intranasal influenza

3. When are vaccines contraindicated in general?
Vaccines are contraindicated when a patient has had previous anaphylactic reactions to them.

4. When is the MMR vaccine also contraindicated?
The MMR vaccine is contraindicated when a patient has neomycin allergies or a previous anaphylactic reaction to the vaccine.

5. When is the influenza virus vaccine also contraindicated?
The influenza virus vaccine is also contraindicated when a patient has egg allergies.

Patients allergic to eggs can be given an egg free trivalent inactivated vaccine (TIV).

6. All live vaccines are contraindicated in immunocompromised patients. True or false?
True.

7. Why is pneumococcal conjugate vaccine (PCV) preferred to pneumococcal polysaccharide vaccine in children?
Polysaccharide antigens in children are not easily recognized by their immature immune system. Administer PCV in all children during infancy.

8. What is the initial test used for cholesterol?

The initial test is the fasting total cholesterol (not fasting lipid profile). Only when total cholesterol is >200 mg/dl is the fasting lipid profile (total cholesterol, high-density lipoprotein [HDL], low-density lipoprotein [LDL], and triglycerides) used.

9. When should healthy patients start screening for total cholesterol?

Healthy male patients should start screening at age 34, every 5 years, and women aged 45 and older should start screening if they are at increased risk for CAD.

10. When should patients be screened for diabetes?

Only patients with documented hypertension should be screened for diabetes with fasting blood glucose. Also consider screening patients with dyslipidemia for diabetes.

11. When should healthy patients start screening for blood pressure?

Healthy patients should start screening for blood pressure at age 18 and every 2 years thereafter except if it is higher than 120-139/80-89, which requires a yearly check.

12. What determines treatment for cholesterol?

LDL levels (not total, not HDL) determine treatment.

13. What is the most important lipid used to determine risk for coronary artery disease (CAD)?

LDL is the most important in determining risk. Why? Studies have shown that treating LDL will reduce a patient's risk of developing CHD.

14. What are the major risk factors that determine risk for CAD?

The major risk factors are HDL <40 mg/dl, age ≥45 years if male, age ≥55 years if female, family history of premature CAD (defined as first-degree male relative ≤55 years of age and first-degree female relative ≤65 years of age), smoking, and hypertension.

What conditions are CAD equivalent?

15. What medical conditions are CAD equivalent?

Diabetes, peripheral arterial disease, carotid arthrosclerosis, abdominal aortic aneurysm, Framingham risk factor >20%, and chronic kidney disease with creatinine >1.5 mg/dl or GFR <60 ml/min are CAD equivalent.

16. What is primary prevention?

Primary prevention prevents the development of a disease and reduces its incidence (e.g., aspirin in the prevention of coronary artery disease).

What type of prevention reduces incidence rate?

17. What is secondary prevention?

Secondary prevention detects the early development of a disease (e.g., colonoscopy in the screening of colon cancer) and applies interventions to prevent the progression of a disease (e.g., aspirin in the progression of coronary heart disease after acute coronary syndrome).

18. What is tertiary prevention?

Tertiary prevention rehabilitates patients or alleviates the progression of an established disease (e.g., physical therapy and rehabilitation in patients with motor deficits from a stroke).

19. What is the drug of choice given preoperatively to those with cardiovascular disease or at high risk for CAD to prevent cardiovascular complications?

Beta-blockers are the drug of choice. Why? Studies have shown that they are the most effective in preventing cardiovascular complications in patients with CAD or at high risk for CAD.

20. What determines whether antibiotics should be administered?

The propensity for infection determines whether antibiotics should be given.

21. What types of antibiotics are recommended preoperatively for patients with valvular heart disease?

Amoxicillin is recommended for most dental (oral) procedures and surgeries to prevent endocarditis.

What antibiotics are given to patients who are allergic to amoxicillin for preoperative prophylaxis?

22. What antibiotics are given preoperatively to patients with valvular disease who are allergic to amoxicillin?

Clindamycin or azithromycin is given preoperatively.

23. What should be discussed with the elderly population (>65 years) at some point?

Advance directives should be discussed with the elderly.

24. What should be ruled out as a cause of weight loss in the elderly population?

Nutrition due to poor dentition should be ruled out.

25. What is the treatment for the elderly who have poor dentition?
The treatment is frequent, small soft meals.

26. List the screening tests for adults.
See Table 18-1.

Table 18-1. *Screening Tests and Adult Vaccines*

Age or Risk Factors	Screening Test	Frequency	Comments
≥11-26 years old male and female	HPV vaccine	3 doses	
≥21 years old, female	Pap smear	Annually or 1-2 years	
≥25 years old sexually active female or women at high risk[a]	*Chlamydia* and *gonorrhea*	Annually	
≥35 years old plus male or female ≥ 45 years old with risk factors for CAD	Screening total cholesterol as initial test, only if ≥200 mg/dl is fasting lipid is obtained	Every 5 years	
≥40 years old, male if high risk[b] or ≥50 years old	Ask about PSA		
≥50 years old, female	Mammogram	1-2 years	
≥50 years old or 10 years younger than when first-degree relative acquired it or at 40 years old in a patient with family history	Colonoscopy, sigmoidoscopy	Every 10 years	Always do a colonoscopy at age 50, then either sigmoidoscopy or colonoscopy after that. Which is better? Colonoscopy examines the entire colon, while sigmoidoscopy looks at only the distal third. If given a choice on the boards, select colonoscopy.

Influenza vaccine recommendation 2012: all persons age 6 months or older should receive influenza vaccine annually.	Influenza vaccine	Annually	Why annually? The virus is highly variable
≥60 years old with risk factors[c] or ≥65 years old plus female sex.	DEXA (bone density test) T score of < −2.5 standard deviations is osteoporosis	Every 2-5 years	
≥65 years old or chronic lung disease, chronic alcoholism, chronic liver disease, diabetes, kidney failure, asplenia, immunocompromised, chronic long-term care facilities, special environment such as Alaskan natives or native Americans	Pneumococcal polysacch aride vaccine	For age 19-64 years, one-time revaccination is recommended after 5 years in those with asplenia, chronic renal failure or nephrotic syndrome, or immunocompromised conditions.	For age ≥65 years, one-time revaccination is recommended in those who received the first dose >5 years earlier and were younger than 65 at the time.
65-75 years old plus male sex and smoking history.	Abdominal ultrasound	Once	To detect abdominal aortic aneurysm
Adult or after 18 years old	Tetanus, diphtheria booster (toxoid)	Every 10 years	For previously fully immunized

Adult	Tetanus vaccine (toxoid)	>5 years if unclean wound	For previously fully immunized
Adult	Tetanus immunoglobulin and toxoid; start initial primary series	Conta-minated or unclean wound	For nonimmunized or unknown status
Adult: traveling to a foreign country, daycare center, chronic liver disease, MSM, illicit drug users, workers in healthcare	Hepatitis A	Within 4 weeks of traveling; if not, give immuno-globulin instead. 2 doses given within 6 months	Consider anywhere you can acquire the virus (fecal-oral route)
Adult: Traveling to a foreign country more than 6 months, chronic liver disease, high risk,[d] diabetes, working with blood, immunocompromised	Hepatitis B	3 doses within 6 months	Consider anywhere you can acquire the virus (via semen or blood products)
HIV patients, asymptomatic, CD4 count >200	MMR vaccine, varicella		If CD4 count <200, do not give

DEXA, dual-energy X-ray absorptiometry; HIV, human immunode- ficiency virus; HPV, human papillomavirus; IV intravenous; MMR, measles-mumps-rubella vaccine; MSM, men who have sex with men; PSA, prostrate-specific antigen; STD, sexually transmitted disease.

[a] High risk includes multiple sexual partners, MSM, having previous chlamydia or gonorrhea infection or other STDs, using condoms inconsistently, using drugs.

[b] High risk includes African American race and family history of prostate cancer.

[c] High risk includes family history of osteoporosis, Asian or Caucasian female, and low body weight (female <70 pounds).

[d] Adult with multiple sexual partners, STDs, IV drug use, HIV, end-stage renal disease, MSM, household contacts of those with hepatitis B.

27. What disease should be ruled out in patients with CAD?

Make sure you rule out hypothyroidism in patients with CAD.

28. What does it mean if HDL is >60 mg/dl?

If HDL >60 mg/dl, subtract one risk factor, which means it is protective. If a person has hypertension and smokes, which is a risk factor of 2, and HDL is 60 mg/dl, then the person has only one risk factor.

29. What is a cohort study?

A cohort study is a **long observational study** used to study a risk factor for an outcome, especially from a segment of a population with several variables in common (cohort). For example, a group of patients with a commonality (e.g., nurses) and a variable risk factor (e.g., dietary intake) are followed over time for an outcome (e.g., colon cancer) to study the effect of that risk factor. The type of diet in the group can be assessed (e.g., high- vs low-fiber diet) and the **relative risk** of colon cancer evaluated in those with a high- versus a low-fiber diet.

30. What is a case control study?

A case control study is a retrospective study used to study a risk factor associated with a **rare outcome**. Those with the condition (cases) are compared with those without it (controls). A common example is the study of tobacco as a risk factor for lung cancer. For example, a group of patients with lung cancer and a matched group from a population without lung cancer are identified and observed; the use of tobacco in each group would then be compared.

Case control is used to study rare outcomes.

31. What is a randomized controlled trial?

A randomized controlled trial is a **randomized prospective** study in which the efficacy of various interventions is tested in a patient population. This is the **gold standard** for trials. It is the best trial used to prove causality. For example, a group of patients is **randomly** assigned to the intervention arm (e.g., aspirin) and another to a control group (placebo) and followed over a period of time to determine whether the intervention (aspirin) results in the desired outcome (prevents MI). The risk of MI in those with aspirin is then calculated **relative** to those without aspirin and MI.

An OR is used in case control studies, and ARR is used in cohort and RCT

32. What is a meta-analysis trial?

A meta-analysis trial is a combination or pooling of various randomized controlled trials to identify common patterns or divergent results among studies.

33. What is the concept of relative risk reduction (RRR)?

This is the **ratio** of the **difference in outcomes** experienced by those exposed to the event and by the controls relative to the outcome experienced by the controls, or the risk of an event developing compared with exposure. For example, if the probability of developing cancer is 80% in those exposed to X-rays and 20% among those not exposed to X-rays, then the RRR is 0.6/0.2 = 3, which means that those exposed to X-rays are 3 **times** more likely than those not exposed to develop cancer. RRR is used in **randomized controlled trials and cohort studies**.

34. What is an odds ratio (OR)?

An OR describes the ratio of the odds occurring in an exposed group compared with the odds of it occurring in a control group. It is used in **uncommon diseases** in which it is difficult to estimate the true proportion of patients exposed to a risk factor and the relative risk cannot be calculated. Relative risk and OR are interpreted relative to one. For example, an OR of 0.4 suggests that the patients exposed to a risk factor are 60% less likely to develop a specific outcome compared with the control group. Similarly, an OR of 1.5 suggests that the patients exposed have an increased risk of 50%. An OR is used in **case control studies.**

35. What is the concept of absolute risk reduction (ARR)?

This is the difference in outcomes experienced by those exposed to the event and by those not exposed. For example, the ARR for the previous example is 60%, which means that there is a 60% chance of developing cancer if you are exposed to X-rays. Note that RRR and odds ratio (OR) are expressed as comparisons with a standard as opposed to ARR. ARR is used in **cohort and randomized controlled trial studies.**

36. What is the number needed to treat (NNT)?

This is the number needed to treat to prevent one bad outcome (**1/ARR**). For example, if the ARR of a certain drug is a 20% mortality rate, then NNT is 1/0.2 = 5. Thus, this suggests that only 5 patients need to be treated to prevent one death.

37. What is the concept of confidence interval?
A 95% confidence interval means that if a study is repeated a hundred times, 95% of the time this range of values will be expected for the population, e.g., 3.5 (3.0-4.0). If the confidence interval includes 1, it is statistically insignificant.

38. Draw a table of sensitivity, specificity, positive predictive value, and negative predictive value.
See Table 18-2.

Table 18-2. *Sensitivity, Specificity, and Positive and Negative Predictive Values*[a]

	Disease	No Disease	Total
Tests (+)	TP	FP	TP + FP
(-)	FN	TN	FN + TN
Total	TP + FN	FP + TN	Total patients

FN, false negative; FP, false positive; TP, true positive; TN, true negative.

a Sensitivity = TP/ (TP + FN); Specificity = TN/ (FP + TN); Positive predictive value = TP/ (TP + FP); Negative predictive value = TN/ (TN + FN).

39. How does prevalence affect sensitivity, specificity, positive predictive value, and negative predictive value?
Sensitivity and specificity are not affected by prevalence, positive predictive value increases with prevalence, and negative predictive value decreases with prevalence.

40. What is the definition of a likelihood ratio (LR)?
This is a function of **sensitivity**, or the likelihood that a positive test "rules in" a diagnosis. LR = sensitivity/1-specificity. The farther away the result is from 1.0, the more useful it is. The likelihood that a negative test "rules out "a diagnosis = 1-sensitivity/specificity.

41. What is the definition of power?
Power is the ability to detect the difference between two groups (power = 1-beta).

42. What is a type I error?
In a type I error, the null hypothesis is incorrectly rejected (also known as alpha).

43. What is a type II error?
In a type II error, one fails to reject a false null hypothesis (also known as beta).

44. What is the definition of ethical autonomy?
This is the right of a competent and appropriately informed patient to make choices regarding his or her health; it is the right to decline treatment or a procedure.

Always find a patient a provider prior to discharging him/her.

45. What is the concept of the ethical principle of respect for justice?

This means to treat like things alike; respect for autonomy should not be bridged because of sex or pregnancy.

46. What is the recommended approach to a patient who wishes to choose a different therapy?

You should try to understand the reason for the patient not wanting a certain therapy and to address any concerns that a patient may have. If after doing this, the patient still insists, then go with the patient's chosen plan even if it means finding the patient a different physician; do not abandon the patient until you find a different physician.

Chapter 19

Psychiatry

1. **What is the definition of a psychotic disorder?**
A psychotic disorder is a combination of delusions, hallucinations, and thought disorders.

2. **What is the definition of schizophrenia?**
Schizophrenia is two or more psychotic symptoms for 6 months or more.

3. **What is the definition of schizoaffective disorder?**
Schizoaffective disorder includes the criteria for schizophrenia and mood disorder.

4. **What is the definition of schizophreniform disorder?**
Schizophreniform disorder consists of psychotic symptoms that last <6 months.

5. **What is the definition of a brief psychotic disorder?**
A brief psychotic disorder is a psychosis secondary to stress or postpartum onset that lasts at least 1 day but less than a month.

6. **What are treatment options for schizophrenia?**
Prior to treatment, make sure to assess for extrapyramidal symptoms, tardive dyskinesia, and metabolic syndrome, and obtain an EKG in those with cardiac disease or if antipsychotic medication may cause a prolonged QT interval. The first line of treatment can be any antipsychotic except olanzapine because of the adverse effects of weight gain and metabolic syndrome, or clozapine because of the adverse effects of agranulocytosis.

What is the first-line drug for patients with schizophrenia?

What antipsychotic drugs can be used via the parenteral route?

7. Which antipsychotics may cause a prolonged QT syndrome?

Clozapine, thioridazine, iloperidone, and ziprasidone may cause this.

8. What are the two types of antipsychotic drugs?

Antipsychotic drugs can be typical (first generation) or atypical (second generation).

Typical antipsychotic drugs are traditional antipsychotics that inhibit the dopamine receptor, causing an extrapyramidal effect. Haloperidol and fluphenazine are common high-potency typical antipsychotics. Examples of low-potency typical antipsychotics are thioridazine and chlorpromazine.

9. How do atypical antipsychotics work?

Atypical antipsychotics work by inhibiting the serotonin receptor, preventing extrapyramidal effects and suppressing negative symptoms (flat affect, anhedonia). Atypical antipsychotics such as risperidone are the first-line drugs of choice for patients with schizophrenia if extrapyramidal side effects are not desired.

Other atypical antipsychotics are clozapine and olanzapine.

10. Clozapine is effective and recommended in patients with refractory symptoms despite trials of other first-line antipsychotics. True or false?

True.

11. Haloperidol and fluphenazine are the only drugs available for the parenteral route in the treatment of schizophrenia. True or false?

False. In addition to haloperidol and fluphenazine, second-generation antipsychotics, including risperidone, paliperidone, and olanzapine, are currently available in the United States for use via the parenteral route. They are injected over 2-4 weeks in those patients who are nonadherent to oral therapy, as nonadherence can cause relapse and frequent hospitalizations.

12. What are extrapyramidal effects?

- Akathisia: Movement disorder causing restlessness and an inner urge to move. Treatment: Beta-blockers. The second-line drug is benzodiazepine.
- Dystonia: Abnormal contraction of the head and neck muscles and tongue, ocular spasms, and

laryngeal spasms. Treatment: A muscarinic antagonist (benzatropine)

- Tardive dyskinesia: Oral-facial choreoathetoid movement disorder due to the use of a high-dose antipsychotic. Treatment: Discontinue the drug. No treatment is known.
- Neuroleptic malignant syndrome: Tachycardia, hypotension, fever, and weakness due to a hypercontractile state caused by the use of a high-dose antipsychotic. Treatment: Discontinue the drug and administer dantrolene (a muscle relaxant) and/or dopamine agonists.

13. What is a major complication of schizophrenia?

Thirty percent of patients with schizophrenia will attempt suicide.

Prognosis: A favorable prognosis is aided by family support and little or no stress.

Disorganized behavior suggests a worse prognosis.

14. What are the criteria for the diagnosis of major depression?

SIGECAPS:

Sleep disturbance
Loss of interest in activities
Guilt or hopelessness
Low energy level
Loss of concentration
Loss of appetite
Psychomotor retardation
Suicidal

Five or more of these criteria lasting for >2 weeks is diagnostic.

15. What is the definition of atypical depression?

Atypical depression includes symptoms of excessive sleepiness, increased appetite, or weight gain in addition to the criteria for depression. Treat with a monoamine oxidase inhibitor (MAOI).

16. What is the definition of dysthymic disorder?

Dysthymic disorder is a less severe form of depression that is chronic and recurrent and lasts for 2 years or more.

17. What is the definition of bipolar disorder?

Bipolar disorder comprises manic episodes (pressured speech, insomnia, grandiosity, flight of ideas, increased activity, distractibility, thoughtlessness, shopping spree,

What is the mechanism of neuroleptic malignant syndrome?

What is a major complication of schizophrenia?

SIGECAPS is a mnemonic for major depression.

Know the criteria needed to diagnose major depression.

Know the treatment of an acute manic episode vs. stabilization of bipolar disorder.

What is the first-line drug for major depression?

Acute panic disorder is usually associated with agoraphobia.

promiscuity) associated with alternating episodes of major depression.

18. What are the treatment options for mood disorders?
Treat depression with selective serotonin reuptake inhibitors (SSRIs), serotonin-norepinephrine reuptake inhibitors (SNRIs), bupropion, MAOIs, and psychotherapy. First-line treatment is typically with an SSRI with or without psychotherapy; if not responsive after 2-4 weeks, then consider alternatives. Treat acute mania disorder with benzodiazepine and lithium for bipolar stabilization.

19. What are the most reported favorable and unfavorable complications of SSRI?
Weight loss is a favorable adverse effect, whereas **sexual dysfunction** is a commonly reported unfavorable one.

20. How do patients present with anxiety disorder?
Patients present with excessive fear that is unreal. The patient can also present with acute panic disorder as palpitations, paresthesias, chest pain, shortness of breath, fear of choking, and fear of impending doom. These symptoms must impair the patient's daily life to be diagnostic. A source for the fear may not be found.

Acute panic disorder is usually associated with agoraphobia (fear of public places).

21. What is the treatment of acute panic disorder?
Acute panic disorder is treated with a short-acting benzodiazepine (alprazolam, clonazepam). Treat recurrent panic disorder with an SSRI.

22. What is the definition of specific phobia?
A specific phobia is excessive fear that does not match a specific object or situation, for example, fear of heights or fear of lizards. Treat with flooding or systemic desensitization therapy.

23. What is the definition of social phobia?
Social phobia is fear of speaking in a public gathering because one is afraid of being criticized.

First-line treatment is an SSRI and desensitization therapy.

24. How may acute stress disorder present?
Patients present with symptoms similar to those with PTSD. Symptoms can appear after traumatic injury

or near-death experience, but these symptoms last a minimum of 2 days and a maximum of 4 weeks. Treatment is reassurance that this is normal and will self-resolve.

25. What is the definition of generalized anxiety disorder?
Generalized anxiety disorder consists of worrying over various aspects of life (school, family, financial stability), which impairs daily living. Treat with SNRIs or SSRIs. They are both first-line drugs. Second-line medications are benzodiazepines, buspirone, and tricyclic antidepressants.

26. What is the definition of posttraumatic stress disorder (PTSD)?
PTSD consists of re-experiencing an event because of a severe traumatic incidence (near-death experience). The patient presents with hyperarousal, flashbacks, and an attempt to avoid recall. Treat with beta-blockers (hyper-responsiveness) or an SSRI and psychotherapy.

Hyperarousal, flashbacks, and an attempt to avoid recall characterize PTSD.

27. What is the definition of obsessive-compulsive disorder (OCD)?
OCD involves intrusive thoughts (obsessions) that cause one to perform recurrent physical or mental actions (compulsions). Treat with an SSRI as the first-line drug and desensitization therapy. The second-line drug is the tricyclic antidepressant (TCA) clomipramine.

What is the first-line drug for OCD?

28. SSRIs are the first-line treatment for major depression. True or false?
True. An example is fluoxetine.
Adverse effects: Anxiety, neuromuscular restlessness, sexual dysfunction

29. How is a TCA typically used for depression?
A TCA is second-line therapy.
Adverse effects: Anticholinergic symptoms such as dry mouth, dry skin, hyperthermia, agitation, and blurry vision

30. How is an MAOI typically used for depression?
An MAOI is used for atypical depression or for depression that is refractory to treatment. Examples are phenelzine and tranylcypromine.
Complication: Tyramine-releasing foods (red wine, cheese, and meat) can cause sympathetic activation and an MAOI crisis.

What is the most common ECT complication?

31. What are the indications for electroconvulsive therapy (ECT) for depression?

ECT is indicated when depression is refractory to other treatment and in elderly patients with comorbidities.

Complication: Memory loss is the most common complication.

32. What is the action of trazodone in depression?

Trazodone is similar in action to a TCA. Trazodone is used to treat depression as a second-line agent, especially in those with insomnia. Do not give it to patients with sexual dysfunction.

33. Why is trazodone used as a last resort in the treatment of depression?

Trazodone causes priapism.

34. What is a first-line agent against bipolar disorder?

Lithium monotherapy is used as a first-line agent to stabilize bipolar disorder.

Adverse effects: Tremor, polyuria (renal insufficiency), hypothyroidism, weight gain

Prevention of side effects: Monitor levels of thyroid-stimulating hormone, blood urea nitrogen/creatinine levels, and lithium. For those unable to tolerate lithium or unresponsive to it, lamotrigine or long-acting injectable risperidone can be given. Second-line medications include divalproex, aripiprazole, quetiapine, and olanzapine.

What personality disorder is associated with splitting?

What is the difference between schizoid and avoidant personality disorders?

35. What are the types of personality disorders and their characteristics?

Paranoid: The patient is suspicious of others' intent and thinks that other people are out to get or harm him or her.

Schizoid: The patient wants to be alone or left alone. Differentiate this disorder from avoidant personality disorder.

Schizotypal: The patient has odd thinking (magical thinking that words can move objects).

Narcissistic: The patient is arrogant and pompous with a sense of entitlement and importance.

Borderline: The patient has recurrent suicidal threats, hypersensitivity to rejection, and fear of abandonment. This disorder is associated with defense mechanisms such as splitting.

Histrionic: The patient presents as the center of attention, with superficial emotion (suicide bluff) and sexual and flirty behavior.

Dependent: The patient depends on others for decision making.

Avoidant: The patient ends up being alone to avoid anxiousness. The patient does not want to be alone.

Obsessive-compulsive personality disorder: The patient is very orderly and pays attention to the last bit of detail.

Treatment of personality disorders: Combination of psychotherapy and pharmacological therapy

36. What is the definition of alcohol abuse?

Alcohol abuse is the recurrent use of alcohol regardless of its interference with job, family, and friends.

What is the difference between alcohol abuse and dependence?

37. What is the definition of alcohol dependence?

Alcohol dependence consists of withdrawal symptoms, tolerance, and alcohol abuse. Withdrawal symptoms are nausea, vomiting, tremors, and seizures.

38. How do patients present with delirium tremens?

Delirium tremens (DTs) is a severe manifestation of alcohol withdrawal. It occurs 3-10 days following the last drink. The patient presents with fever, autonomic hyperactivity, and confusion.

Treatment of DTs: Administer thiamine, benzodiazepines (chlordiazepoxide), multivitamins, vitamin B12, and folate; correct electrolytes; and administer intravenous fluids. The use of thiamine is to prevent Wernicke encephalopathy and Korsakoff syndrome, and benzodiazepines are used to treat the symptoms and signs of alcohol withdrawal.

Disulfiram can be used to maintain sobriety by inhibiting acetaldehyde dehydrogenase and retaining acetaldehyde, which causes nausea and vomiting when alcohol is ingested.

Naltrexone, an opiod antagonist similar to naloxone, can also be used to treat alcohol dependence in addition to being used to treat opiod dependence.

39. What are the major risk factors for suicide?

The major risk factors are prior suicide attempt, age >55 years, and male sex.

40. What is the definition of bereavement?

Bereavement is a constellation of symptoms that lasts for 6 months after the death of a loved one. The patient will present with shock, disbelief, trouble accepting reality,

What is the treatment for somatoform disorders?

and visual and auditory hallucinations. Symptoms will usually resolve in months. Do not treat.

41. What is the definition of complicated bereavement?
This is a syndrome of persistent or prolonged bereavement >6 months, which includes difficulty moving on, detachment, denial of death, a feeling of emptiness, agitation, and trouble trusting others. Social withdrawal may also be seen. Psychiatry referral should be made for evaluation and treatment.

42. What is the definition of bereavement-related depression?
This is defined as symptoms of depression for at least 2 weeks at 6 to 8 weeks after a major loss. Treat for depression.

43. What is the definition of somatoform disorders?
Somatoform disorders are physical manifestations of a nonorganic disorder. Somatization disorder, hypochondriasis, conversion disorder, factitious disorder and malingering, and body dysmorphic disorder are examples. Treatment of somatoform disorders consists of regularly scheduled office visits, and psychotherapy. Consider antidepressants in those with pain syndromes and depression.

44. How do patients present with somatization disorder?
The patient can present with pain in four different sites, two gastrointestinal problems, one sexual symptom, and one pseudo-neurological symptom (hemiparalysis).

45. What is the definition of adjustment disorder?
Adjustment disorder is excessive emotional response to a stressor that is out of proportion and not sufficient to meet a diagnosis of major depression or dysthymic disorder. The patient can present with anxiety and symptoms of depression, including loss of appetite and lack of energy in response to a stressor (divorce, moving).

46. Conversion disorder is characterized by acute onset of a neurological symptom (e.g., unilateral weakness) in response to excessive stress. True or false?
True.

47. Hypochondriasis is the constant fear of developing a serious medical condition. True or false?
True. **Differentiate this from body dysmorphic disorder,**

which is preoccupation with an exaggerated or imagined body defect.

48. Factitious disorder is faking medical illness for the sole purpose of assuming the sick role. True or false?

True. Differentiate this from **malingering,** which is feigning medical illness for the purpose of monetary gain.

49. What is the definition of Munchausen syndrome?

This is a type of **factitious disorder** in which patients present with self-induced illness, e.g., surreptitious insulin injection.

50. How do patients present with parasomnia?

The patient presents with sleep disturbances during sleep. Sleep terror and sleep nightmares are examples.

Sleep terror: The patient screams out during sleep, usually occurring during stage 3 and 4 (delta). The patient is not usually awake and the episodes are not recalled.

Nightmare: The patient can have frightening dreams and scream out during sleep, usually occurring during rapid-eye-movement sleep. However, the patient may not be able to go back to sleep and the episodes are recalled.

What is the difference between sleep terror and nightmares?

51. When is a do-not-resuscitate form (DNR) needed?

A DNR form is needed for terminal disease that is not reversible. A written DNR form is valid. If a DNR is not available and the patient is not able to make competent decisions, then the spouse is the legal next of kin who should make the decision, followed by the children, and then siblings, in that order.

What is the order of hierarchy for a surrogate decision maker?

52. When is an ethics committee consulted for patients with terminal disease?

One example is if persons at the same level of hierarchy (e.g., children of the patient) disagree on the type of care that should be pursued, try to resolve the conflict with an ethics committee while continuing aggressive therapy.

53. Confidentiality of treatment in adolescents should be kept in what situations?

Most states do not require parental consent for treatment of sexually transmitted diseases and drugs in adolescents. However, it is important to encourage adolescents to talk to their parents about issues affecting their health. Emancipated minors do not require consent from parents to be treated for any medical condition.

Adults have similar exceptions to confidentiality as in children except in the case of abuse.

In adults, abuse is not reported except in the elderly.

54. What are exceptions to adolescent confidentiality?

- Child abuse
- Violent injuries: Gunshot or stab wounds, regardless of patient age
- Sexually transmitted diseases: Need to notify public health, regardless of patient age
- Suicidal ideation or attempt, regardless of patient age
- Homicidal ideation, regardless of patient age

55. What is the definition of an emancipated minor?

Emancipated minors are those who are able to provide their own consent for medical services because of the following:

- Married
- Independent financially from parents
- Run away
- Have a child

Chapter 20

Renal System

1. What are three causes of acute renal failure (ARF)?
The three causes are prerenal, postrenal, and intrinsic.

The patient may present within hours to weeks with nausea and vomiting, uremia, pericarditis, and peripheral neuropathy.

2. What is the definition of uremia?
Uremia is the combination of symptoms because of accumulation of toxic substances leading to itching, nausea, vomiting, and bleeding.

3. What are the three stages of ARF?
The three stages are oliguria, anuria, and polyuria. **Polyuria is due to tubular damage.**

4. What is the first step in the evaluation of ARF?
The first step is to acquire the blood urea nitrogen (BUN)/creatinine ratio and serum and urine electrolyte levels. Why? It is important to find out the type of renal failure and the severity of electrolyte imbalances. Next, obtain a urinalysis (UA). An elevated urine protein level (proteinuria), urine white blood cell (WBC)-positive result, and urine red blood cell (RBC)-positive (hematuria) result may be seen.

5. What are prerenal causes of ARF?
- Hypovolemia
- Heart failure
- Postsurgery
- Hemorrhage
- Liver disease

Why is the fractional excretion of sodium very low in prerenal ARF?

- Nephrotic syndrome
- Sepsis
- Iodinated contrast (glomerular capillary pressure decrease)
- Hypercalcemia

Laboratory tests will show a BUN/creatinine ratio of >20 and a fractional excretion of sodium of <1%. Why? **This is caused by volume depletion,** as the kidneys are trying to conserve as much sodium as possible because excreting it causes loss of fluid.

6. What are postrenal causes of ARF?

The patient may present with low abdominal pain and fullness in the hypogastric region.

Causes are as follows:

- Bladder obstruction
- Urethral obstruction
- Ureter obstruction
- Benign prostatic hyperplasia

Treatment: Transurethral bladder (Foley) catheter for bladder outlet and urethral obstruction, ureteral stents for distal ureteral obstruction, and nephrostomy tube placement for midureteral or proximal ureteral obstruction. Surgical intervention may be needed for urethral obstruction.

7. Renal ultrasound should be part of the evaluation for all patients with ARF. True or false?

True. This is used to rule out **hydronephrosis**, which is present in most patients with obstruction of the renal system.

8. What are intrinsic renal failure causes of ARF?

- Acute interstitial nephritis caused by drugs
- Acute tubular necrosis caused by ischemia, an aminoglycoside, or cyclosporine
- Rhabdomyolysis
- Polycystic kidney disease
- Glomerulonephritis
- Nephrotoxicity by IV contrast and drugs

Treatment: Discontinue toxic drugs and treat IV contrast-induced nephritis by administering IV fluids before administering contrast. Dialysis is needed for complications such as pericarditis and peripheral neuropathy.

Adequate hydration is the preventive therapy against contrast-induced nephritis.

9. Drugs can cause tubular renal obstruction. True or false?

True. At the microscopic level, tubular obstruction can be caused by **calcium oxalate crystals** that are formed from **ethylene glycol** crystals, **uric acid** from tumor lysis syndrome, and **light chains** from multiple myeloma. Other crystal-forming drugs are indinavir (protease inhibitor), acyclovir, methotrexate, and sulfasalazine.

10. How do patients present with acute interstitial nephritis?

The patient may present within weeks to months of toxin exposure (e.g., drugs such as proton pump inhibitors, NSAIDs, rifampin, penicillin, cephalosporins) with rash, fever, and acute renal dysfunction. Interstitial nephritis can also be caused by infections, immune-mediated disease, and glomerular disease, or it can be idiopathic. UA may show elevated WBCs (sterile pyuria), WBC casts, and proteinuria; urine microscopy alone or with specific stains may show eosinophils; and serum may reveal eosinophilia.

Treatment: Remove inciting agent or treat underlying infection. If this fails, consider corticosteroids.

WBC casts and eosinophilia are very important laboratory results used in diagnosing interstitial nephritis on the exam.

11. What are the characteristic clinical and laboratory features of rhabdomyolysis?

This usually occurs after prolonged immobilization, **extreme physical activity**, or exposure to some drugs. It causes myalgias, **CK elevation**, and **low calcium** levels with **elevated uric acid** and metabolic acidosis. Urine results are positive for blood but not RBCs, suggesting **myoglobinuria**. Treat with isotonic IV fluids.

12. What is the most common cause of chronic kidney disease (CKD) in the United States?

The most common cause is diabetes, followed by hypertension. Others are glomerulonephritis and nephrotic syndrome.

13. How is CKD due to hypertension differentiated from that caused by diabetes?

CKD due to hypertension usually presents with proteinuria of <1 g/24 hours, whereas CKD due to diabetes is a nephrotic range **proteinuria** of >3 g/24 hours.

14. What is the first step in the evaluation of asymptomatic microscopic hematuria (>3 RBC/hpf)?

After ruling out an infectious cause of hematuria, the first step is analysis of urine under the microscope to determine whether there are **dysmorphic** (glomerular damage) or **nondysmorphic** (nonglomerular cause) RBCs.

15. What is the first step in the evaluation of nonglomerular hematuria?

First obtain CT urography, if imaging is unrevealing for occult stones or a mass, rule out **bladder malignancy** with urine cytology for all. If urine cytology is unrevealing, obtain cystoscopy in those ≥50 years of age or at high risk for bladder malignancy. If urine cytology is unrevealing, workup ends in those <50 years of age without risk for bladder cancer.

16. What are the risk factors for bladder cancer?

Risk factors are cigarette smoking, analgesic abuse, benzene exposure, and abnormal voiding history.

What is the most common cause of painless urinary bleed?

17. How do patients present with gross hematuria?

The patient may present with a painless urinary bleed. The most common cause of a painless urinary bleed is bladder cancer (not renal cancer).

Know the causes of papillary necrosis.

18. How do patients present with papillary necrosis?

The patient can also present with painless hematuria. The most common causes are diabetes, analgesic nephropathy (NSAIDs), and sickle cell anemia. It is characterized by coagulopathic **ischemia** of the renal medullary pyramids and papilla leading to necrosis. **Urography** study may reveal abnormalities in renal papillae including hooks, spurs and ring-shaped filling defects.

What medication must be discontinued in patients with renal failure? Metformin, as it causes lactic acidosis

19. How do patients present with CKD?

The patient may present within months to years with uremic signs and symptoms and serum electrolyte abnormalities:

- Asterixis
- Pericarditis
- Bleeding
- Hypertriglyceridemia
- Hypocalcemia
- Hyperphosphatemia (vitamin D loss)
- Hyperkalemia

- Anemia (erythropoietin loss)
- Peripheral or generalized edema (intravascular retention)
- Heart failure (intravascular retention)
- Hypertension

20. What is the mnemonic for indications of acute dialysis?
The mnemonic is AEIOU: acidosis, electrolyte abnormality, ingestion of toxins, refractory volume overload, uremia.

21. Autosomal dominant polycystic kidney disease (APKD) is the most frequently inherited kidney disease and causes end-stage renal disease. True or false?
True. Numerous cysts in the kidneys damage the renal parenchyma, leading to **kidney hypertrophy** and **renal failure**, **hypertension**, **flank pain**, and **hematuria** in the fifth decade of life.

22. What extrarenal findings are present in APKD?
Cerebral aneurysm, liver cysts, pancreatic cysts, diverticular colon disease, and aortic aneurysms can be found.

23. Multiple renal cysts that are asymptomatic and associated with UTI, hypercalciuria, and hemihypertrophy suggest what condition?
These suggest medullary sponge kidney, a benign condition that does not cause renal failure.

24. How is end-stage renal disease (ESRD) treated?
ESRD is treated by dialysis while the patient waits for a kidney transplant, as well as with erythropoietin, phosphate binders, and vitamin D supplements.

Angiotensin-converting enzyme inhibitors and reduction of protein in the diet reduce the progression of kidney disease in patients with CKD or microalbuminuria.

What therapies reduce the progression of CKD?

25. What are the complications of hemodialysis?
One complication is disequilibrium syndrome: dizziness, nausea, and vomiting that can progress to confusion, seizures, coma, and death. It can occur during or after dialysis. The pathogenesis is serum urea nitrogen that decreases too rapidly, causing osmotic shifts that lead to cerebral edema. Treatment is slow dialysis to remove serum urea more slowly, especially in new dialysis patients who are at highest risk.

Other complications of hemodialysis are infection of the access catheter or fistula/graft, and hypotension.

26. What is the cause of secondary hyperparathyroidism in CKD?

Hypocalcemia and 1,25 OH vitamin D deficiency stimulates PTH. Phosphate is retained, which contributes to hypocalcemia and hyperparathyroidism. Treatment is phosphate binders and vitamin D supplements.

27. For all patients with CKD, what is the effect of blood pressure control on the progression of CKD?

BP control slows the progression of CKD. Renin-angiotensin system inhibitors have been shown to be more likely to reduce the progression of CKD compared with other antihypertensives.

28. What is the definition of nephritis?

Nephritis is a disease of ruptured glomeruli capillary wall (mesangial cells or proliferative mesangial cells), leading to hematuria and proteinuria, **hypertension,** and **renal failure**. The first step in nephritis and nephrotic syndrome is to obtain a UA.

29. What is the definition of Wegener glomerulonephritis?

In Wegener glomerulonephritis, self-antibodies are directed against the neutrophil cytoplasm (C-ANCA), **a granulomatous inflammation**. In addition to the kidneys (glomerulonephritis), it affects the upper respiratory system (sinusitis, rhinorrhea, nasal crusting), lungs (cough, dyspnea, hemoptysis) and less commonly affects other organs (GI, eyes, nervous, heart)..

30. What are the diagnostic features of analgesic nephropathy?

The features are chronic analgesic use, renal failure, bland urine sediment, and occasional leukocyte and granular casts. Renal ultrasound will show **small kidneys**.

Wegener glomerulonephritis is associated with C-ANCA, while Goodpasture syndrome is associated with anti-GBM.

31. List two common pulmonary renal syndrome in glomerulonephritis.

- Anti-glomerular basement membrane (GBM) antibody (Goodpasture syndrome)
- Wegener granulomatosis

Note that C-ANCA is associated with **proteinase** and P-ANCA is associated with **myeloperoxidase**.

32. What is the presentation of post-streptococcal glomerulonephritis?

Post-streptococcal glomerulonephritis occurs 3-4 weeks after having a streptococcal sore throat (streptococcal pharyngitis). The patient presents with nephritis. Why? Immune complex antibodies are deposited in the basement membrane. Laboratory tests show elevated anti-streptolysin-O or anti-DNase B levels and low C3 levels.

33. Post-streptococcal glomerulonephritis does seem to be prevented by antibiotic treatment of streptococcal pharyngitis. True or false?

False.

34. What is the presentation of IGA nephropathy?

This is the most common cause of **asymptomatic microscopic hematuria**. It is due to a thin basement membrane. The patient presents with hematuria preceding a viral respiratory illness. The workup is UA and urine microscopy to look for RBCs and RBC casts from glomeruli injury, as well as assessment of proteinuria by 24-hour protein collection or by using a spot urine protein/creatinine ratio (normal ratio is <0.1). The serum IgA level may be elevated, but insensitive and nonspecific.

Treatment is prednisone for delay in renal failure progression and an angiotensin-converting enzyme (ACE) inhibitor for hypertension.

35. What is the definition of Alport syndrome?

Alport syndrome is an X-linked recessive defect due to collagen IV deficiency, which is present in the ear (cochlear) and glomerular basement membrane. The patient presents with hearing loss, glomerulonephritis (hematuria, proteinuria), and **progressive renal failure**.

36. What are hereditary syndromes that may mimic the effect of loop (Na-K-2Cl carrier) and distal tubule (Na-Cl carrier) diuretics?

- Barter's syndrome: Na-K-2Cl transporter mutation
- Gitelman's syndrome: Na-Cl transporter mutation

These conditions are usually found in children and can present as **musculoskeletal symptoms**. Furosemide is an example of loop tubule inhibitor, while a thiazide diuretic is an example of a distal tubule inhibitor.

What is the key distinguishing factor for Wegener glomerulonephritis compared with other systemic vasculitis diseases such as Goodpasture syndrome? The presence of upper respiratory signs (e.g., sinusitis)

With hearing loss and glomerulonephritis, consider Alport syndrome.

37. What is an X-linked disease that causes accumulation of alpha-glucosidase in multiple tissues including the kidneys?

This is **Fabry's disease**, associated with **progressive renal failure, premature CAD, paresthesias**, and cutaneous disease (**angiokeratomas**). Acarbose, an oral antidiabetic medication, is an example of alpha glucosidase inhibitor.

38. What is the definition of nephrotic syndrome?

Nephrotic syndrome is increased permeability of the epithelial cells or glomerular basement membrane. The patient presents with proteinuria (>3.5 g of protein per 24 hours), hypoalbuminemia, and hyperlipidemia. Hypoalbuminemia can cause anasarca and generalized edema, or the patient may present with periorbital edema.

How does hypercoagulopathy occur in patients with nephrotic syndrome?

39. What are the complications of nephrotic syndrome?

Patients are prone to hypercoagulopathy due to urinary loss of fibrinolytic factors and can present with renal vein thrombosis (flank pain and hematuria), peritonitis (abdominal pain and fever), hypocalcemia due to loss of vitamin D, and anemia due to loss of erythropoietin and transferrin.

With hepatitis B and nephritis, consider membranous glomerulopathy.

40. What is the most common primary cause of nephrotic disease in adults?

Membranous glomerulopathy is the most common nephrotic disease. It is common in white men and in those with hepatitis B, syphilis, and malignancies. Treat with steroids.

41. Membranous nephropathy is an immune complex-associated nephrotic syndrome. True or false?

True. Immune complex deposits on the GBM lead to increased permeability to proteins.

42. Normal C3 and low C4 with positive hepatitis C in the setting of membranoproliferative glomerulonephritis is suggestive of what condition?

This suggests **cryoglobulinemia**, an immune complex formation that leads to membranoproliferative glomerulonephritis.

43. What is the most common secondary cause of nephrotic syndrome in adults?

Diabetes is the most common secondary cause in adults.

44. What is seen under the microscope in minimal change disease (MCD)?

MCD is the most common cause of nephrotic syndrome in **children**. In MCD, under the light microscope, you will see nothing (normal), but under the electron microscope, you will see effacement of foot processes of podocytes. Treatment is steroids. The recurrence rate is very high.

Know the light microscope and electron microscope findings in MCD.

45. What is unique about patients with focal segmental glomerulosclerosis (FSGS)?

Patients present with nephritic and nephrotic syndrome. FSGS is associated with **viruses** and **drugs**, HIV, IV drug use, and being African American (associated with worse outcomes). Treat the underlying causes.

IV drug use, being African American, and HIV are associated with glomerulosclerosis.

46. What is the definition of renal tubular acidosis (RTA)?

RTA is defined as hyperchloremic metabolic acidosis or impaired urinary acidification that occurs as a result of renal tubular dysfunction, without urea or anion retention. RTA can be proximal or distal. Usually bicarbonate is reabsorbed proximally in the renal tubules and secreted distally (via hydrogen excretion). If bicarbonate is not absorbed proximally, proximal RTA results (type 2). Type 2 RTA is usually associated with multiple proximal tubular transport defects, causing excretion of glucose, amino acids, phosphate and uric acid, and organic acids (e.g., citrate): this is referred to as Fanconi syndrome, which occurs in multiple myeloma. RTA here is associated with **non-anion gap** metabolic acidosis, **hypokalemia**, and eventually, **acidotic urinary pH**.

47. If hydrogen is not secreted distally, distal RTA results (type 1). True or false?

True. RTA here is manifested by **non-anion gap** metabolic acidosis, **hypokalemia**, and **alkalotic urinary pH**. Nephrocalcinosis results from bone buffering with calcium, which can result in kidney stone formation. Calcium losses this way can also result in diminished bone growth and osteoporosis.

Distal tubular acidosis can cause hypokalemia.

48. Type 4 RTA, a type of distal RTA, occurs in diabetic patients and can be due to aldosterone deficiency or resistance. True or false?

True. These patients present with persistent hyperkalemia.

What is the most common cause of kidney stones?

49. What are the treatment options for RTA?

Treat the underlying causes (e.g., Fanconi syndrome is a cause of proximal renal acidosis; therefore, treat underlying multiple myeloma), or use an alkalinizing agent (bicarbonate). If not contraindicated, diet restriction of potassium, avoidance of iatrogenic offenders (e.g., beta-blockers, ACE), and use of mineralocorticoid therapy are some treatment options for type 4 RTA.

50. What are the different types of nephrolithiasis?

- Calcium
- Uric acid
- Struvite stones
- Cystine
- Oxalate

51. How do patients with kidney stones present?

Patients present with flank pain that radiates to the genitals. The pain peaks at about 20 minutes (rapidly).

The first step is to obtain a plain abdominal X-ray or intravenous urogram (delayed excretion of contrast material and dilated renal pelvis seen on X-ray is diagnostic). An ultrasound can also be used for diagnosis. The best and definitive test to confirm diagnosis is a computed tomography scan. Why? It shows the stone in more detail than does an X-ray or ultrasound. UA is also performed, which may show hematuria.

52. What are the risk factors for the development of kidney stones?

Risk factors are high levels of **stone promoters**, such as calcium, uric acid, and oxalate, and low levels of **stone inhibitors**, such as citrate.

53. What are the causes of calcium stones?

These stones can form as calcium phosphate or calcium oxalate. Calcium oxalate is the most common type of stone. The most common metabolic abnormality is hypercalciuria, which can be caused by hyperparathyroidism, metastatic cancer, and a high-protein diet. A thiazide diuretic can reduce hypercalciuria.

54. What are the causes of oxalic acid stones?

Oxalic acid stones can develop with increased urinary excretion of oxalic acid (hyperoxaluria):

a) Primary hyperoxaluria is a genetic defect of oxalic acid metabolism that manifests as nephrolithiasis, nephrocalcinosis, kidney failure, and early death.
b) Secondary hyperoxaluria includes malabsorption diseases such as Crohn disease, as well as small bowel resection. Other causes of secondary hyperoxaluria are ethylene glycol ingestion, high dietary intake of oxalic acid, high doses of ascorbic acid, and pyridoxine deficiency. Dietary restriction of oxalic acid is the mainstay of treatment, but increased dietary intake of calcium, which precipitates oxalate, or cholestyramine, which binds oxalate, can prevent free oxalic acid from being absorbed and hyperoxaluria, leading to less stone formation.

55. What are the causes of hyperuricosuria?
Hyperuricosuria can be caused by myeloproliferative cancers or conditions that causes increased production of uric acid. Hyperuricosuria acts as a precipitant for calcium-oxalate stone formation and patients with overproduction of uric acid and gout are at risk for uric acid stones. Allopurinol should be given to these patients to prevent formation of stones.

56. Which bacteria cause struvite stones?
Struvite stones develop because bacteria (Proteus) that possess an enzyme break down ammonium to ammonia, making urine alkalotic.

57. What is the definition of cystine nephrolithiasis?
Cystine nephrolithiasis is a hereditary disease characterized by a lack of amino acid transporters. A positive family history is usually present.

58. What is the treatment for acute kidney stones?
Treat a kidney stone by hydrating the patient and managing pain if the stone is relatively small (<1.0 cm or 10 mm). If the stone is large (≥1.0 cm or 10 mm), it is treated by shock wave lithotripsy to break it up, or percutaneous removal. **Struvite stones** form relatively large staghorn calculi and thus are treated with either shock wave lithotripsy or percutaneous removal. Antibiotics are also used to suppress bacteria responsible for the formation of struvite stones. Use urine alkalinization

Size determines the management of kidney stones.

MUDPILES is a mnemonic for causes of anion gap metabolic acidosis.

for uric acid and cysteine stones. The recurrence rate of kidney stones is very high; thus, perform an abdominal X-ray for the first year, and if negative, then every 2 years.

59. What is the definition of respiratory acidosis?

Respiratory acidosis is elevated PCO2 and low pH levels. Compensation by bicarbonate buffer causes serum HCO3 to increase by 1 mEq/L for every 10 mm Hg elevation in PCO2.

60. What is the definition of metabolic acidosis?

Metabolic acidosis is low bicarbonate (HCO3) and low pH levels.

61. What is the definition of respiratory alkalosis?

Respiratory alkalosis is low PCO2 and high pH levels. Compensation occurs by the serum HCO3 falling by 2 mEq/L for every 10 mm Hg reduction in PCO2.

62. What is the definition of metabolic alkalosis?

Metabolic alkalosis is elevated HCO3 and high pH levels. Respiratory compensation occurs by increasing PCO2 by 0.7 mm Hg for every 1 mEq/L elevation in serum HCO3.

63. What is the formula for the calculation of metabolic acidosis compensation?

$PCO2 = 1.5 \times (HCO3) + 8 \pm 2$

64. What is the calculation of anion gap?

$Na - HCO3 + Cl = 12$

65. What are the causes of anion gap metabolic acidosis?

MUDPILES:

- Methanol
- Uremia
- Diabetic ketoacidosis/ketosis
- Propylene glycol
- Isoniazid or iron
- Lactic acidosis
- Ethylene glycol (antifreeze)
- Salicylates

66. Rapid compensation for metabolic and respiratory acid-base disorders occurs how?

It occurs by **respiratory** means for metabolic acid-base disorders and **bicarbonate adjustments for respiratory acid-base** disorders, whereas long-term (3-4 days) compensation for respiratory acid-base disorders occurs by renal adjustments of bicarbonate. Note that the compensation occurs in the **same direction** of the acid-base disorder.

67. What are the causes of non-anion gap metabolic acidosis?

The general causes of non-**anion gap metabolic acidosis** are usually due to excess bicarbonate loss (diarrhea, intestinal losses, RTA, posttreatment of ketoacidosis, carbonic anhydrase inhibitors, ureteral diversion [ileal loop]) or decreased renal excretion (RTA, CKD).

68. What are some causes of metabolic alkalosis?

It is usually due to excessive bicarbonate intake or loss of H+:

- Bicarbonate infusion
- Milk: Alkali syndrome
- Citrate
- Vomiting
- Renal losses: Diuretics

69. What are the causes of respiratory acidosis?

It is generally due to factors that cause retention of PCO2:

- Airway obstruction (obstructive sleep apnea)
- Neuromuscular disorders (myasthenia gravis, morbid obesity)
- Central respiratory depression (drugs, opiates, sedatives, central apnea)
- Respiratory disorders (COPD, pulmonary edema)

70. A normal pH (7.366 to 7.44) or overcompensated pH suggests a mixed acid-base disorder. True or false?

True. An example is aspirin toxicity, which can cause metabolic acidosis and respiratory alkalosis. The general causes of respiratory alkalosis are **hyperventilation syndromes**, including pulmonary embolism, acute coronary syndrome, metabolic syndrome (ketoacidosis, hypoglycemia, hypercalcemia), heart failure, arrhythmia, asthma, COPD, pneumothorax, seizures, and hyperthyroidism.

Aspirin toxicity causes both metabolic acidosis and respiratory alkalosis.

71. What are the different types of IV fluids?

- Crystalloid: Normal saline, lactated Ringer solution
- Colloid: Albumin, fresh frozen plasma (FFP), blood synthetics, dextran

What is the initial fluid type used to replace fluid deficits?

Remember the 3:1 rule.

- Normal saline consists of sodium and chloride. This is usually the initial type of fluid used to replace deficits. Lactated Ringer solution consists of sodium, chloride, potassium, and calcium.
- It takes 3 ml of crystalloid to replace 1 ml of blood (3:1 rule).

72. What are some electrolyte disturbances?

- Hyponatremia
- Hypernatremia
- Hyperkalemia
- Hypokalemia

73. How does a patient present with hyponatremia?

The patient can present with fatigue, brain edema, and seizures. Coma can occur depending on the severity.

74. What are some causes of hyponatremia?

It is generally due to impaired renal water excretion plus free water intake:

- Hypovolemia (diuretics, gastrointestinal losses)
- Euvolemia (syndrome of inappropriate ADH [SIADH])
- Hypervolemia (congestive heart failure, liver failure, kidney failure)
- Normovolemia (hyperglycemia, hyperlipidemia, hyperproteinemia)
- Psychogenic polydipsia

Rapid correction of hyponatremia may cause central pontine myelinosis.

75. How is hyponatremia treated?

Replenish with IV fluids if there is hypovolemia. Restrict fluid if SIADH is mild or give 3% Na if SIADH is severe (SIADH with neurological symptoms).

Treat underlying systemic disease for other causes. Do not correct hyponatremia too quickly. Why? It will cause central pontine myelinosis.

When you see elderly, debilitated, or very young patients, consider hypernatremia.

76. How does a patient present with hypernatremia?

The patient can present with lethargy or coma depending on the severity.

77. What are the causes of hypernatremia?

Hypernatremia usually presents in patients who are elderly or debilitated or in children who have restricted fluid intake and do not drink enough fluids. Diabetes insipidus is an important cause of hypernatremia.

Treatment: Rehydration with IV fluids with normal saline

78. How do patients present with hypokalemia?
The patient can present with arrhythmias, ileus, muscle weakness, and hyporeflexia (decreased deep tendon reflexes). Why? The potassium gradient is increased so that relaxation is increased.

Decreased DTR occurs in hypokalemia.

79. What are the causes of hypokalemia?
It is generally due to excess aldosterone secretion or abnormality in reabsorption and secretion of potassium:
- Shifts of potassium (insulin, beta agonists)
- Adrenal aldosterone tumor
- Thiazide or other diuretics (renal losses)
- Distal tubular acidosis (RTA)
- Gastrointestinal losses

80. What is seen in laboratory tests for hypokalemia?
The EKG reveals flat T waves.

81. How is hypokalemia treated?
Treat hypokalemia with oral or parenteral replacement of potassium depending on its severity. If this fails, check for low serum magnesium levels and administer magnesium. Why? Potassium is not well absorbed in low magnesium states.

Why is potassium low in the presence of low magnesium?

82. What are the causes of hyperkalemia?
- Shifts of potassium (beta antagonists)
- Addison disease
- Kidney failure
- Drugs (amiloride, spironolactone, renin-angiotensin inhibitors, NSAIDs)
- Rhabdomyolysis (increased creatine kinase and epithelial casts)
- Type IV RTA

83. What are some EKG findings in patients with hyperkalemia?
There are peak T waves, a wide QRS, small P waves, and sinusoidal waves.

84. How is hyperkalemia treated?
The first step is to obtain an EKG; if abnormal (peak T waves, wide QRS, small P waves, sinusoidal waves), administer IV calcium gluconate to protect the membrane

Why administer calcium gluconate as the initial therapy for hyperkalemia?

of the heart, and then insulin and glucose, or bicarbonate, to shift potassium into the cell.

Kayexalate and cholestyramine resin are the only drugs that will eliminate potassium by binding.

85. What common medication is used for a kidney transplant?

Cyclosporine is used for immunosuppression.

86. How do patients present with acute renal allograft rejection after an organ transplant?

The patient may present with tenderness of the graft secondary to lymphocytic cell destruction.

Treatment is IV steroids or anti-T-cell antibody therapies.

87. What are some common side effects of cyclosporine?

Side effects include kidney failure, glucose intolerance, hypertension, and gingival hypertrophy.

Why does left testicular varicocele occur in patients with renal cancer?

88. How do patients present with renal cell cancer?

Invasion of the inferior vena cava (IVC) occurs. Because the gonadal vessel on the left branches off the left renal vein, which drains into the IVC, a left testicular varicocele can present in these patients.

On laboratory tests, the serum erythropoietin level is elevated (paraneoplastic syndrome).

Chapter 21

Respiratory System

What is the difference between blue bloaters and pink puffers?

1. What is the definition of chronic obstructive pulmonary disease (COPD)?

COPD is irreversible obstructive lung disease. Mucus hypersecretion, ciliary dysfunction, and airway obstruction leads to cough, sputum production, dyspnea, and hemoptysis. The patient with end-stage COPD may present with cyanosis, distended jugular veins, leg edema, and weight gain (**blue bloater's** chronic bronchitis), or alternatively may present with weight loss, a barrel chest, and acyanosis (**pink puffer's** emphysema). Most patients have a combination of chronic bronchitis and emphysema.

2. What are risk factors for the development of COPD?

Risk factors are tobacco smoke, heavy exposure to occupational dust and chemicals, indoor and outdoor air pollution, and genetics (alpha-1 antitrypsin deficiency).

3. What are complications of COPD?

Complications include frequent acute exacerbations. These are more common with chronic bronchitis.

4. What is the preventive therapy in COPD?

The preventive therapy is use of muscarinic antagonists: An ipratropium inhaler (not beta agonist) is preferred to reduce exacerbations. It is the first line for prevention.

5. What is the first step in the diagnosis of COPD?

The first step is to perform spirometry, a pulmonary function test. A forced expiratory volume/forced vital capacity (FEV1/FVC) ratio of 0.75-0.8 is normal. A

COPD FEV1/FVC ratio is < 0.7. Lung volumes such as total lung capacity (TLC), and residual volume (RV) are also increased (Figure 21-1).

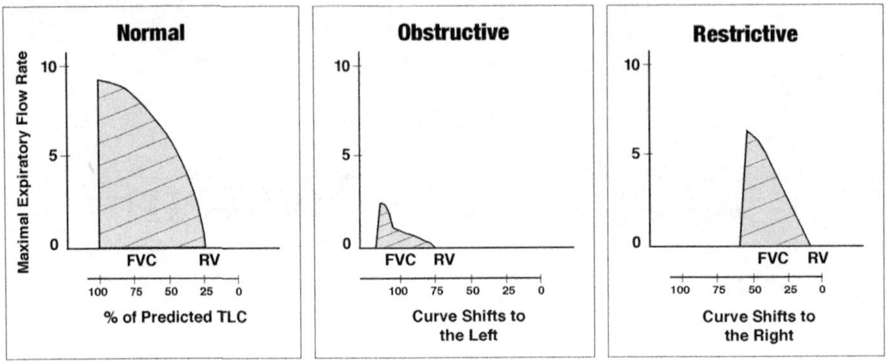

Figure 21-1. *Spirometry*

6. What is the significance of DLCO in COPD?

This is diffusing capacity of carbon monoxide, which is usually low in emphysema and mildly reduced in chronic bronchitis.

7. In moderate COPD (FEV1 less than 80% predicted but more than 50%), addition of what therapy improves lung function?

Therapy with long-acting beta agonists or long-acting anticholinergic agents improves function compared with short-acting bronchodilators alone.

8. In severe COPD (FEV1<50% predicted), inhaled corticosteroids are effective in reducing COPD exacerbations. True or false?

True. However, a combination of inhaled corticosteroids and long-acting beta agonists in severe COPD will further reduce exacerbations.

What treatment options reduce the mortality rate in patients with COPD?

9. Oxygen therapy and smoking cessation are the only treatments that will reduce mortality in COPD patients. True or false?

True.

10. Oxygen is indicated in patients who have COPD. When?

Oxygen is indicated when PO2 is <55 mm Hg and oxygen saturation is <90% or PO2 is <59 mm Hg if the patient has cor pulmonale or pulmonary hypertension.

You can start by giving a facial oxygen mask, and then intubation if that does not work in severe cases of COPD exacerbation.

In chronic bronchitis, hypoxia drives ventilation; therefore, do not give too much oxygen because it will eliminate the hypoxic drive.

Why should too much oxygen be avoided in patients with COPD?

11. How do patients present with acute exacerbation of COPD?

The patient may present with productive cough, sputum, and dyspnea.

Treatment: Antibiotics against common bacteria and atypicals (azithromycin), bronchodilator, and oral steroids. Common bacteria in COPD patients are *Streptococcus pneumoniae, Haemophilus influenza,* and *Moraxella catarrhalis.*

12. What is the definition of restrictive disease?

Restrictive disease is a group of lung diseases characterized by low lung volumes and reduced diffusion capacity (DLCO).

Lung volumes in COPD are high.

Lung volumes in restrictive lung diseases are low.

The patient will present with exertional dyspnea and nonproductive cough with no history of smoking. The patient may have occupational risks (e.g., fiber glass car industry worker).

The first step is to order pulmonary function testing. The FEV/FVC ratio in these patients is normal (0.8) or high. RV and TLC are low (Figure 21-1). The next step is to look for an underlying cause by working closely with a pulmonary specialist.

13. List common causes of restrictive lung disease.

Common causes are primary restrictive lung diseases (e.g., idiopathic pulmonary fibrosis; a chest X-ray [CXR] finding of bilateral reticular infiltrates with lower lobe predominance is suggestive of diagnosis) and systemic diseases (e.g., sarcoidosis, polymyositis, and dermatomyositis).

14. In Caucasian Americans, sarcoidosis may present asymptomatically with an abnormal CXR finding. True or false?

True. It may present only with a CXR finding as **hilar lymphadenopathy**. Asymptomatic sarcoidosis does not require treatment unless there is organ involvement or lung parenchyma.

15. What are some examples of extrapulmonary involvement in sarcoidosis?

These include parotid swelling, uveitis, hypercalcemia, neurological disease, erythema nodosum, and cardiac disease.

16. Symptoms of cough, dyspnea, and myalgias occurring acutely after exposure to a particular antigen without extrapulmonary manifestations and a radiograph with interstitial infiltrates are suggestive of what lung disease?

These suggest **hypersensitivity pneumonitis**, especially if the removal of the antigen results in resolution of symptoms. Examples of antigens are avian proteins (e.g., bird fancier's **lung**), gardens **or** farms (farmer's lung by thermophylic actinomycetes), vaporizers, air conditioners (microbial, aerosols), and mold. Presence in a hot tub can cause "**hot tub**" pneumonitis caused by *Mycobacterium avium* complex. Avoidance of antigens is the mainstay of treatment, or steroids in severe cases.

What is the key difference between COPD and asthma? Reversibility

Why is silent chest an ominous sign in patients with obstructive lung disease?

How do NSAIDs cause asthma?

Why are ABG results different for mild and severe asthma?

17. What is the definition of asthma?

Asthma is reversible hyperactive obstructive lung disease that involves chronic inflammation.

In acute exacerbation, the patient will present with wheezing, dyspnea, cough, and possibly allergy history. On the physical examination, intercostal retractions are present, as well as nasal flaring (in children) and use of accessory muscles in severe exacerbation. Over time, the patient's muscles may be fatigued to the point where there is inadequate breathing, leading to hypercapnia and silent chest on auscultation (this is an ominous sign in severe acute exacerbation).

18. What are factors that precipitate asthma?

Cold air, exercise, allergens, dust mites, molds, NSAIDs, and beta-blockers precipitate asthma.

NSAIDs can cause asthma by causing a shift to leukotrienes.

19. What is the first step in the evaluation of asthma?

Obtain the peak expiratory flow rate to characterize the severity of the asthma attack. A severe attack is <20% of normal and a mild attack is >60% of normal. Arterial blood gas (ABG) results for mild asthma may show respiratory alkalosis (hyperventilation), whereas for a severe case, ABG results may reveal respiratory acidosis (because of hypercapnia from fatigued muscles).

20. What are the four types of asthma?

- Intermittent: Symptoms ≤2 days a week in the daytime and ≥2 times a month at night. Normal FEV1 between exacerbations, or FEV1 >80% of predicted
- Mild: Symptoms >2 days a week in the daytime and >2 times (3-4 times) a month at night, FEV1 ≥80% of predicted
- Moderate: Symptoms every day and nighttime symptoms >1 time a week. FEV1 > 60, but <80% of predicted
- Severe: Symptoms every day several times a day and every night 7 times a week. FEV1 <60% of predicted

21. How is intermittent asthma treated?

A short-acting beta-2 agonist inhaler (albuterol) is the treatment for intermittent asthma.

22. How is mild asthma treated?

Albuterol and a low-dose steroid inhaler is the treatment for mild asthma.

23. How is moderate asthma treated?

Albuterol, a high-dose steroid inhaler, and a long-acting beta agonist (salmeterol) is the treatment for moderate asthma.

24. How is severe asthma treated?

Treat as moderate asthma, with intermittent oral steroids. Consider omalizumab (an anti-IgE monoclonal antibody) for severe persistent asthma.

25. Why use cromolyn sodium for prophylaxis of asthma?

Cromolyn sodium stabilizes mast cells; therefore, it works well before exposure to an asthma precipitant such as exercise. It is very useful for patients with other allergies (allergic rhinitis and atopic dermatitis).

26. When is a leukotriene inhibitor (montelukast) used?

Montelukast is used as an alternative therapy for inhaled steroids in mild to moderate asthma, especially in young children. It can also be used as an add-on therapy to inhaled steroid in severe asthma in adults. Montelukast can be given prophylactically 2 hours prior to exercise

Asthma classification is based on daytime and nighttime symptoms.

Why are asthma symptoms worse at night? Cortisol drops and histamine rises.

Cromolyn sodium is used in patients with asthma who have other allergic disorders.

in exercise-induced asthma and is very useful in those with allergic rhinitis.

27. When are leukotriene modifiers (e.g., zileuton) used?

Leukotriene modifiers can be used as add-on agents in moderate asthma or as an alternative to long-acting beta antagonists. Persons with obesity, who smoke cigarettes, and who have aspirin sensitivity may benefit from leukotriene modifiers. Patients with triad asthma (asthma, aspirin sensitivity, and nasal polyposis) have been shown to benefit more with leukotriene modifiers than with leukotriene antagonists.

28. What is allergic bronchopulmonary aspergillosis?

This is a known complication of asthma. Patients develop a reaction to *Aspergillus fumigatus* in their airways, leading to inflammation, airway damage, and central bronchiectasis that eventually leads to pulmonary fibrosis. The characteristic features are moderate to severe **asthma**, CXR with **lung infiltrates**, bronchiectasis, **elevated IgE level**, **eosinophilia**, and skin reaction to *Aspergillus fumigatus*. Treatment is steroids.

Pulmonary embolus can cause both a transudative and an exudative pleural effusion.

29. What is the definition of pleural effusion?

Pleural effusion is excess fluid accumulating in the pleural cavity.

Transudate: Causes are congestive heart failure, nephrotic syndrome, liver cirrhosis, and pulmonary embolus

Exudate: Causes are pneumonia, tuberculosis (diagnostic pleural adenosine deaminase), pulmonary embolus, and malignancy

30. Asbestos exposure is a risk factor for what pleural cancer?

It is a risk factor for mesothelioma (irregular, nodular pleural thickening with pleural effusion).

31. A pulmonary embolus can cause both a transudative and an exudative pleural effusion. True or false?

True. Increased hydrostatic pressure is the pathogenesis of a transudate, whereas alteration of pleural membrane is the pathogenesis of an exudate.

32. How do patients with an exudative pleural effusion present?

Pneumonia is the most common cause of exudates. Malignancy is also a known cause.

The patient will present with the underlying disease or dyspnea.

The physical examination may reveal dullness on percussion, decreased breath sounds, and a shift of the mediastinum to the opposite side if there is massive pleural effusion.

The next step is to obtain a CXR, standing and lateral decubitus, to show the effusion. A CXR may show blunting of the costophrenic angle on the involved side (Figure 21-2).

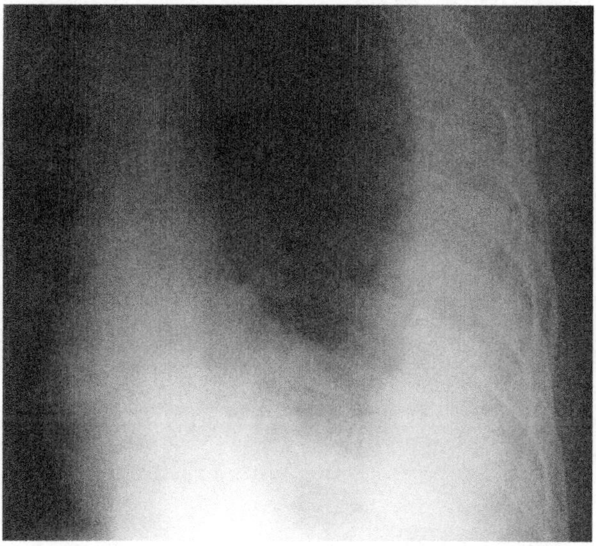

Figure 21-2. *Left-sided pleural effusion. There is blunting of the left costophrenic angle.*

Pneumonia is the most common cause of a pleural exudate.

33. What is the next step after a pleural effusion has been localized on a CXR?

The next step would be to tap the effusion to define it (thoracentesis). Laboratory tests that show pleural lactate dehydrogenase (LDH) >200 IU, pleural-to-serum LDH >0.6, and pleural-to-serum protein >0.5 are indicative of an exudative effusion. A serum-to-pleural fluid albumin >1.2 suggests transudate if it is discordant exudate (an exudate that meets criteria by protein only). This is usually due to a diuretic effect.

34. What is the definition of a parapneumonic exudate?

A parapneumonic exudate is an infected exudate. The characteristics on laboratory tests usually reveal pH <7.0, positive gram stain, gross pus, and glucose <60 mg/dl. Treat with antibiotics and a tube thoracostomy.

What is the difference between a transudative and an exudative effusion?

35. How do patients present with a transudative pleural effusion?

A common cause is congestive heart failure.

The patient will present similarly to those with an exudate. Laboratory tests will reveal an LDH of <200 IU, pleural-to-serum LDH of <0.6, and pleural-to-serum protein of <0.5.

What is a Pancoast tumor?

Which lung cancer is central and which is peripheral? Small cell and squamous are central. Adenocarcinoma is peripheral.

36. How do patients present with lung cancer?

Lung cancer is the number one cause of cancer-related death.

The patient may present in later stages with systemic symptoms (fever, weight loss, loss of appetite), symptoms as a consequence of physical compression of the mass (shoulder pain radiating to the arm), Horner syndrome (ptosis, anhidrosis, meiosis), or SVC syndrome from a Pancoast tumor. The patient will usually have a long history of smoking (30 pack years) and may have COPD. However, the most common symptom is **chronic cough.**

On examination, the patient may have signs of hypertrophic osteoarthropathy, including finger clubbing and proliferation of bone tissue (periostosis).

The first step will be to get a CXR to look for a mass. If a mass is present, other tests, including a CT scan or bronchoscopy, will be done.

37. What are the risk factors for lung cancer?

The risk factors are smoking, asbestos exposure, radon gas exposure, family history, personal history of malignancy, and advanced age.

What type of lung cancer is common in nonsmokers? Bronchioloalveolar

38. Which types of lung cancers are associated with smoking?

Squamous cell and non-small cell lung cancer are associated with smoking. Adenocarcinoma is less likely to be associated with smoking.

38. Which type of lung cancer frequently metastasizes at an early stage?

Small cell lung cancer often metastasizes early.

39. What is the most important genetic test to perform after diagnosis of metastatic lung adenocarcinoma?

Testing for EGFR tyrosine kinase mutation is most

important because patients can be treated with anti-EGFR drugs (gefitinib).

40. How is lung cancer treated?

Small-cell cancer can be treated with combination chemotherapy. Why? Studies have shown that small-cell cancer is very responsive to chemotherapy. For localized non-small cell cancer, resection is the treatment.

For severe, metastatic non-small cell cancer, palliation with radiation is the treatment.

41. What is the workup for a solid pulmonary nodule?

If a solid pulmonary nodule is accidentally found in a patient, the first step is to obtain an old CXR to compare. Why? Increasing size represents malignancy and should be biopsied. Any solid nodule that is stable over 2 years can be considered benign.

What is the first step in the evaluation of an incidental pulmonary nodule?

42. What is the next step in the workup of a solid pulmonary nodule that does not meet the criteria above (q41)?

Examine the clinical and radiological features. Smoking, , a certain calcification pattern (asymmetric calcification), an irregular border, and increased density all increase the likelihood of malignancy of a pulmonary nodule.

43. What is the next step after identifying benign clinical and radiological features?

If the probability of malignancy is low, follow up with serial CT scans.

44. What is the next step in patients with a high probability for malignancy?

The next step is surgical excision.

45. A bronchogenic mass with "popcorn calcifications" is indicative of what lung mass?

It indicates a benign lung mass such as a **pulmonary hamartomas**. Popcorn calcification and most calcifications in a solitary pulmonary nodule represent a benign feature. It can be resected if it is symptomatic.

46. What is presentation of cystic fibrosis (CF) in adults?

CF is characterized by the loss of a chloride channel transporter, leading to the lack of chloride in the lung membranes, which causes dryness and consequent infection of the lung with Pseudomonas. The patient will present with frequent lung infections: cough,

What should one consider in treating pulmonary infections in patients with CF?
Pseudomonas

dyspnea, and constitutional symptoms that are recurrent. However, multiple organs are affected.

The first step is to obtain a sweat chloride test. The result will be high in CF (>60 mEq/l).

Treatment: Antibiotics against Pseudomonas (imipenem) and against gram-negative bacteria (gentamycin) are used for acute exacerbations.

47. What are the complications of CF in adults?

Multiple organs are affected, including genitourinary (infertility) and upper and lower airways, leading to frequent sinusitis and bronchiectasis thick and dilated airways).

48. What are some specific pneumonia organisms and their treatment?

- Streptococcus pneumoniae (localized consolidation signs): Most common cause of community acquired pneumonia is Streptococcus pneumoniae. Treat with penicillin if Streptococcus has been identified (Figure 21-3).

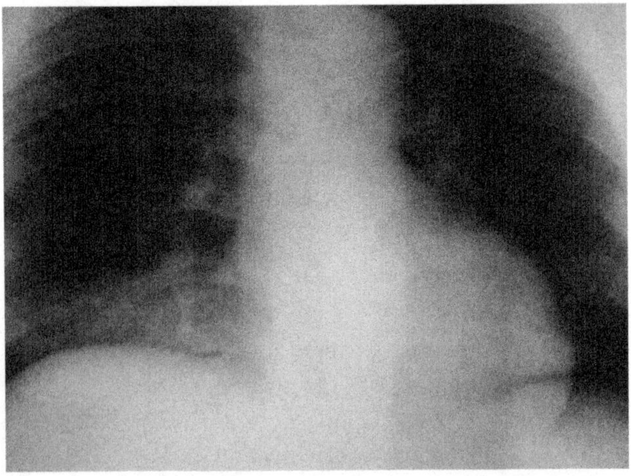

Figure 21-3. *Right-lobar pneumonia. There is consolidation on the right middle lobe (silhouette sign). The silhouette sign is the blurring of the right heart border, which indicates middle-lobe pneumonia.*

- Mycoplasma pneumoniae (upper respiratory signs and nonproductive cough): Prolonged cough is a common feature, as well as positive test results for cold agglutinins antibody. Treat with azithromycin, erythromycin, doxycycline, or a pulmonary quinolone. Why? This organism lacks a cell wall, and so the antibiotic needs to work in the cell.

- Klebsiella pneumoniae (currant jelly sputum or mucoid): Treat with a third-generation cephalosporin. Why? This organism is a gram-negative rod. However, recent extended spectrum beta-lactamase strains are resistant to third-generation cephalosporins and treatment is guided by susceptibility testing.
- Legionella: Usually presents with pneumonia signs plus gastrointestinal symptoms (vomiting and diarrhea). Transmitted by cooling systems, humidifiers, and respiratory therapy equipment. Treat with azithromycin. Why? This is an intracellular organism.
- *Staphylococcus aureus*: Pneumonia is usually preceded by a viral influenza illness. Treat empirically with vancomycin.

49. What is the most common physical sign in patients with diaphragmatic dysfunction?

The most common sign is an **abdominal paradox**: inward movement of the abdomen with inspiration. This occurs due to compensatory use of the accessory muscles of the rib cage and neck.

50. What is the cause of acute respiratory distress syndrome (ARDS)?

ARDS can be caused by sepsis and trauma that result in pulmonary edema without affecting the heart. Pulmonary capillary wedge pressure is normal (**less than 18 mm Hg**), jugular venous pressure is normal, and preload is normal. The **PO2/FIO2 ratio** is ≤200. The CXR will show diffuse interstitial infiltrates.

Treatment: Treat with mechanical ventilation via low tidal volume ventilation; extracorporeal membrane oxygenation (ECMO) for severe and or refractory ARDS.

51. What is the definition of obstructive sleep apnea (OSA)?

OSA is an obstruction of the airway as a result of a hypertrophied upper airway. The patient will present with excessive daytime sleepiness, frequent night awakenings, and morning headache. Secondary elevation of erythropoietin may occur. Diagnosis is with **polysomnography** (sleep studies).

Why may erythropoietin increase in patients with OSA? Hypoxic compensatory response

52. What is a major complication of OSA?

OSA can be complicated by pulmonary hypertension, which can lead to right-sided heart failure (cor pulmonale).

Treat with continuous positive airway pressure (CPAP) or loss of weight for obese patients.

53. What is the first step in the evaluation of pulmonary hypertension?

It is usually first detected by an **echocardiogram**; obtain a right heart and pulmonary artery catheterization to confirm diagnosis. Also obtain pulmonary function tests, polysomnography, and, if indicated, serologic tests for HIV and connective tissue disease since COPD, OSA, HIV, and connective tissue disease (e.g., scleroderma) are all possible causes of secondary pulmonary hypertension. Initially treat the underlying cause before it becomes irreversible.

54. What are possible treatment options for idiopathic pulmonary arterial hypertension (primary pulmonary hypertension) and irreversible secondary hypertension)?

Prostacyclin analogues (epoprostenol, iloprost), vasodilators (sildenafil), endothelin receptor antagonists (bosentan), or certain calcium blockers can be used to treat primary pulmonary hypertension after confirming response to treatment with right heart catheterization. Always try to treat the underlying secondary causes in secondary pulmonary hypertension initially; however, therapy may be directed at the pulmonary hypertension in more advanced cases.

55. What is the correct placement of an intubation tube?

The tube should be between the vocal cords and the carina.

Check with a CXR after insertion to verify the location.

Know the complications of incorrect endotracheal tube placement.

56. What is an ominous complication of an incorrect endotracheal tube placement?

The tube can enter the right-stem bronchus (right-stem bronchus intubation), leading to hyperinflation in the ipsilateral lung or hypoinflation (decreased breath sounds) in the contralateral lung.

Memorize extubation criteria.

57. When is a patient fit to be extubated after endotracheal intubation for respiratory failure?

The patient can be considered for extubation when the rapid shallow breathing index is <105, spontaneous respiration >30 beats/minute, negative inspiratory force >–20 cm, positive end-expiratory pressure <5-8 cm H20, and minute ventilation <10 L/min.

58. What is the definition of the rapid shallow breathing index?

The rapid shallow breathing index is the ratio of the respiratory rate to the tidal volume.

60. What is CPAP?

CPAP is used to provide respiratory support, for example in ARDS or OSA.

What is the goal of oxygen therapy with a CPAP?

The goal of oxygen therapy is to keep PaO2 >50 mm Hg; therefore, set FiO2 to the level that achieves this. However, FiO2 should not exceed 60% to prevent barotrauma.

If FiO2 exceeds 60% to reach the goal of PaO2 (>50 mm Hg), then intubation is needed.

61. What is a major complication of mechanical ventilation?

A major complication is barotrauma (emphysema, pneumothorax), which can be minimized by using low FiO2.

62. What is the most common cause of primary and secondary pneumothorax?

Primary pneumothorax occurs in normal lungs in thin, young men who smoke, whereas secondary pneumothorax occurs in those with abnormal lungs, COPD, and intubation of the right stem bronchus.

63. Obstructive atelectasis is common in children and patients on high FIO_2. True or false?

True. Children have less well-developed collaterals, and so a foreign object easily causes an obstructed airway. In patients on high FIO2, nitrogen in the airways is minimal and does not keep airways opened.

64. Differentiate atelectasis from pleural effusion on a CXR or lung examination.

In atelectasis (collapse of lung tissue), there is **hyper-resonance and lack of breath sounds** on the affected side, and on CXR, the hemithorax is partially or completely white and there may be a shift of the **mediastinum to the side of the lesion**. In pleural effusion, there is **dullness** and **lack of breath sounds** on the affected side and CXR may also show a partial or completely white hemothorax, but there is a shift of the **mediastinum to the contralateral side.**

65. What are the first signs of nonexertional heat stroke?

The first signs are anhidrosis (absence of sweating), warm and dry skin, and **hyperthermia** (>41° C), and then **altered sensorium** such as hallucinations, seizures, delusions, and coma. Multiple organ dysfunctions such as renal failure, rhabdomyolysis, hepatic injury, pulmonary edema, and DIC can occur.

Anhidrosis is usually present in nonexertional heat stroke, which is common among the **elderly population** after a prolonged heat wave and who are taking medications that impair sweating (e.g., anticholinergic and psychiatric drugs). However, **young athletes** with exertional heat stroke can present with sweating and altered sensorium (including syncope). **Heat cramps** (muscle pains) and **heat exhaustion** (presence of sweating only) are a continuum of heat stroke.

DUMBELS-Diarrhea, Urination, Miosis, Bronchorrhea/Bronchospasm/Bradycardia, Emesis, Lacrimation, Salivation, is another mnemoic for cholinergic toxicity.

Organophosphates are present in nerve agents and insecticides.

66. What is the treatment of cholinergic crisis?

Cholinergic crisis may result from "nerve agents," which are organophosphates, causing bronchorrhea, miosis, salivation, lacrimation, and respiratory failure from diaphragmatic paralysis. Treatment is atropine and pralidoxime.

67. What is a mnemonic for symptoms of cholinergic crisis?

A mnemonic is **SLUGE**: salivation, lacrimation, increased urination, gastrointestinal upset, and emesis.

68. What conditions can precipitate neuroleptic malignant syndrome?

Such conditions include abruptly discontinued levodopa or anticholinergic drugs, or those taking neuroleptic agents such as haloperidol or fluphenazine or other antipsychotic agents. It is characterized by fever, muscular rigidity, and altered sensorium due to dopamine inhibition in the brain. Dopamine agents, muscle relaxants, and supportive care are the mainstay of treatment.

69. What are the clinical features of serotonin syndrome?

Symptoms are agitation, ataxia, tremor, hyperreflexia, myoclonus, and hyperthermia, with a history of taking a selective serotonin reuptake inhibitor (SSRI) and a recent increase in the dose of SSRI or the addition of a serotonergic agent such as monoamine oxidase inhibitors, TCA, trazodone, serotonin-norepinephrine reuptake inhibitors, lithium, opioids (meperidine), amphetamines/stimulants, cocaine, or herbal and dietary supplements (St. John's wort).

Meperidine can precipitate a serotonin or MAOI crisis.

70. What is the definition of malignant hyperthermia?
Malignant hyperthermia is an **inherited muscle disorder** that causes a hypermetabolic state from increased intracellular calcium, leading to tachycardia, hypotension, and fever, as well as **muscular rigidity** from exposure to drugs (**inhaled anesthetics** and depolarizing muscle relaxants) during anesthesia.

Treatment: Discontinue the anesthetic and administer dantrolene (a muscle relaxant).

71. Which toxic ingestions cause miosis versus mydriasis?
Narcotics and cholinergics cause miosis, whereas sympathomimetics and anticholinergics cause mydriasis.

72. List common chemical irritants and their consequences.

- Hydrogen sulfide: Respiratory irritant that can cause metabolic acidosis
- Hydrogen cyanide: Can cause metabolic acidosis by inhibiting mitochondrial oxidation, causing headache, seizure, coma, and death

73. List toxic ingestions and the antidotes used.

- Acetaminophen: *N*-Acetylcysteine
- Amphetamines: Benzodiazepine
- Arsenic: EDTA, dimercaprol
- Aspirin (salicylates): Urine alkalinization
- Benzodiazepines: Flumazenil
- Beta-blockers: Glucagon, calcium chloride, pacing
- Calcium channel blocker: Calcium, glucagon, pacing
- Cocaine: Benzodiazepine
- Cyanide: Amyl nitrite/sodium nitrite, thiosulfate, hydroxocobalamin
- Digoxin: Digoxin immune Fab
- Ethylene glycol: Ethanol, fomepizole
- Heparin: Protamine sulfate
- INH: Pyridoxine (vitamin B6)
- Lithium: Hemodialysis
- Methanol: Ethanol, fomepizole

- Methemoglobin: Methylene blue
- Opioids: Naloxone
- Organophosphates: Atropine, pralidoxime
- TCA: Alkalinization
- Warfarin: Vitamin K, fresh frozen plasma(FFP)

Recognize the symptoms of mild to severe carbon monoxide poisoning in those susceptible to it.

74. Cognitive deficits such as memory loss, poor judgment, and other nonspecific symptoms can occur after exposure to which common chemical agent?

Mild forms of carbon monoxide poisoning can present with nonspecific myalgias, dizziness, and **memory lapse**, while severe deficits can present with **memory loss or other neuropsychologic deficits**, confusion, and coma, which can occur in firefighters, coal miners, and commercial vehicle operators or in the household (e.g., from a chronic leak). Measurement of the **carboxyhemoglobin level** (>3% in nonsmokers and >10% in smokers) and a finding of metabolic acidosis can confirm diagnosis. Give 100% oxygen or hyperbaric oxygen as treatment.

Chapter 22

Surgery

1. Define diverticulosis.

Diverticulosis is a protrusion of the mucosa through the muscle wall of the colon.

Risk factors are a low-fiber diet and constipation.

The patient usually presents with rectal bleeding or asymptomatically.

Diagnosis: It is usually found incidentally on colonoscopy. Diverticulosis is the most common cause of a lower gastrointestinal (GI) bleed. Bleeding usually self-resolves; otherwise, angiography and embolization can be performed. Surgical resection of the colon is an option for recurrent bleed.

2. Define diverticulitis.

Diverticulitis is an inflammation of a diverticulosis. The risk factors are constipation and a low-fiber diet. The patient will present with abdominal pain, nausea and vomiting, and fever. On the physical examination, left lower quadrant tenderness is present.

The first step is to treat acutely with antibiotics and bed rest (nothing by mouth).

When the patient is stable, obtain a computed tomography (CT) scan to confirm the diagnosis.

Surgery is indicated when there is a perforation, obstruction, and fistula.

High consumption of fiber in the diet may reduce the recurrence of diverticulitis.

3. How does the patient present with angiodysplasia?

The patient presents with rectal bleeding. Diagnosis is usually done via endoscopy including upper endoscopy, colonoscopy, capsule endoscopy, and small bowel

Always perform an appendectomy in a patient with typical signs and symptoms of appendicitis.

Ulcerative colitis involves the rectum most of the time.

Oxalate accumulation from ileocecal involvement can cause nephrolithiasis.

enteroscopy during evaluation of GI bleeding. Imaging such as CT scan angiography is also diagnostic.

4. How do patients present with appendicitis?

The patient presents with periumbilical pain that progresses to right lower quadrant pain with nausea and vomiting.

The patient may have low-grade fever and laboratory tests may show leukocytosis.

On examination, the patient may display localized rigidity, distention, and a positive psoas and obturator test.

The first step before laboratory testing or imaging if the symptoms are highly suspicious is to perform an appendectomy. If you are not sure or the symptoms are not typical, a CT scan can be diagnostic.

In female patients, ultrasound can rule out female pathological findings.

5. What is the surgical treatment for complications of peptic ulcer disease (PUD)?

Those with gastric outlet obstruction, perforation, or refractory bleed can be treated with a **vagotomy plus drainage procedure**, highly selective vagotomy, or vagotomy with gastrectomy.

6. What are the two types of drainage procedures for PUD surgery?

The two procedures are gastroduodenostomy (Billroth I) and gastrojejunostomy (Billroth II).

7. How do patients present with appendicitis abscess?

A bulging mass is felt on the examination in addition to right lower quadrant tenderness. The patient reports a history of right lower quadrant pain of >24 hours.

8. How do patients present with cholecystitis?

Cholecystitis is a cystic duct occlusion by a stone or sludge. The patient presents with epigastric abdominal pain, nausea, and vomiting initially; hours later, the pain migrates to the right upper quadrant, and a low-grade fever may be present. Risk factors are obesity, mid-40s, female (a mnemonic is fat, forty, and fertile), rapid weight loss (stasis), hemolytic crisis, and Crohn disease (decreased enterohepatic circulation).

On the physical examination, a positive Murphy sign is observed.

9. What is the first step in the evaluation of cholecystitis?

Obtain an ultrasound that shows a thickened gallbladder (3 to 4 mm) and peri-cholecystosis fluid, which is diagnostic. A hepatobiliary iminodiacetic acid(HIDA) scan and cholangiography can be used to further delineate the anatomy of the biliary system.

Treatment is cholecystectomy after treating with antibiotics. Cholecystotomy is performed in the elderly or in those with comorbidities, and ursodeoxycholic acid is given to those who are candidates for surgery but refuse it.

10. How do patients present with acalculous cholecystitis?

Patients undergoing parenteral therapy, those who are **acutely ill** in the ICU, and those with hypokinetic gallbladder have increased risk because the gallbladder is not being stimulated by food in the intestine.

Ultrasound shows pericholecystitis fluid, but the gallbladder wall is not thickened.

Treatment: Cholecystotomy (not cholecystectomy) is the treatment because most patients have associated comorbidities and are not surgical candidates; otherwise treat with urgent cholecystectomy.

11. How do patients present with biliary colic?

Biliary colic is an obstruction of the cystic duct without inflammation or infection. The patient presents with right upper quadrant pain that radiates to the right scapula, secondary to the irritation of the diaphragm by the liver. No fever is present. Schedule a cholecystectomy regardless. Why? Biliary colic will eventually lead to cholecystitis.

12. What is the pathogenesis of emphysematous cholecystitis?

Emphysematous cholecystitis is a complication of cholecystitis due to bacterial infection such as Clostridium perfringens, which causes air in the wall or lumen of the gallbladder.

Treat with antibiotics and cholecystectomy.

13. What is the significance of a porcelain gallbladder?

This is a calcified gallbladder, which has the risk of developing into cancer. Treatment: Treat with a cholecystectomy to prevent gallbladder cancer.

Cholecystitis in Crohn disease is the result of what?

What are indications for a cholecystotomy?

What are the risk factors for acalculous cholecystitis?

Why schedule an elective cholecystectomy for patients with biliary colic?

Why should you treat a porcelain gallbladder?

Why is sigmoidoscopy the diagnostic test of choice for volvulus?

Why is the left testicle mostly affected in a varicocele?

14. What are the risk factors for large bowel obstruction?

The risk factors are diverticulitis, scarred colon, volvulus, and cancer.

The patient will present with nausea, vomiting, abdominal pain, obstipation, and constipation. The first step for suspected obstruction is to obtain an abdominal series: get a chest X-ray (CXR) (look for air under the diaphragm) and an abdominal X-ray (look for dilated loops of bowel and air-fluid levels).

15. What is the definition of a volvulus?

It is torsion of a segment of the intestine, usually the sigmoid or cecum colon.

16. What is the typical presentation of volvulus?

This usually occurs in elderly patients with debilitated neurological and psychiatric conditions and can present as continuous and severe colicky abdominal pain, nausea, and constipation and obstipation. It can also present in younger patients as recurrent attacks of abdominal pain. A plain abdominal X-ray of a distended large bowel proximal to the sigmoid colon can be diagnostic.

17. Volvulus can be diagnosed and uncoiled by flexible sigmoidoscopy. True or false?

True. Flexible sigmoidoscopy should be attempted in those without gangrene or perforation to detorse the twisted segment.

18. What is the pathogenesis of a varicocele?

A varicocele is a dilated pampiniform plexus (testicular veins), especially of the left testicle. Why the left testicle? The left testicular vein drains via the left renal vein, which is angulated and predisposed to obstruction. The patient presents with ipsilateral testicular swelling (bag of worms), especially with increased intra-abdominal pressure (Valsalva maneuver) and standing.

19. How is head injury classified?

Head injury is classified according to the Glasgow coma scale. The patient with increased intracranial pressure (ICP) may present with nausea, vomiting, and headaches.

20. What is the first step in the treatment of elevated ICP?

The first step is rapid reduction of ICP by hyperventilation and elevation of the head. The next step is to initiate medical treatment with mannitol, a carbonic anhydrase inhibitor, and diuretics.

21. How does hyperventilation reduce ICP?
Hyperventilation causes low carbon dioxide levels, leading to vasoconstriction of the brain vessels.

22. What are the zones of the neck?
The zones of the neck are zones I, II, and III.

Zone 1 is below the cricoid cartilage, zone II is between the angle of the mandible and the cricoid cartilage, and zone III is above the angle of the mandible.

23. Why is mandatory exploration indicated for a zone II injury?
Zone II is easy to manipulate operatively, and so if an injury occurs in this region, mandatory exploration is advised. In zones I and III, an immediate arteriogram or other tests (bronchoscopy, esophagram) are ordered and patients are managed accordingly because these zones are difficult to manipulate operatively.

24. How do patients present with a reducible inguinal hernia?
A reducible inguinal hernia is one that is still reducible on examination. The patient presents with a groin bulge that is exacerbated by activity and relieved by lying down.

A reducible hernia is not treated unless the patient insists.

25. How do patients present with a strangulated inguinal hernia?
The contents of a strangulated inguinal hernia have been twisted about, leading to obstruction and ischemia. The patient presents with pain, fever, constipation, and bowel obstruction. Laboratory tests show an elevated white blood cell (WBC) count.

Treatment: Surgery. The hernia is reduced and the bowel resected if indicated.

26. How do patients present with an incarcerated hernia?
Bowel ischemia and necrosis has occurred. The patient presents with pain and fever. Laboratory tests show an elevated WBC count.

Treatment: Surgery. The hernia is reduced and the bowel resected if indicated.

Why is mandatory surgical exploration indicated for zone II injuries regardless of hemodynamic stability?

What are indications for surgery in patients with an inguinal hernia?

Why are there no reflux symptoms in patients with type II esophageal hernia?

What is a major risk factor for Zenker diverticulum?

What are the predisposing factors in Boerhaave syndrome?

HIV can cause esophagitis.

27. What is the definition of a type I esophageal hernia?

A type I esophageal hernia involves a slipping of the gastroesophageal junction toward the fundus of the stomach. Risk factors are obesity and pregnancy. The patient presents with heartburn that is worse on lying down.

A known complication is foul-smelling breath secondary to dysphagia.

28. What is the definition of a type II esophageal hernia?

A type II esophageal hernia involves movement of the gastric fundus adjacent to the gastroesophageal junction. It does not involve the gastroesophageal junction, however, and so there are no reflux symptoms.

29. What is the definition of esophageal diverticula (also Zenker diverticula)?

Esophageal diverticula are caused by herniation of the esophageal mucosa through the esophageal wall. A major risk factor is a weak cricothyroid muscle.

The patient will present with dysphagia, regurgitation, and foul-smelling breath. Endoscopy and barium enema can diagnose it.

Treat with resection of the diverticula.

30. What is the definition of Boerhaave syndrome?

Boerhaave syndrome is the rupture of the esophagus due to trauma caused by excessive retching. The patient will present with nausea, vomiting, chest pain, shock, and sepsis.

On the physical examination, a pleural effusion is present and imaging may reveal subcutaneous emphysema on CXR.

The next step is to stabilize the patient.

Treat the symptoms; for example, perform a tube thoracostomy for a pleural effusion.

31. Esophagitis can predispose an individual to esophageal rupture. True or false?

True. HIV-positive and immunocompromised patients are predisposed to esophagitis.

32. What are common indications for esophageal gastroduodenoscopy (EGD)?

EGD is indicated during complications of reflux disease or alarming features (dysphagia, excessive vomiting, iron-deficiency anemia, weight loss, older age) to rule out esophageal cancer; if there is hematemesis, EGD can be performed to rule out causes of upper gastrointestinal bleed.

33. What is an ominous complication of EGD?
An ominous complication is esophageal rupture. You can confirm the diagnosis with an esophagram (Gastrografin contrast study of the esophagus).

34. How do patients with a small bowel obstruction (SBO) present?
The causes of SBO are masses, adhesions, hernias, and gallstones.

The patient with SBO presents with nausea, vomiting, obstipation, constipation, and abdominal distention. Dilated loops of bowel are seen in supine and upright abdominal X-ray, but are not needed to confirm diagnosis. History and physical examination alone are used in most cases to diagnose SBO.

The most common cause of SBO in the United States is a hernia, followed by adhesions. Look for a mass in a young patient with SBO or a patient with no history of previous surgeries, hernia, or adhesions.

35. How is SBO treated?
If no signs of peritonitis are present, give the patient nothing by mouth, perform nasogastric decompression, and administer IV saline fluids. If peritonitis is present (rebound tenderness, abdominal rigidity), an exploratory laparotomy is indicated immediately.

36. What are the clinical features of intestinal ileus?
It usually occurs after abdominal surgery. It can occur after neurological trauma such as spinal cord injury, metabolic abnormality, sepsis, or use of anticholinergic medications. Patients may present with acute abdominal pain, distention, and nausea or vomiting. On imaging, there is gas throughout the intestine. Treatment is a conservative approach with nasogastric tube decompression.

37. How do patients with a carcinoid tumor present?
When the tumor occurs in the small bowel (distal ileum), the patient presents with carcinoid syndrome (flushing, wheezing, and diarrhea) due to the action of serotonin in the blood. Tryptophan levels may be low because serotonin is made from it.

What is the most common cause of SBO in the United States?

When is an exploratory laparotomy indicated in patients with SBO?

Why may tryptophan levels be low in patients with carcinoid cancer?

Mnemonic for narcotic equivalency = **C**ornel **M**edical **D**octor

Mnemonic for corticosteroids equivalency = Cornel **P**resbyterian **M**edical **D**octor

What are the three possible causes of postoperative oliguria?

Why is urinary tract infection the most common postoperative nosocomial infection?

38. What is the pathogenesis and presentation of gallstone ileus?

This is an important cause of mechanical bowel obstruction in the elderly population with comorbidities. Gallstones from the common bile duct can fall into the small bowel to cause partial obstruction. The patient's ultrasound shows air in the biliary tree (pneumobilia).

Treatment: Remove the stone from the intestine via surgery.

39. What is the equivalency for narcotics?

Mnemonic: Cornel Medical Doctor:

Codeine 130 mg
Morphine 30 mg
Dilaudid (hydromorphone) 7.5 mg

40. What is the equivalency for corticosteroids?

The mnemonic is Cornel Presbyterian Medical Doctor:

Cortisone 25 mg
Prednisone 5 mg
Methylprednisolone 4 mg
Dexamethasone 0.75 mg

41. What is the IV equivalent of oral morphine?

It is 2:1. IV morphine is 2 times that of oral morphine.

42. What is a commonly tested side effect of meperidine?

Meperidine can cause tachycardia; therefore, avoid it in patients who are taking a monoamine oxidase inhibitor or other serotonergic agents to prevent the serotonin syndrome.

43. How does an epidural and spinal block cause hypotension?

Hypotension occurs by diminishing the sympathetic response.

44. What are the three causes of postoperative oliguria?

Postoperative oliguria can be caused by mechanical factors such as a Foley obstruction (postrenal), dehydration (prerenal), or intrinsic renal failure. Normal urine output is 0.5 ml/kg/hour.

45. What is the most common nosocomial infection postoperatively?

The most common nosocomial infection is a urinary tract infection from a Foley catheter insertion. Organisms responsible are Staphylococcus aureus and Escherichia coli.

46. What is a common complication on the first postoperative day?

A common complication is atelectasis (wind).

47. What is a common complication on the second postoperative day?

A common complication is a wound infection (wound).

48. What is a common complication on the third postoperative day?

A common complication is pneumonia (water).

49. How do narcotics (morphine, meperidine) cause postoperative ileus?

Narcotics have an inhibitory action in the GI tract. Treatment is to first minimize postoperative opioids.

Remember the mnemonic wind, wound, and water as causes of postoperative complications.

Why do narcotics cause postoperative ileus?

Index

B

C

D

E

F

G

H

I

J

K

L

M

N

O

T

U

V

W

X

Y

Z

Reference List

New England Journal of Medicine, S. Nizam Ahmed, James Scozzafava, Meningioma, Volume 356, Page 16. Copyright © (2013) Massachusetts Medical Society. Reprinted with permission from Massachusetts Medical Society.

New England Journal of Medicine, Gary L. Gallia, Michael H. Sobotta, Traumatic Epidural Hematoma, Volume 360, Page 6. Copyright © (2013) Massachusetts Medical Society. Reprinted with permission from Massachusetts Medical Society.

New England Journal of Medicine, Barbara J. Bain, Diagnosis from the Blood Smear, Volume 353, Page 5. Copyright © (2013) Massachusetts Medical Society. Reprinted with permission from Massachusetts Medical Society.

New England Journal of Medicine, Puneet Bhargava, Jeffrey H. Maki, "Cotton Wool" Appearance of Paget's Disease, Volume 363, Page 6. Copyright © (2013) Massachusetts Medical Society. Reprinted with permission from Massachusetts Medical Society.

New England Journal of Medicine, Casey Grover, "Thumb Sign" of Epiglottitis, Volume 365, Page 5. Copyright © (2013) Massachusetts Medical Society. Reprinted with permission from Massachusetts Medical Society.

New England Journal of Medicine, Saweera Sabbar, Eric James Nilles, Deep Sulcus Sign, Volume 366, Page 6. Copyright © (2013) Massachusetts Medical Society. Reprinted with permission from Massachusetts Medical Society.

New England Journal of Medicine, Chun-Chao Huang, Shin-Lin Shih, Steeple Sign of Croup, Volume 367, Page 1. Copyright © (2013) Massachusetts Medical Society. Reprinted with permission from Massachusetts Medical Society.

New England Journal of Medicine, Joanne Monterroso, Sreenivasa Chandana, Massive Splenomegaly in Hairy Cell Leukemia, Volume 367, Page 22. Copyright © (2013) Massachusetts Medical Society. Reprinted with permission from Massachusetts Medical Society.

New England Journal of Medicine, Meike W. Vernooiji, M. Arfan Ikram, Herve L. Tanghe, et al., Incidental Findings on Brain MRI in the General Population, Volume 357, Page 18. Copyright © (2013) Massachusetts Medical Society. Reprinted with permission from Massachusetts Medical Society.

Printed in Dunstable, United Kingdom

91218900R00228